Case-based Reviews in
Dermatology

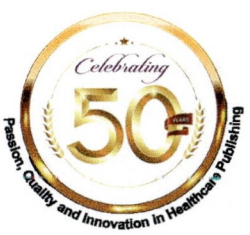

Case-based Reviews in
Dermatology

Editor

Rashmi Sarkar MD MNAMS
Professor of Dermatology, STD and Leprosy
Maulana Azad Medical College and
Lok Nayak Jai Prakash Narayan Hospital
New Delhi, India

Co-Editors

Anupam Das MD
Assistant Professor
Department of Dermatology
KPC Medical College and Hospital
Kolkata, West Bengal, India

Isha Narang MD (MAMC) MRCP (SCE)
Specialist Registrar (Dermatology)
University Hospitals of Derby and Burton
United Kingdom

Indrashis Podder MD DNB
RMO cum Clinical Tutor
Department of Dermatology
College of Medicine and Sagore Dutta Hospital
Kolkata, West Bengal, India

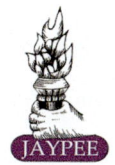

JAYPEE BROTHERS MEDICAL PUBLISHERS
The Health Sciences Publisher
New Delhi | London

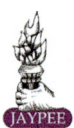 **Jaypee Brothers Medical Publishers (P) Ltd**

Headquarters
Jaypee Brothers Medical Publishers (P) Ltd
4838/24, Ansari Road, Daryaganj
New Delhi 110 002, India
Phone: +91-11-43574357
Fax: +91-11-43574314
Email: jaypee@jaypeebrothers.com

Overseas Offices
J.P. Medical Ltd
83 Victoria Street, London
SW1H 0HW (UK)
Phone: +44 20 3170 8910
Fax: +44 (0)20 3008 6180
Email: info@jpmedpub.com

Website: www.jaypeebrothers.com
Website: www.jaypeedigital.com

© 2020, Jaypee Brothers Medical Publishers

The views and opinions expressed in this book are solely those of the original contributor(s)/author(s) and do not necessarily represent those of editor(s) of the book.

All rights reserved. No part of this publication may be reproduced, stored or transmitted in any form or by any means, electronic, mechanical, photocopying, recording or otherwise, without the prior permission in writing of the publishers.

All brand names and product names used in this book are trade names, service marks, trademarks or registered trademarks of their respective owners. The publisher is not associated with any product or vendor mentioned in this book.

Medical knowledge and practice change constantly. This book is designed to provide accurate, authoritative information about the subject matter in question. However, readers are advised to check the most current information available on procedures included and check information from the manufacturer of each product to be administered, to verify the recommended dose, formula, method and duration of administration, adverse effects and contraindications. It is the responsibility of the practitioner to take all appropriate safety precautions. Neither the publisher nor the author(s)/editor(s) assume any liability for any injury and/or damage to persons or property arising from or related to use of material in this book.

This book is sold on the understanding that the publisher is not engaged in providing professional medical services. If such advice or services are required, the services of a competent medical professional should be sought.

Every effort has been made where necessary to contact holders of copyright to obtain permission to reproduce copyright material. If any have been inadvertently overlooked, the publisher will be pleased to make the necessary arrangements at the first opportunity. The **CD/DVD-ROM** (if any) provided in the sealed envelope with this book is complimentary and free of cost. **Not meant for sale.**

Inquiries for bulk sales may be solicited at: jaypee@jaypeebrothers.com

Case-based Reviews in Dermatology / *Rashmi Sarkar*

First Edition: **2020**

ISBN: 978-93-5270-705-8

Printed at Replika Press Pvt. Ltd.

Dedicated to

My late mother, Mrs Chhobi Sarkar
(We need more of her kind to make this world a better place)
— **Rashmi Sarkar**

My parents,
for their constant support and encouragement
— **Anupam Das**

To my brother,
husband and our parents
— **Isha Narang**

All my teachers, family and
the wonderful patients I have encountered
— **Indrashis Podder**

Contributors

EDITOR

Rashmi Sarkar MD MNAMS
Professor of Dermatology, STD and Leprosy
Maulana Azad Medical College and
Lok Nayak Jai Prakash Narayan Hospital
New Delhi, India

CO-EDITORS

Anupam Das MD
Assistant Professor
Department of Dermatology
KPC Medical College and Hospital
Kolkata, West Bengal, India

Isha Narang MD (MAMC) MRCP (SCE)
Specialist Registrar (Dermatology)
University Hospitals of Derby and Burton
United Kingdom

Indrashis Podder MD DNB
RMO cum Clinical Tutor
Department of Dermatology
College of Medicine and Sagore Dutta Hospital
Kolkata, West Bengal, India

CONTRIBUTING AUTHORS

Aayushi Mehta MBBS FCPS
Consultant, Tvak Laser Clinic
New Delhi, India

Anand Toshniwal MD
Consultant Dermatologist
Aesthetic Aura Skin and Hair Clinic
Hyderabad, Telangana, India

Bela J Shah MD
Professor and Head
Department of Dermatology
BJ Medical College, Civil Hospital
Ahmedabad, Gujarat, India

Bhavya Swarnkar MBBS
Postgraduate
Maulana Azad Medical College
New Delhi, India

Debabrata Bandyopadhyay MD
Professor and Head
Department of Dermatology,
Venereology, and Leprosy
Medical College and Hospital
Kolkata, West Bengal, India

Deval B Mistry MBBS
Third Year Resident Doctor
Department of Dermatology
BJ Medical College, Civil Hospital
Ahmedabad, Gujarat, India

Geeti Khullar MD DNB
Specialist
Department of Dermatology and STD
Vardhman Mahavir Medical College and
Safdarjung Hospital
New Delhi, India

Kavita Poonia MD
Senior Resident
Dermatology of Venereology and Leprology
Government Medical College and Hospital
Chandigarh, Punjab, India

Komal Agarwal MBBS
Final Year Postgraduate Student (MD Dermatology)
Assam Medical College and Hospital
Assam, Guwahati, India

Lalit K Gupta MD
Senior Professor
Department of Dermatology
RNT Medical College
Udaipur, Rajasthan, India

Mahima Agrawal MD DNB MRCP
Senior Resident
Department of Dermatology and STD
Lady Hardinge Medical College and Associated Hospitals
New Delhi, India

Mala Bhalla MBBS MD
Professor
Dermatology of Venereology and Leprosy
Government Medical College and Hospital
Chandigarh, Punjab, India

Monica Chahar MD
Consultant Dermatologist and Hair Transplant Surgeon
AK Clinics
New Delhi, India

Nilay Kanti Das MD
Associate Professor
Department of Dermatology
Medical College
Kolkata, West Bengal, India

Nitin Nadkarni MBBS MD
Professor, Department of Dermatology
DY Patil School of Medicine
Navi Mumbai
Maharashtra, India

Paschal D'Souza MD
Professor
Department of Dermatology and Venereology
Employees' State Insurance-Postgraduate Institute of Medical Sciences and Research
New Delhi, India

Poonam Puri MD
Professor
Department of Dermatology and STD
Vardhman Mahavir Medical College and Safdarjung Hospital
New Delhi, India

Sanjeev Handa MD FAMS FAAD FRCP (Edin)
Professor and Head
Department of Dermatology, Venereology and Leprology
The Postgraduate Institute of Medical Education and Research
Chandigarh, Punjab, India

Sheetanshu Kumar MD
Senior Resident
Department of Dermatology, Venereology and Leprology
The Postgraduate Institute of Medical Education and Research
Chandigarh, Punjab, India

Shrikant Kumavat MBBS DDVL
Senior Resident
Dr Vasantrao Pawar Medical College, Hospital and Research Centre
Nashik, Maharashtra, India

Somodyuti Chandra MD DNB SCE-UK
Consultant Dermatologist
Fellow
The Venkat Centre for Skin and Plastic Surgery
Bangalore, Karnataka, India

Sudheer K Arava MD
Associate Professor
Department of Pathology
All India Institute of Medical Sciences
New Delhi, India

Sushruta Kathuria MD
Specialist Dermatology
Department of Dermatology and STD
Vardhman Mahavir Medical College and
Safdarjung Hospital
New Delhi, India

Taru Garg MD
Professor
Department of Dermatology and STD
Lady Hardinge Medical College and
Associated Hospitals
New Delhi, India

V Ramesh MD
Professor
Department of Dermatology and
Apex STD Centre
Vardhman Mahavir Medical College and
Safdarjung Hospital
New Delhi, India

Vijay P Zawar MD DNB DVD FRCP (Edin)
Professor
Department of Dermatology
Dr Vasantrao Pawar Medical College
Nashik, Maharashtra, India

Preface

Dermatology is a discipline, which has become one of the most favorite options for residents, when it comes to choosing an area of specialization. It is an ever expanding field with introduction of newer entities, therapeutic regimens, newer drugs and many other interesting observations. The field is nowadays greatly flanked by the esthetic and cosmetic counterpart, which has made the specialty even more lucrative to the youngsters.

However, the importance of learning the basics of clinical dermatology cannot be overemphasized. It is the three years of postgraduation when the building blocks of clinical dermatology are laid down. Our book is a first of its kind attempt, on the methodology of approaching case scenarios in daily OPDs and admitted patients. It is nice to know numerous entities (common as well as uncommon) in isolation, but the actual challenge lies in utilizing the association fibers of our brains, correlating the clinical findings and the laboratory investigations and arriving at a diagnosis for further management.

We have focused on the common case scenarios and presentations and how to approach the same, both in exams and day-to-day practice. The chapters have been designed in a reader-friendly format and the authors have been hand-picked in terms of their teaching experience and their dedication toward the subject. Most of the senior authors who have contributed to this book, bring to the table their experience and therefore, their insights and thoughts on how to approach a case, which is immensely valuable. The younger authors have collaboratively added their thoughts as well. This book is surely going to be a ready reckoner and easy reference for everyone.

All four of us, introduced to the senior editor and getting to know each other at different stages of one's life have tried to bring together their enthusiasm for knowledge in this book and hope that it would be immensely valuable to the readers.

Rashmi Sarkar
Anupam Das
Isha Narang
Indrashis Podder

Content

1. **Oral Ulcers with Joint Pains** — 1
   Sanjeev Handa, Sheetanshu Kumar

2. **Genital Ulcer** — 28
   Somodyuti Chandra, Nilay Kanti Das

3. **Generalized Pruritus** — 43
   Debabrata Bandyopadhyay

4. **Diffuse Hyperpigmentation** — 57
   Komal Agarwal, Anupam Das, Rashmi Sarkar

5. **Fever with Rash in a Child** — 72
   Nitin Nadkarni, Aayushi Mehta

6. **Nerve Thickening with or without Hypoesthetic Patch** — 80
   Mala Bhalla, Kavita Poonia

7. **Papulonodular Lesions of Face** — 96
   Anupam Das, Anand Toshniwal

8. **Vesiculopustular and Bullous Disorders in Children** — 104
   Indrashis Podder, Rashmi Sarkar

9. **Vesiculobullous Disorder in Middle Age** — 121
   Monica Chahar, Paschal D'Souza, Lalit K Gupta, Sudheer Kumar

10. **Erythroderma** — 149
    Vijay P Zawar, Shrikant Kumavat

11. **Vaginal Discharge** — 156
    Poonam Puri, Sushruta Kathuria

12. **Urethral Discharge** — 172
    Taru Garg, Mahima Agrawal

13. **Granulomatous Disorders** — 183
    Geeti Khullar, V Ramesh

14.	**Diffuse Hair Loss**	196
	Bela J Shah, Deval B Mistry	
15.	**Scalp Pruritus**	207
	Poonam Puri, Sushruta Kathuria	
16.	**Facial Melanosis**	219
	Rashmi Sarkar, Isha Narang, Bhavya Swarnkar	

Index — 233

CHAPTER 1

Oral Ulcers with Joint Pains

Sanjeev Handa, Sheetanshu Kumar

INTRODUCTION

Oral ulcers can be a manifestation of a myriad of mucocutaneous and systemic disorders. Joint symptoms with oral ulcerative lesions is not an uncommon association, seen by dermatologists, rheumatologists and family practitioners alike. Association of joint pain and oral ulcers in a patient warrants exhaustive clinical and laboratory evaluation as it can herald the presence of multiple systemic diseases. This case-based review is an attempt to discuss the diagnosis and management of patients presenting with oral ulcers and joint pain.

CASE 1

A 30-year-old male presented with complaint of recurrent painful oral ulcers mostly over inner labial and buccal mucosa from the last 4 years which persisted for 1–3 weeks on an average and then healed spontaneously, never lasting beyond 1 month. From last 1 year, he also complained of painful ulcers over scrotum and penis which typically persisted longer than a month, before healing spontaneously. He denied any involvement of nasal or anal mucosa. He also complained of accompanying joint pains for last 1 year involving left knee and ankle with morning stiffness lasting more than half an hour. For last 6 months, he complained of recurrent painful bluish red nodules lasting for 7–10 days over both lower legs, especially over shins. Apart from these nodules over lower legs, he denied history of any other cutaneous lesions. He also complained of photophobia, blurring of vision, floaters and periorbital pain from last 6 months and occasional episodes of diarrhea and abdominal pain from last 3 months. He had no neurological or cardiovascular complaints. He denied any history of photosensitivity or Raynaud's phenomenon.

On examination, multiple, round to oval ulcers with sharp borders surrounded by erythematous halo covered with whitish pseudomembrane and greyish yellow fibrinous base, with size ranging from few mm to 2–3 cm, were observed. Over scrotum, there was a solitary ulcer of similar morphology, but deeper than the oral ulcers.

> On closer examination, there were few round to oval atrophic scars over the scrotum. There were round to oval tender subcutaneous nodules of 2–3 cm diameter with bluish red discoloration of overlying skin on both the shins. Apart from these lesions, mucocutaneous examination was unremarkable. Panuveitis was detected after thorough ophthalmological evaluation. Ileocecal ulceration was found in colonoscopy.
>
> **Diagnosis:** Behçet's disease.

■ INTERACTIVE TOPIC REVIEW

Q.1 What are the clinical features of Behçet's disease?

Ans: Behçet's syndrome is a multisystem disease. Major clinical features are summarized as follows:

Oral Ulcers
- Prevalence: 92–100%
- Prognosis: Favorable
- Common sites: Labial, gingival and buccal mucosa, tongue. May also involve soft and hard palates, pharynx and tonsils
- Earliest disease manifestation in majority of the patients
- May be the sole clinical feature for years
- Round to oval painful lesions, with sharp borders surrounded by erythematous halo covered with whitish pseudomembrane and greyish yellow fibrinous base, with size ranging from few mm to 2–3 cm (Fig. 1)
- Lesions develop rapidly from a superficial to deep ulcer
- May occur as solitary or multiple ulcers in crops
- Typically heal without scarring although minimal scarring can be seen occasionally
- Minor ulcers: Size <1 cm in diameter, heal in 4–14 days, less painful

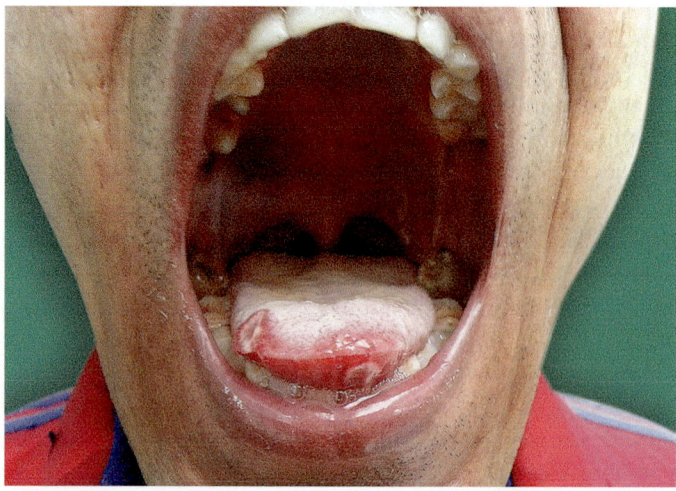

Fig. 1: Aphthae like oral ulceration over tongue in Behçet's disease.

- Major ulcers: Size >1 cm in diameter, heal within 2–6 weeks, more painful
- Herpetiform ulcers: Painful grouped small ulcers, 0.2–0.3 cm in diameter occurring in recurrent crops
- Treatment: Symptomatic, favorable prognosis.

Genital Ulcers
- Common sites:
  - Males: Scrotum, penis, perineum, perianal region and groin, may also involve epididymis
  - Females: Vulva, vagina and cervix. Rarely, fistula may develop secondary to perforation of deep vaginal lesions into bladder.
- Painful and morphologically similar to oral ulcers, but lesions are relatively larger, deeper and margins are more irregular when compared to oral ulcers (Fig. 2)
- Lesions heal leaving characteristic atrophic scars which may help in reaching diagnosis retrospectively
- Prognosis is guarded if fistulae and internal lesions develop and risk of infections if not managed properly.

Cutaneous Lesions
- Prevalence: 38–99%
- Prognosis: Favorable
- Leukocytoclastic vasculitis or neutrophilic vascular reactions are seen in biopsy from early cutaneous lesions although lymphocytic vasculitis prevail in mature lesions
- Lesions considered to be diagnostically relevant are:
  - Papulopustular lesions (28–96%): Sterile, folliculitis-like or acneiform lesions seen commonly over trunk, buttocks or lower limbs which start as erythematous papular lesion and rapidly evolve into pustule after

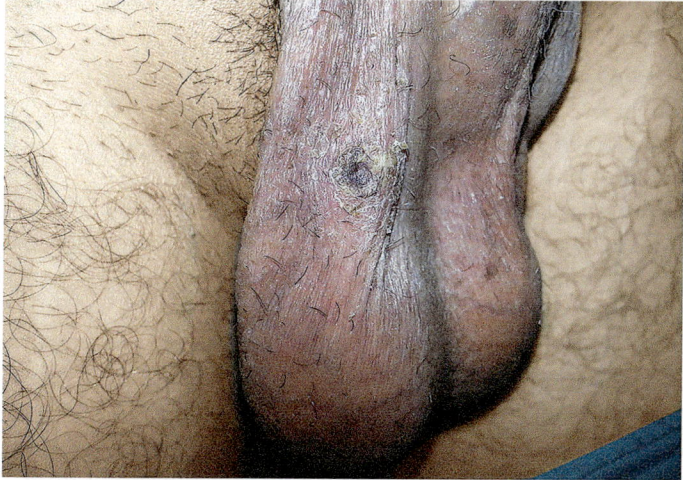

Fig. 2: Scrotal ulceration in Behçet's disease.

1–2 days. Papulopustular lesions are seen to be associated with positive pathergy test and arthritis in patients
- Erythema nodosum like lesions (15–78%): Mostly over lower limbs in females. Bilateral, warm, tender, pretibial, subcutaneous nodules with erythematous overlying skin which gradually turn bluish and heal spontaneously typically in 2–3 weeks leaving mild hyperpigmentation in pigmented skin type. The lesions never ulcerate. Recurrence is common. Although lesions are morphologically similar to erythema nodosum, vasculitis is seen on histopathology which differentiates these lesions from erythema nodosum
- Superficial thrombophlebitis: Classified as variable vessel vasculitis, Behçet's disease can involve vessels of any size and type. Veins are involved most commonly and superficial thrombophlebitis is the most common venous manifestations. The veins become inflamed, thrombosed, sclerosed and palpable as a string-like hardening with erythema of the overlying skin. Erythematous, tender, subcutaneous nodules overlying the veins can also be palpated and seen. The thrombophlebitis can be migratory because of involvement of multiple veins and multiple segments of same vein. Superficial thrombophlebitis can frequently be associated with other forms of vascular disease in Behçet's disease.
- Other cutaneous manifestations of Behçet's disease:
  - Positive pathergy test
  - Sweet syndrome lesions
  - Pyoderma gangrenosum like ulcerative lesions
  - Palpable purpuric lesions
  - Extragenital ulcers resembling aphthous ulcers of the disease seen over legs, axillae, breast and interdigital skin of the foot and neck
  - Erythema multiforme-like lesions
  - Subungual infarctions
  - Hemorrhagic bullae.

Ocular Manifestations
- Prevalence: 38–99%
- Prognosis: Poor
- Associated with more severe disease
- May progress to blindness in around 25% of patients despite aggressive treatment with corticosteroid. With the use of aggressive immunosuppressant therapy, prognosis improving gradually
- Symptoms reported more frequently in males
- Usually develops 2–3 years after the onset of oral or genital involvement
- May be the first manifestation of disease in around 10–20 % of patients
- Chronically relapsing bilateral nongranulomatous uveitis involving the anterior segment, the posterior segment or both segments (panuveitis-worse prognosis, more common in males)

- Iridocyclitis, keratitis, episcleritis, scleritis, vitritis, vitreous hemorrhage, retinal vasculitis, retinal vein occlusion, retinal neovascularization and optic neuritis
- Ocular symptoms: Blurred vision, photophobia, lacrimation, periorbital pain, floaters and hyperemia
- Secondary complications may arise secondary to recurrent inflammatory attacks—posterior and peripheral anterior synechia, iris atrophy, cataract, secondary glaucoma, etc.

Articular Manifestations
- Prevalence: 16–84%
- Prognosis: Favorable
- Arthralgia, monoarthritis, or polyarthritis
- Usually nonerosive, nondeforming oligoarthralgia
- Progression to deforming arthritis: Rare
- Knees, ankles, elbows and wrists: Most frequently involved joints
- Neutrophilic and mononuclear cell infiltrates in the synovium and small vessel lesions with thrombosis typically characterize articular disease.

Cardiovascular Manifestations
- Prevalence: 7–49%, more frequent in males
- Prognosis: Poor
- Involvement of arteries and veins, as well as the heart
- Veins involved most commonly: Superficial thrombophlebitis and deep venous thrombosis, thrombosis of superior and inferior vena cava, dural sinuses and suprahepatic veins
- Artery: Pulmonary arterial aneurysms, occlusion or rupture of aneurysm in major arteries may lead to bleeding, infarction or organ failure, especially in lungs and brain
- Cardiac involvement: Pericarditis, myocarditis, endocarditis, mitral valve prolapse, valve lesions, intracardiac thrombosis, endomyocardial fibrosis, cardiomyopathy, and coronary artery lesions.

Gastrointestinal Manifestations
- Prevalence: 3–26%
- Prognosis: Poor
- Mucosal inflammation and ulceration of the gastrointestinal tract especially in the ileocecal region
- Anorexia, vomiting, dyspepsia, diarrhea, melena, abdominal pain.

Neurological Manifestations
- Prevalence: 5–10%
- Prognosis: Poor
- Usually manifests after 5 years of onset of disease
- More frequent in males
- Central nervous system (CNS) involved more frequently than the peripheral nervous system
- Headache: Most common neurological symptom

- Parenchymal (80% of patients), nonparenchymal or mixed brain disease
- Parenchymal brain disease: Involvement of brainstem and/or basal ganglia– poor prognosis
- Nonparenchymal brain disease: Associated with sinister prognosis. Cerebral venous thrombosis, notably dural sinus thrombosis, arterial vasculitis and aseptic meningitis may lead to neurological deficits, coma and death.

Q.2 What is the diagnostic criteria for Behçet's disease?

Ans: Revised ICBD (International Criteria for Behçet's Disease) is based on point score system (Table 1). Total score of 4 or more is required for establishing the diagnosis.

TABLE 1: Revised ICBD (International Criteria for Behçet's Disease) for diagnosis of Behcet's disease.

Sign/symptom	Points
Oral aphthosis (recurrent)	2
Genital aphthosis (recurrent)	2
Ocular lesions (recurrent)	2
Skin lesions	1
Neurological manifestations	1
Vascular manifestations	1
Positive pathergy test*	1

* Primary scoring system in Behçet's disease does not include pathergy testing. Pathergy test is optional, but if pathergy testing have been performed, one extra point may be assigned for a positive result.

Q.3 What is MAGIC syndrome?

Ans: The entity "mouth and genital ulcer with inflamed cartilage (MAGIC)" syndrome has been used for those patients who have features fulfilling the diagnostic criteria of both Behçet's disease and relapsing polychondritis.

Q.4 What is oral and skin pathergy testing?

Ans: Pathergy phenomenon is a nonspecific, abnormal skin response to minor trauma. Pathergy skin or oral test is an easy bedside procedure to test for presence of pathergy phenomenon.
- Oral pathergy testing: Inner labial mucosa and submucosa is pierced by 20 gauge blunt needle. The site is evaluated after 48 hours and test is considered positive if a pustule or ulcer develops at the prick site
- Skin pathergy testing: Hairless volar surface of forearm is pricked with a 20 gauge needle obliquely at an angle of 45° upto a depth of 3–5 mm with or without injection of 0.1 mL saline. The development of papule or pustule of induration of >2 mm diameter after 48 hours is considered positive.

Q.5 What are the disorders in which pathergy test is positive?

Ans:
- Behçet's disease
- Pyoderma gangrenosum

- Sweet's syndrome
- Eosinophilic pustular folliculitis
- Interferon alpha-treated chronic myeloid leukemia patients
- Inflammatory bowel disease
- Sometimes in healthy individuals.

Q.6 What are the prognostic factors and usual clinical course in Behçet's disease?

Ans: Salient features of the course of the disease:
- There may be delay in diagnosis of Behçet's disease which may adversely affect the prognosis
- Chronic course with unpredictable spontaneous exacerbations and remissions
- The prevalence rates of the clinical features have been mentioned earlier. Oral ulcers are most common manifestations followed by genital ulcers, cutaneous, ocular and articular complaints
- Oral ulcers are usually the first manifestation of disease followed by genital ulcers, cutaneous and ocular involvement, but exceptions can be there
- In around 15% of cases, combination of symptoms can be the presenting features of disease, combination of oral and genital ulcers being most common.

Prognostic factors:
- Risk factors for the development of superficial thrombophlebitis and vision loss, HLA-B51 positivity, recurrent erythema nodosum like lesions
- Risk factors for the systemic involvement: Male gender, superficial thrombophlebitis and ocular lesions
- Presence of posterior uveitis warrants early and aggressive treatment to prevent blindness
- Poor prognostic markers: Male gender, HLA-B51 positivity, and early systemic involvement
- Leading cause of morbidity: Ophthalmological and neurological involvement followed by gastrointestinal and vascular involvement.

Q.7 What is seen in the histopathology from cutaneous lesions of Behçet's disease?

Ans:
- Cutaneous lesions from patients with Behçet's disease on histopathology demonstrates primarily vasculitis and thrombosis
- In early cutaneous lesions, either of the two patterns specified below can be seen:
  - Leukocytoclastic vasculitis (karyorrhexis of neutrophils, extravasation of erythrocytes and fibrinoid necrosis of postcapillary venules)
  - Neutrophilic vascular reaction (neutrophilic infiltrate, nuclear dust and extravasation of erythrocytes without fibrinoid necrosis).
- Late lesions and autopsy demonstrates–primarily lymphocytic perivasculitis
- Histopathology of pathergy reaction shows leukocytoclastic vasculitis/neutrophilic vascular reaction.

Q.8 What investigations would you recommend in a case of Behçet's disease?

Ans:
- Complete blood count (anemia of chronic disease can be seen, platelet and total leukocyte counts are elevated)
- Liver function test, renal function test (baseline values before starting treatment)
- Inflammatory markers: C-reactive protein, erythrocyte sedimentation rate (ESR) and serum cytokines (TNF-α, IFNc, IL-1b, IL-6 and IL-8) are elevated
- Antinuclear antibody, antineutrophil cytoplasmic antibodies: To rule out connective tissue disease, other forms of vasculitis
- Pathergy testing
- Histopathology
- HLA-B51 typing-Associated with poor prognosis
- Magnetic resonance imaging brain
- Angiography
- Scintigraphy of joints

Q.9 Differentials patient presenting with oral ulcers and joint pain?

Ans: Oral ulcers and joint pain can be seen in myriad of systemic diseases. Sometimes, oral ulcers may be result of medications prescribed for treatment of arthritis (stomatitis secondary to methotrexate or sulfasalazine, fixed drug eruptions secondary to NSAIDs, herpes labialis or oral candidiasis in the setting of immunosuppression due to oral corticosteroids). Few of the major differentials and their differentiating clinical features are discussed in Table 2.

TABLE 2: Major differential diagnoses in patients presenting with oral ulcers and joint pain.

Differentials	Differentiating clinical features	Differentiating laboratory features
Behçet's disease	Presence of oral, genital, cutaneous and systemic features as mentioned above	Positive pathergy, histopathology
SLE	• Presence of photosensitivity, characteristic localized or generalized lupus erythematosus rash, Raynaud's phenomenon, lupus hair, serositis, neurological involvement • Oral ulcers: Painless in contrast to Behçet's disease and located mostly over palate	• ANA, anti-dsDNA antibody, Anti-Smith antibody, Coombs' test positivity • Hematological abnormalities (hemolytic anemia, leukocytopenia, thrombocytopenia), abnormal urinalysis, characteristic histopathology and DIF
Wegener's granulomatosis	Presence of palpable purpura, papulonecrotic lesions, leg ulcers, strawberry gums, epistaxis, nasal mucosal ulceration, nasal septal perforation, dyspnea, cough, hemoptysis, pleuritic glomerulonephritis, musculoskeletal, ocular, neurological, gastrointestinal and cardiac involvement can be seen	• Positive c-ANCA • Irregular infiltrate or nodules on chest X-ray • Abnormal urinalysis • Leukocytoclastic vasculitis and/or granulomatous inflammation can be seen in histopathology

Continued

Continued

TABLE 2: Major differential diagnoses in patients presenting with oral ulcers and joint pain.

Differentials	Differentiating clinical features	Differentiating laboratory features
MAGIC syndrome	Features of relapsing polychondritis (widespread, destructive, inflammatory lesions of cartilaginous structures, including ear, nose, larynx, trachea, bronchi, peripheral joints, eye, heart and skin) along with Behçet's disease	–
Reactive arthritis	• Presence of oligoarticular, asymmetrical arthritis of peripheral joints especially lower limbs, axial arthritis-sacroiliac lumbar spine, Erosive arthritis in contrast to non-erosive arthritis of Behçet's disease and SLE • Enthesitis: Plantar fasciitis, Achilles tendonitis, sausage digits • Cutaneous: Keratoderma blenorrhagicum, circinate balanitis, oral ulcers are painless in contrast to Behçet's disease, geographic tongue • Sterile pyuria, urethral discharge	• Enthesitis and erosive arthritis on radiological investigations • Positive PCR for Chlamydia

(SLE: systemic lupus erythematosus; DIF: direct immunofluorescence: c-ANCA: cytoplasmic antineutrophil cytoplasmic antibodies; MAGIC: mouth and genital ulcer with inflamed cartilage; PCR: polymerase chain reaction; dsDNA: double stranded deoxyribonucleic acid).

Q.10 Treatment options in Behçet's disease?

Ans: Management

Several factors like severity of disease and organ involvement, duration of disease and frequency of recurrences, age of disease onset and gender dictate the treatment strategies followed in individual cases of Behçet's disease. Ocular, gastrointestinal, CNS and cardiovascular involvement requires early, aggressive interventions.

No universal consensus over ideal treatment protocol has been reached till now. Treatment options depending upon the site of involvement have been discussed below.

Management of Mucocutaneous Lesions

Topical Modalities

There is paucity of studies evaluating the management of oral ulcers in Behçet's disease. Strategies commonly followed for the topical treatment of oral ulcers in Behçet's disease are based mostly on studies in recurrent aphthous stomatitis considering the similarities in both the entities. Based on limited evidence, treatment algorithm mentioned below can be followed.

First line:
- Topical corticosteroids (triamcinolone mucosal cream, ointment or paste 0.1%; dexamethasone mucosal paste or solution 0.5 mg/5 mL) four times daily
- Antimicrobial agents: Chlorhexidine gel and mouth rinse, penicillin G potassium troches, tetracycline suspension, triclosan mouth rinse
- Sucralfate suspension 1 g/5 mL four times a day for oral aphthous and genital ulcers
- Pimecrolimus (genital ulcers).

Second line:
- 5-aminosalicylic acid (5% cream) three times a day
- 5% amlexanox oral paste.

Third line:
- Topical anesthetics (lidocaine 2–5%, mepivacaine 1.5%, tetracaine 0.5–1% gel or mucosal ointment) twice or thrice a day
- Silver nitrate

Systemic Modalities

There are several randomized studies on systemic modalities in Behçet's disease based on which the following treatment algorithm can be followed. An evidence based treatment algorithm can be followed as described below.

First line:
- Colchicine
- Colchicine in combination with benzathine penicillin.

Second line:
- Prednisolone
- Dapsone
- Azathioprine
- Thalidomide.

Third line:
- Zinc sulfate
- Rebamipide
- Interferon alpha
- Cyclosporine
- Anti-TNF-α antagonists
- Apremilast
- Isotretinoin.

Management of Ocular Involvement
- Ocular involvement in Behçet's disease should be managed aggressively with combination of systemic and topical therapy in early stages to prevent irreversible damage
- Topical corticosteroids in combination with mydriatics and cycloplegic agents can be used in mild anterior uveitis. Systemic corticosteroids, cyclosporine, azathioprine, IFN-α, anti-TNF-α agents, cyclophosphamide and methotrexate have been found to be effective

- Any patient with posterior uveitis should be managed with a treatment regimen which includes systemic corticosteroids and azathioprine. Cyclosporine or infliximab in combination with azathioprine and corticosteroids is recommended for severe eye involvement defined by 2 lines of drop in visual acuity on a 10/10 scale and/or retinal disease. IFN-α with or without corticosteroids can be used alternatively.

Management of Articular Involvement

Colchicine with or without benzathine penicillin or anti-inflammatory analgesics is considered the first line of therapy. Azathioprine, corticosteroids, methotrexate, salazopyrine, IFN-α, anti-TNF agents have also been used successfully.

Management of Vascular Involvement

- Corticosteroids with or without adjuvants like azathioprine, methotrexate, cyclophosphamide are the mainstay of treatment. Anticoagulation and surgical intervention may be required
- Anti-TNF-α agents have also been found to be effective in vascular involvement. Immunosuppressive agents such as corticosteroids, azathioprine, cyclophosphamide or cyclosporine are recommended for the management of acute deep vein thrombosis
- Cyclophosphamide and corticosteroids are recommended for managing the pulmonary and peripheral arterial aneurysms.

Management of Gastrointestinal Involvement

Sulfasalazine and corticosteroids are the most commonly used agents for gastrointestinal involvement. Azathioprine can be used as adjuvant or second line therapy.

Management of Central Nervous System Involvement

Corticosteroids, IFN-α, azathioprine, cyclophosphamide, methotrexate and TNF-α antagonists are used commonly for parenchymal involvement. Corticosteroids are recommended for dural sinus thrombosis. Cyclosporine should not be used in CNS involvement unless intraocular inflammation is there.

CASE 2

A 27-year-old female presented with complaint of pain and swelling involving small joints of hands and wrist with morning stiffness lasting more than half an hour. She also complained of red itchy and scaly lesions over her face, neck and back of hands. She also reported discomfort, itching and redness within few minutes of exposure to sun. She also has been noticing recurrent painless red oral ulcers commonly over mucosa of hard palate for the past few months which typically lasts few weeks and heals spontaneously. She also described pain and pallor followed by bluish discoloration of the tips of her fingers on exposure to cold. She did not complain of fever, weight loss, dysphagia, shortness of breath, chest pain, abdominal, bladder or bowel complaints. She also denied any history of musculoskeletal, neurological, cardiovascular complaints.

> On examination, cutaneous erythema along with mild scaling and edema was noted over photoexposed sites especially malar area, upper chest and dorsum of hands but sparing the knuckles. Shallow erosions with peripheral rim of erythema were noted over hard palate. Ragged cuticles and nail fold erythema were also noticed on examination of nails. On capillaroscopy of nail fold, nail fold telangiectasia and capillary drop outs were appreciated. Apart from these lesions, mucocutaneous examination was unremarkable.
>
> On musculoskeletal examination, swelling and tenderness of small joints of hands was evident without any deformity. Rest of the systemic examination was unremarkable.
>
> Routine investigations were consistent with anemia, leukopenia and subnephrotic proteinuria. Antinuclear antibody (ANA), double stranded deoxyribonucleic acid (dsDNA) and Coombs' test were found to be positive.
>
> **Diagnosis:** Systemic lupus erythematosus (SLE).

INTERACTIVE TOPIC REVIEW

Q.1 Classification of cutaneous lupus erythematosus.

Ans: James N Gilliam devised a nomenclature and classification for cutaneous lesion associated with lupus erythematosus based on histopathological findings. Lesions associated with characteristic histopathological features were classified as LE specific skin disease while those with histopathological findings not specific for LE are classified as LE-nonspecific lesions.

Lupus Erythematosus-Specific Skin Disease [Cutaneous Lupus Erythematosus (CLE)]
- Acute cutaneous LE (ACLE)
    - Localized ACLE (malar rash; butterfly rash)
    - Generalized ACLE (lupus maculopapular rash, SLE rash, photosensitive lupus dermatitis).
- Subacute cutaneous LE (SCLE)
    - Annular SCLE (Synonyms: Lupus marginatus, symmetric erythema centrifugum, autoimmune annular erythema, lupus erythematosus gyratus repens)
    - Papulosquamous SCLE (Synonyms: Disseminated DLE, subacute disseminated LE, superficial disseminated LE, psoriasiform LE, pityriasiform LE and maculopapular photosensitive LE).
- Chronic cutaneous LE (CCLE)
    - Classic discoid LE (DLE)
        - Localized DLE
        - Generalized DLE.
- Hypertrophic/verrucous DLE
- Lupus profundus/lupus panniculitis
- Mucosal DLE
    - Oral DLE
    - Conjunctival DLE.
- Lupus tumidus (urticarial plaque of LE)

- Chilblain LE (CHLE)
- Lichenoid DLE (LE/lichen planus overlap, lupus planus).

Lupus Erythematosus Nonspecific Lesions
- Cutaneous vascular disease
  - Vasculitis
    - Leukocytoclastic
      - Palpable purpura
      - Urticarial vasculitis.
    - Periarteritis nodosa-like cutaneous lesions.
  - Vasculopathy
    - Degos disease-like lesions
    - Secondary atrophie blanche (synonym livedoid vasculitis, livedo vasculitis).
  - Periungual telangiectasia
  - Livedo reticularis
  - Thrombophlebitis
  - Raynaud's phenomenon
  - Erythromelalgia (erythermalgia).
- Nonscarring alopecia
  - Lupus hair loss
  - Telogen effluvium
  - Alopecia areata.
- Sclerodactyly
- Rheumatoid nodules
- Calcinosis cutis
- LE-nonspecific bullous lesions
- Urticaria
- Papulonodular mucinosis
- Cutis laxa/anetoderma
- Acanthosis nigricans (type B insulin resistance)
- Erythema multiforme
- Leg ulcers
- Lichen planus.

Q.2 Diagnostic criteria for systemic lupus erythematosus?

Ans: The 1982 revised criteria for classification of systemic lupus erythematosus: The proposed classification is based on 11 criteria (Table 3). For the purpose of identifying patients in clinical studies, a person shall be said to have systemic lupus erythematosus if any four or more of the 11 criteria are present, serially or simultaneously, during any interval or observation.

The Systemic Lupus International Collaborating Clinics (SLICC) classification criteria for SLE (Table 4): A patient is classified as having SLE if he or she satisfies four of the clinical and immunological criteria, including at least one clinical criterion, or if he or she has biopsy-proven nephritis compatible with SLE in the presence of ANAs or anti-dsDNA antibodies. Criteria are cumulative and need not be present concurrently.

TABLE 3: 1982 revised criteria for classification of systemic lupus erythematosus.	
Criterion	**Definition**
Malar rash	Fixed erythema, flat or raised, over the malar eminences, tending to spare the nasolabial folds
Discoid rash	Erythematous raised patches with adherent keratotic scaling and follicular plugging; atrophic scarring may occur in older lesions
Photosensitivity	Skin rash as a result of unusual reaction to sunlight, by patient history or physician observation
Oral ulcers	Oral or nasopharyngeal ulceration, usually painless, observed by a physician
Arthritis	Nonerosive arthritis involving two or more peripheral joints, characterized by tenderness, swelling or effusion
Serositis	Pleuritis—convincing history of pleuritic pain or rub heard by a physician or evidence of pleural effusion Or Pericarditis—documented by electrocardiogram or rub or evidence of pericardial effusion
Renal disorder	Persistent proteinuria >0.5 g/day or >3+ if quantitation not performed Or Cellular casts—may be red cell, hemoglobin, granular, tubular or mixed
Neurological disorder	Seizures—in the absence of offending drugs or known metabolic derangements (e.g. uremia, ketoacidosis, or electrolyte imbalance) Or Psychosis—in the absence of offending drugs or known metabolic derangements (e.g. uremia, ketoacidosis or electrolyte imbalance)
Hematologic disorder	Hemolytic anemia with reticulocytosis Or Leukopenia <4,000/μL total on two or more occasions Or Lymphopenia <1,500/ μL on two or more occasions Or Thrombocytopenia <1,500/μL in the absence of offending drugs
Immunologic disorder	Anti-DNA antibody to native DNA in abnormal titer Or Anti-Sm antibody to Sm nuclear antigen present Or Positive finding of antiphospholipid antibodies based on: (i) An abnormal serum level of immunoglobulin G or immunoglobulin M anticardiolipin antibodies; (ii) a positive test result for lupus anticoagulant using a standard method, or (iii) a false-positive serologic test for syphilis known to be positive for at least 6 months and confirmed by *Treponema pallidum* immobilization or fluorescent treponemal antibody absorption test
Antinuclear antibody	An abnormal titer of antinuclear antibody by immunofluorescence of an equivalent assay at any point in time and in the absence of drugs known to be associated with "drug-induced lupus" syndrome

TABLE 4: The Systemic Lupus International Collaborating Clinics (SLICC) classification criteria for SLE.

Clinical criteria	Definition
Acute cutaneous lupus	Including: Lupus malar rash (do not include if malar discoid), bullous lupus, toxic epidermal necrolysis variant of SLE, maculopapular rash, photosensitive lupus rash in the absence of dermatomyositis, or subacute cutaneous lupus
Chronic cutaneous lupus	Including: Classic discoid rash, hypertrophic (verrucous) lupus, lupus panniculitis (profundus), mucosal lupus, lupus erythematosus tumidus, chilblain lupus, discoid lupus/lichen planus overlap
Oral ulcers	Palate, buccal, tongue, or nasal ulcers in the absence of other causes
Nonscarring alopecia	Diffuse thinning or hair fragility with broken hair in the absence of other causes
Synovitis	Involving two or more joints characterized by effusion or swelling or tenderness in two or more joints and at least 30 min of morning stiffness
Serositis, pleurisy, or pericarditis	More that 1-day duration of pleural/pericardial effusions or pleural/pericardial rub
Renal disorder	Persistent proteinuria (>0.5 µg/day) or cellular casts
Neurological disorder	Seizures, psychosis, mononeuritis multiplex, myelitis or acute confusional state in the absence of other causes
Hemolytic anemia	–
Leukopenia	Total leukocyte count <4000/mm^3 at least once Or Lymphopenia (<1000/mm^3)
Thrombocytopenia	<100,000/mm^3 at least once
Immunological criteria	
<ul><li>ANA above reference laboratory range</li><li>Anti-dsDNA antibody above reference laboratory range (or >2-fold the reference range if tested by ELISA)</li><li>Anti-Sm: Presence of antibody to Sm nuclear antigen</li><li>Antiphospholipid antibody positivity</li><li>Low complement (low C3, C4 or CH50)</li><li>Direct Coombs' test in the absence of hemolytic anemia</li></ul>	

Q.3 Pathogenesis of lupus erythematosus.

Ans: The role of various environmental factors in the pathogenesis of lupus erythematosus is illustrated below:

Genetic Susceptibility
- The concordance rate for lupus is 25% among monozygotic twins and approximately 2% among dizygotic twins
- MHC: HLA-A1, B8, and DR3

- Complement: Deficiency of one of the early complement components—C1q (decreased clearance of necrotic tissue), C2, or C4 (decreased elimination of self-reactive β-cells)–90% risk.

Ultraviolet Radiation
- Sunlight usually contains only UVA and UVB, because UVC is absorbed by the stratospheric ozone layer
- UVA penetrates through epidermal and dermal layers of the skin and is weakly absorbed by biomolecules but UVB does not penetrate much farther than the epidermal layer and is strongly absorbed by DNA and protein
- UV light causes apoptosis of keratinocyte which makes previously cryptic peptides available for immune surveillance and also causes exaggerated release of immune mediators.

Sex Hormones
- Systemic lupus erythematosus has a marked female predominance, with a 9:1 female to male ratio
- Apart from estrogen other sex hormones and sex-linked genes also play a role.

Hormones implicated:
- Estrogen
- Prolactin
- Androgens
- Dehydroepiandrosterone.

Smoking
- Exposure to tobacco smoke can alter endogenous proteins, including DNA
- Reactive oxidative species produced from the metabolism of tobacco smoke modify DNA and DNA adducts are formed
- Such damaged DNA is more immunogenic than "native" (undamaged) dsDNA and these adducts are found at high levels within immune complexes
- Patients who smoke are less responsive to antimalarial treatment.

Drugs
- Many drugs are implicated in inducing various features of LE (Table 5).

TABLE 5: Drugs implicated in systemic lupus erythematosus.

Class of drugs	High risk	Medium risk	Low risk
Antiarrhythmics	Procainamide (15–20%)	Quinidine (<1%)	
Antihypertensive	Hydralazine		• Methyldopa • Captopril
Antipsychotics	–	–	Carbamazepine
Antibiotics	–	–	• Isoniazid • Minocycline
Anticonvulsants	–	–	Carbamazepine
Antithyroid	–	–	Propylthiouracil

Q.4 Write briefly about clinical features, histopathology and types of cutaneous lupus erythematosus.

Ans: Discoid Lupus Erythematosus
- Definition: DLE is a benign disorder of the skin, most frequently involving the face and characterized by well-defined, red scaly plaques of variable size, which heal with atrophy, scarring and pigmentary changes
- Epidemiology: Female to male ratio—2:1
- Age of onset: Fourth decade
- Localized disease
- Face is most commonly affected and the scalp, ears, nose and neck to a lesser extent
- Scalp is involved in 60% of cases and one-third of patients develop scarring alopecia
- Photosensitivity occurs in about 70% of patients with discoid lupus erythematosus (DLE)
- The circumscribed or discoid type is the most frequent and occurs particularly on the cheeks, the bridge of the nose, the ears, the side of the neck and the scalp
- There is adherent scale in many cases and when this is removed its undersurface shows horny plugs which have occupied dilated pilosebaceous canals—"carpet-tack" sign
- Heal with a thin white scarred area, often with a slightly raised, red border or zone of hyperpigmentation
- Nonitching hyperkeratotic papulonodular lesions on the arms and hands, resembling keratoacanthoma, hypertrophic lichen planus or nodular prurigo, also occur
- Wide follicular pits, sometimes containing scales or blackheads, occur mainly in the concha or triangular fossa of the ear.

Disseminated Discoid Lupus Erythematosus
- Characteristic lesions of DLE may occur in a widespread pattern on the trunk and limbs, or may be localized to other body sites
- Occurs mainly in women and they are usually cigarette smokers
- This variety tends to be persistent, resistant to therapy
- Risk factors for the development of SLE in DLE patients:
    - Disseminated DLE 20%
    - Generalized lymphadenopathy
    - Subacute cutaneous LE/acute cutaneous LE skin lesions
    - Lupus erythematosus nonspecific lesions–vasculitis, diffuse nonscarring alopecia, periungual capillary nail fold telangiectasia
    - Unexplained anemia, marked leukopenia
    - False positive test for syphilis
    - Persistently positive high ANA titers
    - Antisingle stranded DNA antibody
    - Hypergammaglobulinemia

- High erythrocyte sedimentation rate
  - Positive nonlesional lupus band test
  - High levels of elevated IL-2 receptor levels.

Histopathology

Epidermis:
- Focal hyperkeratosis/parakeratosis. Compact stratum corneum
- Follicular plugging
- Atrophy of stratum malpighi
- Focal liquefactive degeneration of basal cells
- Thick band like periodic acid-Schiff positive basement membrane.

Dermal changes:
- Edema in upper dermis
- Destruction of elastic fibers
- Vasculitis with fibrinoid deposit and extravasation of red blood cells
- Mild panniculitis, mucin deposition rarely.

Immunopathology
- Immunohistology shows the presence of immunoglobulins IgG, IgA, IgM and complement at the dermal–epidermal junction, in approximately 80% of patients.

Antinuclear antibody positivity in DLE:
- Positive in 5–60 % of cases
- "Homogeneous" type of antinuclear factor being twice as frequent as the "speckled" type
- They are more common in:
  - Older patients
  - Long duration of disease
  - Extensive skin involvement
  - Chilblains
  - Raynaud's phenomenon
  - Joint pains.

Prognosis
- The risk of a patient with DLE developing overt SLE is 5% in localized and 20% in disseminated type
- Squamous cell and, less commonly, basal cell carcinomas occasionally occur in the scars of DLE, particularly on the scalp, ears, lips and nose. An incidence of 3.3% has been noted.

Treatment of Discoid Lupus Erythematosus
- Photoprotection, sunscreen
- Topical agents:
  - First line: Topical steroids
  - Second line: Calcineurin inhibitors
- Systemic agents:
  - First line: Antimalarials, short-course steroids
  - Second line: Retinoids, methotrexate
  - Third line: Azathioprine, mycophenolate mofetil, dapsone, thalidomide.

Types of Chronic Cutaneous Lupus Erythematosus other than Classic Discoid Lupus Erythematosus

Hypertrophic Discoid Lupus Erythematosus
- Rare (2%)
- Clinical features:
  - Commonly affect the extensor surface of the arms and legs, the upper back and the face
  - Dull, red and indurated lesions that are covered by keratotic multilayered horny white or yellow scales with a central crateriform atrophy.
- Significance:
  - Less chance of progression to SLE.
- Histopathologic findings:
  - Marked acanthosis, hyperkeratosis and hypergranulosis with a pronounced mononuclear infiltrate
  - Histology of hypertrophic DLE lesions reveal pseudoepitheliomatous hyperplasia engulfing elastotic material
  - The CD123 staining can be a useful feature to distinguish hypertrophic LE from SCC and hypertrophic actinic keratosis.
- Immunologic abnormalities:
  - Rarely have positive serologic tests.
- Treatment:
  - Hypertrophic DLE is particularly resistant to treatment, although local cryotherapy, topical high-potency corticosteroids and systemic antimalarials may be useful
  - Topical tretinoin and particularly systemic isotretinoin (1 mg/kg/day in 2 divided doses for 11 weeks) have also been found to be effective, with dramatic improvement in 3 weeks.

Mucosal Discoid Lupus Erythematosus
- Mucosa is involved in approximately 25% of patients
- Morphology:
  - Painless erythematous patches with a depressed center and superficial ulceration occur and have irregular white borders with radiating striae
  - Lesions on the palate often have a honeycomb appearance
  - Healing occurs with some scarring
  - Rarely oral mucosal lesions can degenerate to SCC.
- Histology: Lymphocyte-rich interface mucositis is seen
- Significance:
  - Chronic mucosal plaques seen in patients with LE do not have life-threatening manifestations of SLE
- Treatment:
  - Topical therapy consists of high potency corticosteroids (clobetasol gel 4–5 times a day), with or without topical tacrolimus ointment (2–3 times a day).

Chilblain Lupus (Hutchinson Lupus)
- Chilblain lupus is a rare manifestation of LE characterized by cold-induced lesions localized in acral areas without cold agglutinins and cryoglobulins

- Approximately 6% of patients, predominantly females develop this condition
- Clinical features:
  - Located on fingers, toes, calves, heels, knees, elbows, nose and ears and are generally aggravated by exposure to cold
  - These lesions are represented by papuloerythematous purplish, sometimes infiltrated, pruriginous or painful elements and may ulcerate
- Significance:
  - Approximately 15% of patients develop SLE and this occurs more frequently in those who develop both forms of cutaneous LE simultaneously and in those with erythema multiforme.
- Immunologic abnormalities:
  - Patients are usually Ro antibody positive
  - A homogeneous or speckled pattern of antinuclear antibodies, anti-DNA antibodies and lupus anticoagulant antibodies have been detected in some patients.
- Treatment:
  - Treatment of chilblain lupus is not easy and antimalarials are only slightly or not at all effective
  - Topical or oral corticosteroids, pentoxifylline, dapsone, etretinate, vasodilators, mycophenolate mofetil can be helpful
  - Warm environment and suitable clothes for protection from cold are even more important.

Lupus Erythematosus Profundus (Panniculitis)

- Occurs more frequently in women between the ages of 20 and 60 years (female to male ratio, 2:1)
- Predilection for the face, proximal extremities, buttocks, breasts and trunk
- Presents as indurated, subcutaneous nodules that are usually firm, rubbery, sharply defined and persistent
- Typical lesions of DLE may be found elsewhere, most frequently on the cheeks
- Healing usually leads to the development of depressed areas
- Significance:
  - Positive ANA (70–75%), leukopenia, hypocomplementemia, circulating rheumatoid factor, false-positive syphilis serology and an increased ESR– higher incidence of SLE
  - Incidence of SLE among patients with lupus profundus is 3–30%.
- Histopathologic findings:
  - Typical lobular lymphocytic panniculitis with hyaline necrosis of fat, lymphocytic aggregates or lymphoid nodules associated with lymphocytic nuclear dust
  - Calcification is common and thickened and hyalinized vessels are often present in the subcutaneous fat and septal regions.
- Treatment:
  - Combined therapy corticosteroids (systemic/topical) and antimalarial drugs may be useful
  - Dapsone and also thalidomide are effective in resistant cases.

Lupus Erythematosus Tumidus
- This is a rare subset of CLE and is characterized by remarkable photo-sensitivity, summer exacerbation and preferential male sex and a good prognosis
- Clinical features:
  - Mean age at onset of the disease in 40 years
  - Face, upper back, V-area of the neck, extensor aspects of the arms and shoulders
  - Presents as indurated, subcutaneous nodules that are usually firm, rubbery, sharply defined and persistent
  - Typical lesions of DLE may be found elsewhere, most frequently on the cheeks
  - Healing usually leads to the development of depressed areas.
- Immunologic abnormalities:
  - Results of direct immunofluorescence testing performed on lesional skin are mostly negative
  - Antinuclear antibodies are detected in 10% of patients.
- Histopathologic findings:
  - Minimal follicular hyperkeratosis with basal layer vacuolization, considerable dermal lymphocytic infiltrate and interstitial mucin deposition.
- Significance:
  - Association with systemic disease seems to be very rare in patients with lupus erythematosus tumidus.
- Treatment:
  - Sunscreen and photoprotection
  - Topical steroids
  - Lupus erythematosus tumidus has a rapid and effective response with systemic treatment with antimalarials.

Subacute Cutaneous Lupus Erythematosus
- Etiology:
  - Occurs in genetically predisposed individuals, most often in patients with HLA-B8, HLA-DR3, HLA-DRw52 and HLA-DQ1
  - A strong association exists with anti-Ro (SS-A) autoantibodies (80% of patients)
  - Ultraviolet radiation (UV-B > UV-A) modulation of autoantigens play a role in pathogenesis.
- Drugs causing SCLE:
  - Chlorothiazide
  - Calcium channel blockers
  - Angiotensin converting enzyme inhibitors
  - Phenytoin
  - Terbinafine
  - Tetracycline
  - Beta-blockers
  - Nonsteroidal anti-inflammatory drugs.

- Clinical features:
  - Characterized by recurrent, nonscarring skin lesions occurring in a symmetrical photodistributed pattern
  - Lesions usually occur above the waist and particularly around the V-area of the neck, upper chest and back and shoulders as well as the extensor aspects of the arms and hands
  - Initially presents as erythematous slightly scaly papule/macule which usually evolves into in one of the following two typical morphological forms:
    - Annular (Fig. 3) or polycyclic plaques ($1/3^{rd}$): Initial lesions expand and clear centrally to produce annular lesions that may merge into polycyclic arrays
    - Papulosquamous (psoriasiform) plaques ($2/3^{rd}$): Initial lesions expand and merge producing retiform arrays of papulosquamous lesions that can mimic those of psoriasis.
  - Rarely patients can have lesions of both morphology
  - May heal with pigmentary changes and telangiectasias, but not with dermal atrophy or scarring
  - Other atypical morphological variants of SCLE:
    - Stevens–Johnson syndrome—toxic epidermal necrolysis like
    - Exfoliative erythroderma
    - Pityriasiform.
  - Absence of induration and atrophic scarring helps to distinguish SCLE from DLE.

Acute Cutaneous Lupus Erythematosus
- It can be transient or lasting for several days
- Lesions wax and wane with sun exposure over a period of several hours
- Can be categorized into:

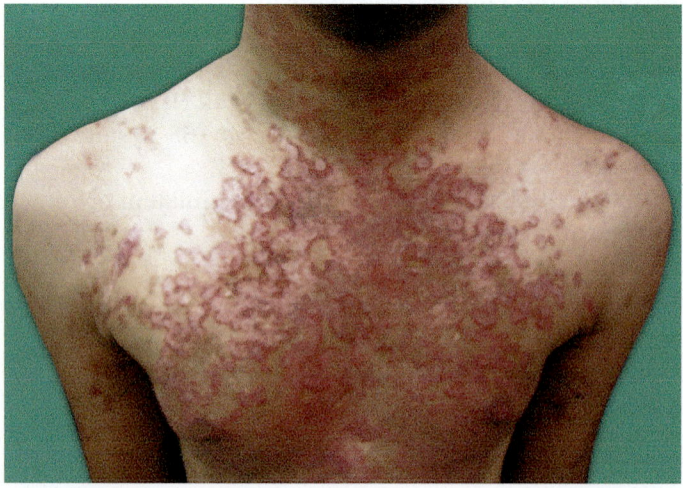

Fig. 3: Annular variants subacute cutaneous lupus erythematosus lesions.

- Localized ACLE: Malar rash, sparing the nasolabial folds. May involve forehead and anterior neck
- Generalized ACLE (Fig. 4): Photosensitive morbilliform rash, spares the knuckles
- Toxic epidermal necrolysis-like ACLE.

Oral Involvement in Lupus Erythematosus
- Painless, shallow, oral ulcers mostly over hard palate palate (Fig. 5). Recurrent apthous stomatitis (Fig. 6) can also be seen in the setting of SLE, but these are different from painless oral ulcers typical of SLE and are not assocoiated with systemic disease activity
- In DLE, three types of lesions:
  - Erythematous lesions

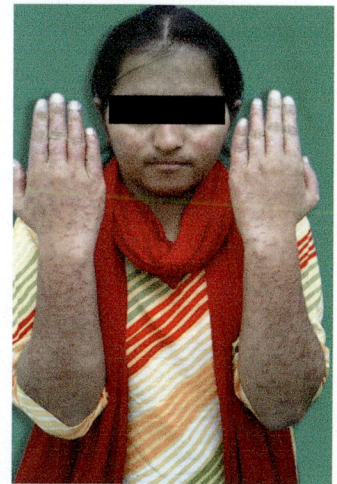

Fig. 4: Generalized acute cutaneous lupus erythematosus.

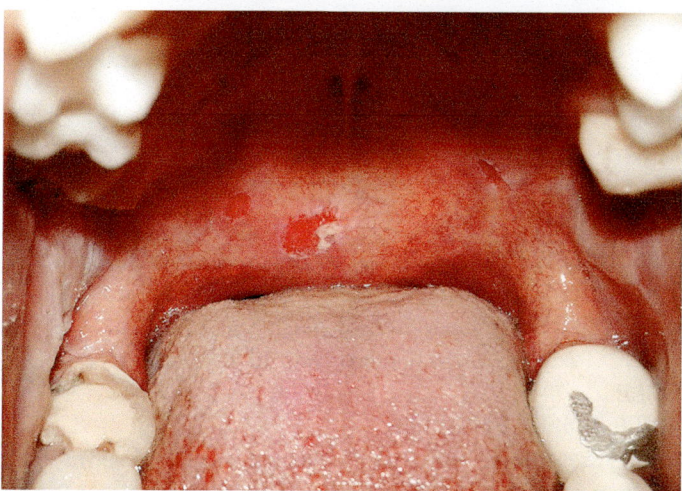

Fig. 5: Painless palatal erosion in lupus erythematosus.

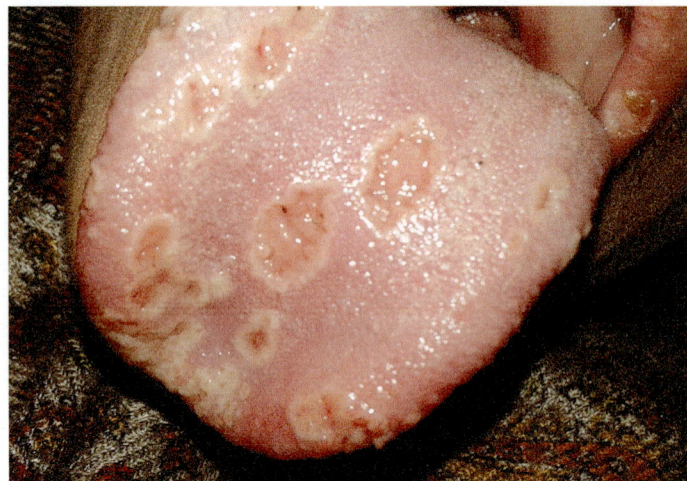

Fig. 6: Extensive aphthous stomatitis like oral ulcers in patient of systemic lupus erythematosus.

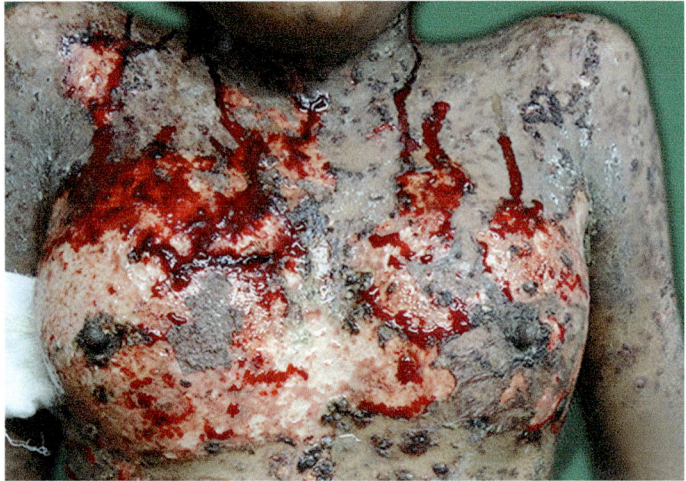

Fig. 7: Toxic epidermal necrolysis-like acute cutaneous lupus erythematosus.

- o Discoid lesions
- o Ulcers.

Vesiculobullous Skin Lesions in Lupus Erythematosus Patients
- Lupus erythematosus specific vesiculobullous lesions:
    - o ACLE: Toxic epidermal necrolysis like ACLE (Fig. 7)
    - o SCLE: Toxic epidermal necrolysis like SCLE, vesiculobullous annular SCLE
    - o CCLE: Bullous discoid LE.
- Lupus erythematosus nonspecific vesiculobullous lesion:
    - o Bullous systemic LE (dermatitis herpetiformis like LE-nonspecific skin disease

- o Epidermolysis bullosa acquisita like LE-nonspecific skin disease.
- Vesiculobullous lesions anecdotally reported to be associated with LE:
  - o Bullous pemphigoid
  - o Dermatitis herpetiformis
  - o Pemphigus erythematosus
  - o Porphyria cutaneous tarda.

Treatment of Acute Cutaneous Lupus Erythematosus/Systemic Lupus Erythematosus

First line:
- Oral hydroxychloroquine (6.5 mg/kg/day)/chloroquine (3.5 mg/kg)
- Short course of oral corticosteroids
- If monotherapy fails add quinacrine (100 mg/day) to hydroxychloroquine or chloroquine.

Second line:
- Azathioprine: 1.5–2.5 mg/kg/day
- Mycophenolate mofetil: 2.5–3.5 g/day
- Methotrexate: 7.5–25 mg/week
- Dapsone: 50–200 mg/day.

Third line:
- Cyclophosphomide: 1.5–2 mg/kg/day.

General Measures
- Photoprotection
  - o Conventional measures:
    - Avoidance of sun exposure
    - Physical protection
    - Broad spectrum sunscreen
    - Elimination of photosensitizing drugs
    - Sunscreens.
  - o Consistent ultraviolet rays protection is recommended by thorough application of light-shielding substances with highly potent chemical/organic or physical/inorganic sunscreens with high sun protection factor (>30). It should be applied in sufficient amounts (approximately 2 mg/cm^2) at least 20–30 minutes before sun exposure.

Topical Treatment
- Topical steroids:
  - o Topical steroids have proven to be a very effective treatment for skin lesions in all subtypes of CLE
  - o The main symptoms, such as redness and scaling, are reduced by steroids
  - o Choice of the steroid class should consider the area of the body and the activity of the skin lesion.
- Calcineurin inhibitors:
  - o Tacrolimus and pimecrolimus
  - o Mechanism of action: Down-regulate T-cell activity by inhibiting the phosphatase calcineurin, responsible for dephosphorylation of the nuclear factor of activated T-cells

- o Advantage: Less atrophy and telangiectasia
- o Disadvantage: Less effective in hyperkeratotic lesions.

Systemic Agents
- Indication for systemic therapy: Skin lesions are widespread, disfiguring, scarring, or refractory to topical agents

Antimalarials
- First line of treatment
- Antimalarials have a variety of effects that may be relevant to their therapeutic benefit in SLE, including interference with TLR signaling
- Hydroxychloroquine, chloroquine, quinacrine
- Can take upon 2–3 months for maximum efficacy
- Smokers often have severe CLE and are more refractory to treatment with antimalarials. Hence, all patients should therefore be counseled for smoking cessation
- Antimalarials are the drug of choice in all subtypes of CLE and elicit a response in 50–90% of patients
- First-line and long-term systemic treatment in all CLE patients with severe or widespread skin lesions, particularly in patients with the risk of scarring and development of systemic disease
- Hydroxychloroquine in a maximum daily dosage of 5 mg/kg real body weight or chloroquine in a maximum daily dosage of 2.3 mg/kg real body weight is recommended. A combination of hydroxychloroquine with chloroquine must be avoided due to the risk of irreversible retinopathy
- In refractory cases, it is recommended to add quinacrine to either hydroxychloroquine or chloroquine
- In cases of contraindication for hydroxychloroquine or chloroquine (e.g. retinopathy), monotherapy with quinacrine is recommended
- Ophthalmological consultation is recommended in all CLE patients treated with hydroxychloroquine or chloroquine at baseline, annually after 5 years of starting treatment or earlier in the presence of risk factors.
    - o Ocular monitoring for hydroxychloroquine:
        - Baseline and regular monitoring (5 yearly) for retinopathy according to latest AAO guidelines
        - It is suggested to measure hydroxychloroquine or chloroquine blood levels in therapy-refractory patients.

CONCLUSION

Oral ulcers with associated joint pain can be a seen in a number of systemic disorders. Occasionally, oral ulcers can be secondary to drugs prescribed for arthritis (methotrexate, NSAIDs, etc). Thorough history and physical examination is of paramount importance for narrowing down the possibilities in such patients. Immunological and other laboratory investigations are usually required to establish the definitive diagnosis. Multidisciplinary approach involving dermatologists, rheumatologists and if required other specialties should be followed for proper management of such cases especially in patients with disorders, like Behcet's disease or SLE as multisystem involvement is fairly common in these disorders. The role of dermatologists is of utmost importance in diagnosis and management of such patients at an early stage.

SUGGESTED READING

1. Al-Araji A, Kidd DP. Neuro-Behçet's disease: Epidemiology, clinical characteristics, and management. Lancet Neurol. 2009;8(2):192-204.
2. Alibaz-Oner F, Sawalha AH, Direskeneli H. Management of Behçet's disease. Curr Opin Rheumatol. 2018;30:238-42.
3. Alpsoy E, Donmez L, Bacanli A, et al. Review of the chronology of clinical manifestations in 60 patients with Behçet's disease. Dermatology. 2003;207:354-6.
4. Alpsoy E, Zouboulis CC, Ehrlich GE. Mucocutaneous lesions of Behçet's disease. Yonsei Medical Journal. 2007;48:573-85.
5. Alpsoy E. Behçet's disease: A comprehensive review with a focus on epidemiology, etiology and clinical features, and management of mucocutaneous lesions. J Dermatol. 2016;43:620-32.
6. Alpsoy E. New evidence-based treatment approach in Behçet's disease. Patholog Res Int. 2012;2012:871019.
7. Borchers AT, Keen CL, Gershwin ME. Drug-induced lupus. Ann N Y Acad Sci. 2007;1108:166-82.
8. Caproni M, Cardinali C, Salvatore E, et al. Subacute cutaneous lupus erythematosus with pityriasis-like cutaneous manifestations. Int J Dermatol. 2001;40(1):59-62.
9. Gilliam JN, Sontheimer RD. Distinctive cutaneous subsets in the spectrum of lupus erythematosus. J Am Acad Dermatol. 1981;4:471-5.
10. Kaneko Y, Nakai N, Kida T, et al. Mouth and genital ulcers with inflamed cartilage syndrome: Case report and review of the published work. Indian J Dermatol. 2016;61(3):347.
11. Kotter I. [EULAR recommendations for the management of Behçet's disease. Report of a task force of the European Standing Committee for International Clinical Studies Including Therapeutics (ESCISIT)]. Z Rheumatol. 2009;68:157-61.
12. Lowell A. Goldsmith SIK, Fitzpatrick's Dermatology in General Medicine, 8 ed, 1909-1926.
13. Mak A, Tay SH. Environmental factors, toxicants and systemic lupus erythematosus. Int J Mol Sci. 2014;15:16043-56.
14. Mendes D, Correia M, Barbedo M, et al. Behçet's disease—A contemporary review. J Autoimmun. 2009;32:178-88.
15. Mok CC, Lau CS. Pathogenesis of systemic lupus erythematosus. J Clin Pathol. 2003;56:481-90.
16. Petri M, Orbai AM, Alarcon GS, et al. Derivation and validation of the Systemic Lupus International Collaborating Clinics classification criteria for systemic lupus erythematosus. Arthritis Rheum. 2012;64:2677-86.
17. Rubin RL. Drug-induced lupus. Toxicology. 2005;209:135-47.
18. Sakane T, Takeno M, Suzuki N, et al. Behçet's disease. N Engl J Med. 1999;341:1284-91.
19. Sequeira F, Daryani D. The oral and skin pathergy test. Indian J Dermatol Venereol Leprol. 2011;77(4):526-30.
20. Tan EM, Cohen AS, Fries JF, et al. The 1982 revised criteria for the classification of systemic lupus erythematosus. Arthritis Rheum. 1982;25:1271-7.
21. The International Criteria for Behçet's Disease (ICBD): A collaborative study of 27 countries on the sensitivity and specificity of the new criteria. J Eur Acad Dermatol Venereol. 2014;28:338-47.
22. Tony Burns SB, Neil Cox , Christopher Griffiths Rook's Textbook of Dermatology, 8 ed, 51.1-51.39.
23. Varol A, Seifert O, Anderson CD. The skin pathergy test: Innately useful? Arch Dermatol Res. 2010;302:155-68.
24. Zeidan MJ, Saadoun D, Garrido M, et al. Behçet's disease physiopathology: A contemporary review. Autoimmunity Highlights. 2016;7:4.
25. Zouboulis CC. Epidemiology of Adamantiades-Behçet's disease. Ann Med Interne (Paris). 1999; 150:488-98.

CHAPTER 2

Genital Ulcer

Somodyuti Chandra, Nilay Kanti Das

■ INTRODUCTION

Genital ulcer is defined as ulcerative, erosive, vesicular or a pustular lesion leading to a breach in the continuity of genital mucosa and/or skin. The global incidence of genital ulcer is estimated to be 20 million cases annually with sexually transmitted infections accounting for about 55% of the ulcers while the rest 45% are due to nonvenereal causes. Determining the etiology of a genital ulcer is complicated by the fact that more than one infection may coexist and the present surge in human immunodeficiency virus (HIV) infection prevalence makes the scenario even more challenging. Early diagnosis and institution of appropriate therapy is of utmost importance not only to the patient but also to the community at large to reduce the risk of transmission to others.

Careful history taking, and meticulous clinical examination are therefore essential for correct diagnosis and management.

CASE REPORT

A previously healthy 25-year-old unmarried man presented to the sexually transmitted diseases (STDs) clinic with asymptomatic lesions over the penis for 5 days. There was no history of pain, dysuria or discharge per urethra or any other complaint. There was no recent drug use. He denied any alcohol or illicit drug use. He did endorse having unprotected intercourse with a commercial sex worker (CSW) about 6 weeks ago.

On examination, a single almost round ulcer measuring 2 cm × 1.5 cm was seen on the shaft of the penis, involving the coronal sulcus (Fig. 1). The ulcer was reddish colored with smooth regular edge and a clean surface. It had nontender but indurated base. Superficial group of inguinal lymph nodes on both sides were found to be enlarged. The lymph nodes were discrete, nontender, firm and had a rubbery consistency, not attached to underlying tissue or overlying skin. All other mucosae and skin were normal and remarkable.

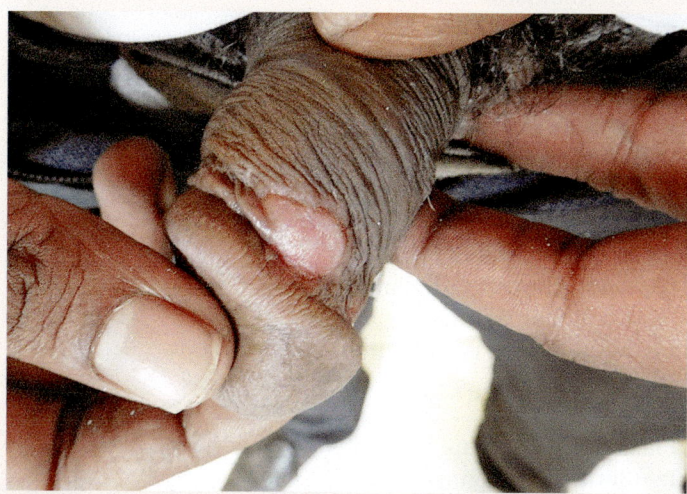

Fig. 1: Solitary well-defined, round, and indurated ulcer on the shaft of penis.

Gram staining of the smear taken from the ulcer was negative. However, dark field microscopy did reveal slender motile spirochetes. Further the authors ordered venereal disease research laboratory (VDRL) test which came to be positive at 1:120 dilution and *Treponema pallidum* hemagglutination (TPHA) was reactive. HIV test was negative.

A diagnosis of syphilitic chancre was made and the patient was treated with a single dose of intramuscular benzathine penicillin.

INTERACTIVE TOPIC REVIEW

Q.1 What are the causes of genital ulcer?

Ans: Genital ulcers may be caused by infectious and noninfectious etiologies:

Infectious Causes

Sexually Transmitted Infection
- Herpes simplex
- Syphilis
- Chancroid
- Lymphogranuloma venereum
- Granuloma inguinale.

Nonsexually Transmitted Infection
- Fungal–*Candida*, deep fungi (rare)
- Viral–Cytomegalovirus, Epstein–Barr virus, Varicella or Herpes Zoster
- Bacterial–*Staphylococcus, Streptococcus, Salmonella, Pseudomonas, Mycobacteria*
- Parasite–Amoebiasis, leishmaniasis, scabies, phthiriasis.

Noninfectious Causes
- Trauma

- Bullous dermatoses:
  - Pemphigus
  - Cicatricial pemphigoid.
- Drug reaction:
  - Erythema multiforme
  - Stevens–Johnson syndrome/toxic epidermal necrolysis
  - Fixed drug reaction
  - Contact dermatitis.
- Inflammatory dermatoses:
  - Nonspecific vulvitis/balanitis
  - Erosive lichen planus
  - Lichen sclerosus et atrophicus
  - Behçet's disease
  - Reiter's disease
  - Plasma cell balanitis
  - Pyoderma gangrenosum
  - Lupus erythematosus
  - Crohn's disease
  - Vasculitis–Wegener's granulomatosis.
- Premalignant or malignant neoplasm:
  - Erythroplasia of Queyrat
  - Extramammary Paget's disease
  - Bowen's disease
  - Squamous cell carcinoma
  - Basal cell carcinoma
  - Lymphoma
  - Leukemia
  - Histiocytosis X.

Q.2 How to approach a case of genital ulcer?

Ans: **History**

Age of Patient
- Children:
  - Trauma
  - Lichen sclerosus et atrophicus
  - Contact dermatitis
  - Scabies.
- Adults:
  - Sexually transmitted infection
  - Other infectious causes (Epstein–Barr virus, tuberculosis)
  - Inflammatory dermatoses (Behçet's, Reiter's, Zoon's balanitis)
  - Pemphigus
  - Contact dermatitis, lichen planus, lupus erythematosus.
- Elderly:
  - Candidiasis, lichen sclerosus et atrophicus, cicatricial pemphigoid
  - Malignancy.

Sex
- Male: Zoon's balanitis
- Female: Lichen sclerosus et atrophicus, lupus erythematosus, extramammary Paget's disease.

Occupation
Sexually transmitted infections are more common in sea men, truck drivers and people with jobs that involve frequent travel.

Onset and Duration of Complaint
- Sudden onset and short duration:
  - Trauma
  - Infectious causes other than syphilis
  - Drug reaction
  - Contact dermatitis
  - Behçet's disease.
- Insidious onset and protracted course:
  - Inflammatory dermatoses like Crohn's disease, lupus erythematosus
  - Erosive lichen planus, lichen sclerosus et atrophicus
  - Pyoderma gangrenosum
  - Zoon's balanitis
  - Pemphigus, cicatricial pemphigoid
  - Malignancy.

Associated Pain
- Painful:
  - Trauma
  - Sexually transmitted infection and other infections other than syphilis
  - Pemphigus, drug reaction, lichen planus, Behçet's disease.
- Painless:
  - Syphilis, granuloma inguinale
  - Lichen sclerosus et atrophicus, lupus erythematosus, papulonecrotic tuberculid
  - Malignancy.

Associated Pruritus
Extreme pruritus is seen in scabies, phthiriasis, lichen sclerosus et atrophicus.

Associated Symptoms
- Retention of urine, meatal stenosis, phimosis: Lichen sclerosus et atrophicus, malignancy
- Dysuria, dyspareunia
- Pain in lower abdomen: Pelvic inflammatory disease (tuberculosis, Chlamydia infection).

Presence of Oral Ulceration
- Pemphigus, lupus erythematosus, lichen planus, Behçet's disease
- Drug reactions.

History of Recurrence
Present in herpes, Behçet's disease, fixed drug eruptions, erythema multiforme/Stevens–Johnson syndrome/toxic epidermal necrolysis, pemphigus, papulo-necrotic tuberculid.

Sexual History
- Detailed sexual history should be enquired in all cases regarding:
    o Sex of the partner
    o Type of exposure (oral, vaginal, anal)
    o Use of condoms
    o Relationship to partner/s (spouse, casual)
    o Problems or symptoms in the partner/s
    o Date of last sexual intercourse
    o Number of partners in the past 3 months
    o Travel to endemic area
    o Serodiscordant partners.

Assessment of High-risk Behavior
- Marital status: Married, living together, single, separated, widowed
- Occupation: Sex workers (male and female), sea men, workers in the hospitality industry, transport workers, migrant workers, etc.
- Unprotected casual sexual encounters (other than with regular partner)
- Previous history of sexually transmitted infection
- History of injections or blood transfusions
- Substance use: Alcohol, drugs (e.g. heroin)
- Tattooing
- Partner with symptoms suggestive of sexually transmitted infection
- Multiple sexual partners.

Drug History
- Whether on immunosuppressants
- History of taking antitubercular drugs in the past
- History of recent drug intake preceding the onset of ulcer.

Examination

General Survey
- Nutrition: Poor in acquired immunodeficiency syndrome, chronic diseases, in oral mucosal involvement, Crohn's disease
- Fever: Human immunodeficiency virus infection, leukemia, lymphoma, tuberculosis, Behçet's disease
- Pallor: Chronic diseases
- Lymph node examination: Number, location, size, tenderness, presence of bubo, consistency and attachment to underlying structure are to be noted
    o Painful, firm, tender and nonsuppurative: Herpes
    o Painless, discrete, shotty, nontender: Syphilis
    o Painful, very tender, suppurative, unilocular: Chancroid
    o Tender, suppurative, soft/firm, multilocular: Lymphogranuloma venereum
    o Matted, nontender, firm or rubbery, fixed to underlying structures: Malignancy

- Bubos: Lymphogranuloma venereum, Chancroid
- Pseudo-bubo-Groove sign: Granuloma inguinale
- Associated with lymphadenopathy elsewhere: Leukemia, lymphoma
- Associated oral lesions may manifest as cervical lymphadenopathy.

Genital Examination
- Examination of the ulcer(s):
  - Site:
    - Glans penis: Fixed drug eruption, pemphigus
    - Glans penis and prepuce: Zoon's balanitis
    - Primary chancre develops on site of primary exposure
    - Scrotum and vulva, anywhere on the perianal skin: Behçet's disease, aphthae
    - Prepucial opening in men and vulval orifice in female: Lichen sclerosus et atrophicus.
  - Size:
    - Small: Herpes, aphthae, Behçet's disease
    - Large erosions: Pemphigus, erosive lichen planus, fixed drug eruption, Stevens–Johnson syndrome/toxic epidermal necrolysis.
  - Number:
    - Numerous: Herpes, aphthae, Behçet's disease, Chancroid
    - Single: Primary chancre, Zoon's balanitis, lymphogranuloma venereum.
  - Edge:
    - Sharply demarcated: Primary chancre, lichen sclerosus et atrophicus, Zoon's balanitis, aphthous, lymphogranuloma venereum
    - Irregular: Coalesced herpes lesions, chancroid, pemphigus, erosive lichen planus, Stevens–Johnson syndrome/toxic epidermal necrolysis.
  - Induration: Present in—primary syphilitic chancre, lichen sclerosus et atrophicus, malignancy
  - Base:
    - Smooth, nonpurulent, covered with serous exudate: Primary chancre
    - Covered with necrotic slough: Chancroid
    - Beefy granulation tissue bleeds easily on touch: Donovanosis
    - Sclerosis with epidermal atrophy: Lichen sclerosus et atrophicus
    - Curdy white material that can be wiped off: Candidiasis.

Oral Examination
- Indurated, painless, button like lesion covered with serous exudate, usually single: Primary chancre
- Snail track mucosal lesions: Secondary syphilis
- Lacy white reticulate, erythematous (atrophic), ulcerative (erosive) lesions: Oral lichen planus
- Painful erosions: Pemphigus
- Ulcers erosions almost always affecting the gingiva: Cicatricial pemphigoid
- Painful erosions on erythematous base: Stevens–Johnson syndrome/toxic epidermal necrolysis, erythema multiforme

- Oral aphthae in Behçet's disease
- Lips and oral mucosa involvement over hyperpigmented/erythematous patch: FDR
- Curdy white membrane that can be wiped off: Oral candidiasis
- Solitary, painless, large ulcer on the hard palate: Systemic lupus erythematosus

Rectal Examination
- Primary chancre depending upon the primary exposure
- Lichen sclerosus et atrophicus—involves perianal area leading to fissures that causes painful defecation
- Traumatic receptive anal sex.

Ophthalmological Examination
Important in Stevens–Johnson syndrome/toxic epidermal necrolysis, Behçet's disease, cicatricial pemphigoid.

Cutaneous Examination
- Thorough cutaneous examination may provide a clue to diagnosis, as:
    - Classic cutaneous lesions of lichen planus present as purple, polygonal, pruritic papule, and plaque and pterygium of nails
    - Behçet's disease: Erythema nodosum, pustules
    - Cicatricial pemphigoid: Occasional dome shaped bullae
    - Pemphigus: Multiple flaccid bullae
    - Target, targetoid lesions typically in palms and soles: Erythema multiforme
    - Macular or atypical targetoid lesions with purpuric centres that coalesce to form bullae and peels off: Stevens–Johnson syndrome/toxic epidermal necrolysis, erythema multiforme
    - Pruritic papular lesions, excoriations, burrows especially in the finger webs: Scabies
    - Red patch that soon evolves an iris or target lesion eventually blisters and erodes healing with hyperpigmentation: Fixed drug eruption
    - Infected genitocrural and pubic eczema: Phthiriasis
    - Diffuse hair loss, Raynaud's phenomenon, photosensitivity, joint pain in systemic lupus erythematosus, discoid lupus erythematosus
    - Swollen lymph nodes, chloromas in a cachectic individual in ulcers associated with leukemia, lymphoma.

Flowchart 1 summarizes approach to genital ulcer.

Q.3   How to confirm diagnosis?

Ans: Diagnosis is clinched by taking into account the clinical presentation along with laboratory findings. The following laboratory tests are done:

Direct Examination
- Dark field microscopy: Slender, motile *T. pallidum* can be seen in chancre
- Gram staining: Gram-negative bacilli in parallel rows having a "school of fish" appearance may be found in chancroid

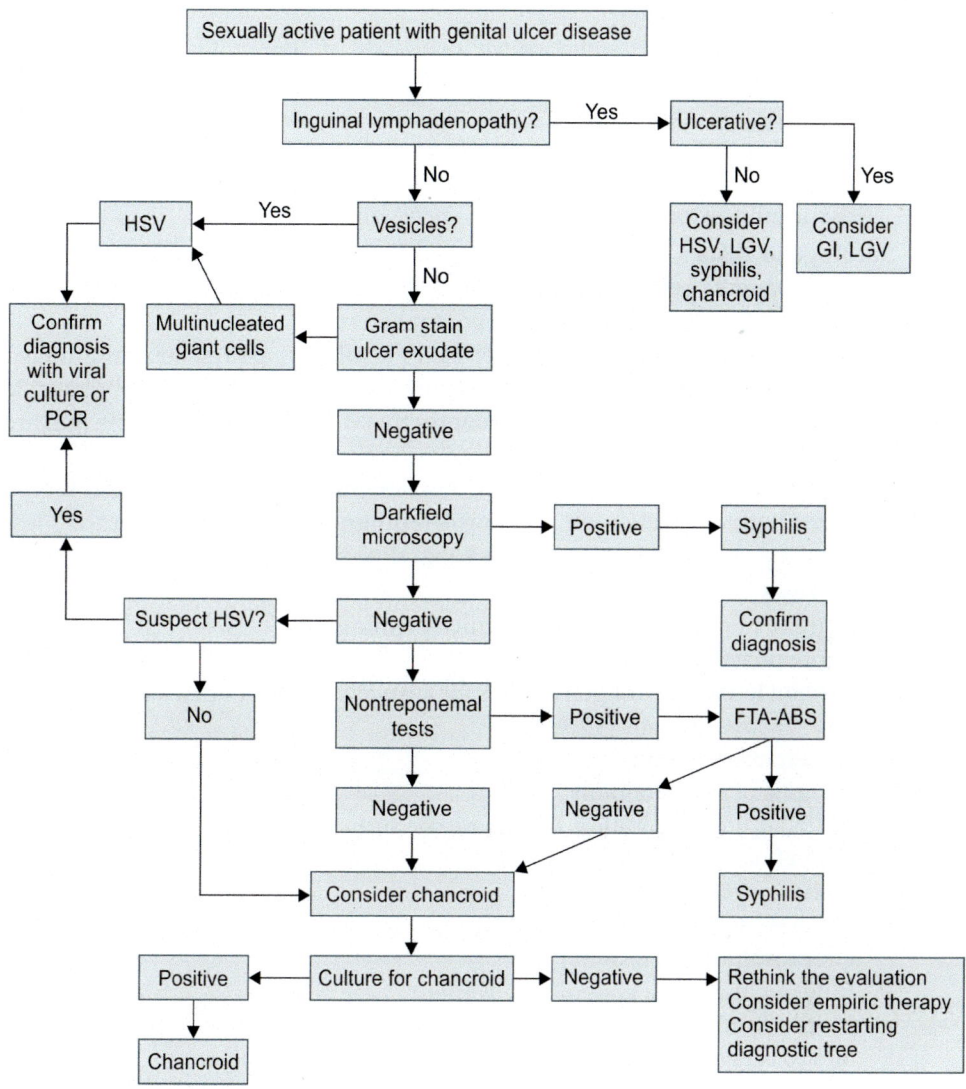

(FTA-ABS: fluorescent treponemal antibody-absorption; GI: granuloma inguinale; HSV: herpes simplex virus; LGV: lymphogranuloma venereum; PCR: polymerase chain reaction).

Flowchart 1: Summary of approach to genital ulcer.

- Tzanck smear: Ballooning degeneration can be seen in herpes simplex virus (HSV) infection
- Giemsa/Leishman stain: Pleomorphic, intracellular (macrophages > neutrophils), gram-negative bacilli surrounded by a well-defined bipolar staining capsule—"Safety pin" appearance seen in chancroid. Dark staining intracellular Donovan bodies are seen in donovanosis
- Potassium hydroxide (KOH) mount: Pseudo-hyphae seen in candidiasis

Culture
- Culture is the gold standard for diagnosis of chancroid and specialized enriched media, Mueller-Hinton agar supplemented with chocolate horse blood agar is used
- Candida can be cultured on a Sabouraud's Dextrose agar
- Lymphogranuloma venereum as well as donovanosis, both need specialized tissue culture techniques.

Serological Tests
- In all patients presenting with genital ulcer HIV testing is mandatory
- Syphilis: Nontreponemal and treponemal test.
- Herpes: Accurate type-specific HSV serologic assays [enzyme-linked immunosorbent assay (ELISA) and immunoblot] based on the HSV-specific glycoprotein G2 (HSV-2) and glycoprotein G1 (HSV-1) are available and are now recommended
- Lymphogranuloma venereum: Complement fixation test, single L-type immunofluorescence test and micro-immunofluorescence (micro-IF) test are used. A titre of 1:64 or more is suggestive of infection.

Other Tests
- Routine hematology and biochemistry workup
- Acute phase reactants
- Human leukocyte antigen studies for suspected Behçet's disease (HLA-B51) and reactive arthritis (HLA-B27)
- Ocular examination
- Imaging of affected joints
- Synovial fluid aspiration biochemistry and cytology in case of significant joint effusion
- Pathergy test
- Patch testing for suspected fixed drug eruptions (may be done at a later date, after resolution of lesions)
- Rule out any organ system involvement
- Biopsy from the ulcer for histopathological examination for donovanosis and to rule out malignancy.

Q.4 How to differentiate between various sexually transmitted disease ulcers?

Ans: The differentiating features of genital ulceration caused by the sexually transmitted infections are tabulated in Table 1.

Q.5 What are the histopathological findings of different sexually transmitted disease ulcers?

Ans:
- Chancre:
  - Dermal edema with dense infiltrate of lymphocytes, histiocytes, plasma cells and sometimes neutrophils
  - Perivascular infiltrate of lymphocytes
  - Endarteritis obliterans.
- Chancroid:
  - Three distinct zones can be seen:

TABLE 1: Differentiating features of sexually transmitted genital ulcers.

Features	Chancre	Chancroid	Herpes	Lymphogranuloma venereum	Donovanosis
Incubation period	9–90 days	1–14 days	2–7 days	3 days–6 weeks	1–4 weeks (upto 6 months)
Pain	Painless	Very tender	Tender	Variable	Uncommon
Number of lesions	Usually single	Usually multiple	Usually multiple, may coalesce	Usually single	Single or multiple
Primary lesion	Papule	Papule or pustule	Vesicle	Papule, pustule or vesicle, evanescent lesion	Papule or nodule
Edge	Sharp, well defined, round or oval, may be raised and rolled out	Irregular, ragged and undermine	Erythematous, polycyclic	Elevated, round or oval	Elevated, irregular
Depth	Deep or superficial	Excavated	Superficial	Usually superficial	Deep
Induration	Button hole induration (Dory Flop sign)	Soft, nonindurated	Nonindurated	Occasionally firm	Firm
Base	Smooth, nonpurulent, covered with serous exudate	Purulent, dirty-grey	Erythematous	Variable	Red, velvety, bleeds easily on touch
Lymph nodes: • Distribution • Tenderness • Fluctuation	• Bilateral • Painless • Firm, rubbery, shotty	• Usually unilateral • Tender • May be fluctuant (unilocular)	• Bilateral • Tender • Nonfluctuant	• Usually unilateral • Tender • May be fluctuant (multilocular)	Pseudobubo formation occurs (subcutaneous granulomas occurring superficially in the inguinal lymph node area)

1. Topmost zone is narrow and consists of neutrophils, red blood cells, fibrin and necrotic tissue
2. Middle zone is wide and consists of newly formed blood vessel with marked endothelial cell proliferation
3. Lower zone consists of dense infiltrate of plasma cells and lymphocytes.

- Herpes genitalis: Ballooning degeneration of epidermis producing multinucleated syncytial giant cells
- Lymphogranuloma venereum: Small areas of necrosis with proliferation of epithelioid cells forming multiple stellate abscess
- Donovanosis:
  - Pseudoepitheliomatous hyperplasia with microabscess in the epidermis at the edge of the ulcer
  - Dense infiltrate of plasma cells throughout the dermis containing intracytoplasmic vacuoles filled with clusters of Donovan bodies
  - Fibrosis and edema variable.

Q.6 How does human immunodeficiency virus coinfection affects the presentation of sexually transmitted disease ulcers?

Ans: There is a strong epidemiological association between sexually transmitted infections (STIs) and HIV infection. STIs that produce genital lesions or evoke an inflammatory response are important risk factors for the acquisition and transmission of HIV. Furthermore, unusual clinical manifestation (Table 2), atypical serological responses, accelerated disease progression and inappropriate response to treatment associated with HIV coinfection, makes diagnosis and management of the STIs a challenge.

TABLE 2: Atypical manifestions of genital ulcers in the presence of HIV coinfection.

Chancre	Chancroid	Herpes	Lymphogranuloma venereum	Donovanosis
• Giant chancre • Multiple lesions • Painful ulcer (due to superinfection) • Concomitant neurological involvement can occur	• Large ulcers • Ulcers persist longer • Multiple inguinal buboes • Giant and phagedenic type of ulcer frequently occur	• Deep progressive ulceration • Hemorrhagic lesions • Ecthyma-like lesions • Hyperkeratotic verrucous lesions resembling condylomata • Disseminated infection	• Acute inflammation with bilateral inguinal bubo which may burst out into ulceration	• Large lesions • Extensive involvement • Pseudobubo formation with ulceration

Q.7 What are the sites where chancre can occur?

Ans: Most chancres are genital (90–95%). Since they are mostly painless, a thorough examination of the genitalia and other mucosae is mandatory.

The usual sites of chancre in males are the coronal sulcus, glans penis, prepuce, frenulum and shaft of penis. In homosexual males, chancre can occur near the anus, or in the anal canal or rectum. Intrameatal chancre has also been reported.

In females chancre can occur on the outer or inner aspect of labia, fourchette, vulva, clitoris, around urethral orifice or vaginal wall. Though cervix is a common site, lesions often remain undetected and patients present later in the secondary stage.

In about 5–10% cases chancres occur at extragenital sites. Lesions can virtually occur anywhere, but are commonly seen on lips, tongue, gum, tonsils, fingers and breasts. Lesions have also been reported on eyelids, bridge of nose, stomach and chest wall.

Q.8 What are the atypical manifestations of chancre?

Ans: Chancre may have the following atypical features:
- Painful lesions
- Multiple lesions
- Ulcers having undermined edge
- Nonindurated lesions
- Phimosis or inflammatory edema
- Tender lymphadenopathy with matting
- Erosive balanitis (Follman's balanitis)
- Perforating lesions of the shaft of penis
- Bubo with balanitis and lymphocele
- Firm, rubbery, unilateral labial swelling (due to deep seated chancre).

Q.9 What is chancre redux and pseudochancre redux?

Ans:
- Chancre redux is the recurrence of a primary chancre at the site of original lesion
- Pseudochancre redux is the occurrence of noninfectious gumma at the site of original chancre.

Q.10 How is dark-field microscopy done?

Ans: The lesion is cleaned with tap water or physiological saline, only if it is encrusted or obviously contaminated. Antiseptics or soaps are avoided as they may kill the treponemes. Minimal amount of liquid is used for cleaning as it may dilute and thus reduce the yield of the organisms. The ulcer is gently squeezed and the clear serous exudate is directly collected on a cover slip or a clean glass slide by pressing directly onto the lesion. For cervical and vaginal lesions, speculum examination is necessary, and the serous exudate is collected using a bacteriological loop or Pasteur pipette and transferred to a slide. If the material is not sufficient, it is mixed with a drop of saline. The edges of the cover slip are sealed with petroleum jelly and examined immediately. If negative at first, dark-field examination should be repeated daily for at least three consecutive days.

Treponema pallidum appear as brightly illuminated objects against a dark background. They are identified by their typical morphology, size, and movement. It is a 0.25–0.3 m wide and 6–16 m long organism with 8–14 regular, tightly wound, deep spirals. It exhibits quick and abrupt movements. The organism rotates slowly along the longitudinal axis (corkscrew motion) accompanied by bending and twisting in the middle.

Q.11 What are the serological tests for syphilis?

Ans: Nontreponemal Tests:
- These are VDRL, rapid plasma reagin card test, automated regain test, reagin screen test, toluidine red unheated serum test (TRUST)
- These tests have high sensitivity and negative predictive value, and hence used as screening tests
- They can be performed as both qualitative as well as quantitative tests. Hence, are used to diagnose current infection as well as to monitor response to treatment
- The standard VDRL antigen contains 0.03% cardiolipin, 0.9% cholesterol and 0.21% lecithin
- These tests measure antilipoid immunoglobulin (Ig) G and IgM antibody (regain antibody)
- Positive test: Indicated by a 4-fold increase in titre
- The VDRL test becomes reactive 2–3 weeks after infection and reverts to negative in one-fourth of the cases during late latency.

Treponemal Tests:
- These tests have high specificity and positive predictive value, and hence used for confirmation
- The antigen used here is either the entire *T. pallidum* (living or dead) or its components to detect specific antibodies
- These tests are: *T. pallidum* immobilization (TPI) test, fluorescent treponemal antibody-absorption (FTA-ABS) tests, TPHA and ELISA.

Q.12 How will you treat this case?

Ans:
- The patient is treated with a single dose of intramuscular injection of benzathine penicillin 2.4 million units divided in two buttocks after prior skin testing
- According to syndromic management, the patient is given Kit 3 for genital ulcer disease (nonherpetic). It contains a single dose of injection benzathine penicillin 2.4 million units and tablet azithromycin 1 g
- For penicillin allergic patients Kit 4 containing tablet doxycycline 100 mg—28 tablets (1 tablet twice daily for 14 days) and tablet azithromycin 1 g is given
- All sexual partners within 90 days preceding the diagnosis are to be treated presumptively with the same drug or kit
- Sexual abstinence is advised during the course of treatment.

Q.13 How will you follow-up this patient?

Ans:
- The patient is reviewed after 7 days
- If HIV test is negative, VDRL titer is repeated after 1, 3, 6 and 12 months. A falling titer indicates adequate response to therapy and it usually becomes nonreactive 1 year after treatment
- If HIV test is positive, cerebrospinal fluid VDRL test becomes mandatory, as neurological involvement can occur in these patients even in the primary stage.

Q.14 How will you differentiate relapse from reinfection?

Ans: Occurrence of chancre at a site different from the previous one or detection of early syphilis lesion in the current sexual partner indicates reinfection.

Q.15 What is syndromic management of sexually transmitted infection?

Ans: A sexually transmitted infection is a public health problem which is made worse by the social stigma that makes the patients hesitant to approach the doctors. It has been noted that by controlling sexually transmitted diseases, not only the health status of the population can be improved, but also HIV transmission can be prevented. To achieve this, the concept of syndromic management was introduced wherein diagnosis is made based on identification of syndromes, which are a combination of symptoms which the clients report and signs which the care giver observes. The recommended treatment includes all the diseases that could cause the identified syndrome and the entire treatment is given on the first visit itself, as it might be the last chance to treat.

Q.16 What are the advantages and disadvantages of syndromic management?

Ans: Advantages of syndromic management are:
- Fast—the patient is diagnosed and treated in the same visit
- Highly effective
- Relatively inexpensive since it avoids the use of laboratory tests
- No need for the patient to return for laboratory results
- All possible sexually transmitted infections causing the particular signs and symptoms are treated at once
- Scientifically tested in many parts of the world
- Easy for health workers to learn and administer
- It can be integrated into the primary health care services effectively.

Disadvantages of syndromic management are:
- Not useful in asymptomatic individuals
- It is too simple for a physician to use; there is no room for a physician's clinical expertise and experience
- Drug wastage
- Over-treatment of a patient having only one sexually transmitted infection causing the syndrome
- It may promote the development of antibiotic resistance.

CONCLUSION

Genital ulcer disease (GUD) is a general term that usually refers to lesions caused by specific STIs. Although GUD is common throughout the world, the specific causes vary widely by geographic region. Genital herpes, syphilis, and chancroid lead the differential diagnosis, but conditions unrelated to STIs should also be considered, such as trauma, Stevens–Johnson syndrome, Beçhet syndrome, Crohn disease, carcinoma and bacterial infection. Careful history taking, meticulous clinical examination and laboratory tests are essential for correct diagnosis and management.

KEY POINTS

- Genital ulcers may be caused by infectious or noninfectious etiologies
- Men and women with GUD are at an increased risk of acquiring and transmitting HIV
- Determining the etiology of a genital ulcer may be complicated by the presence of more than one infection, particularly HIV
- Genital ulcer disease is frequently associated with unilateral or bilateral inguinal lymphadenopathy, even when ulcers are not identified clinically
- Samples for microbiological assessment should be taken from the base and edge of the ulcer and also from the enlarged lymph node (if any)
- Both treponemal and nontreponemal tests should be done for detecting active infections
- The syndromic approach has been a major step forward in rationalising and improving management of STI. However, syndromic algorithms have some shortcomings, and they should be periodically revised and adapted to the epidemiological patterns of STI in a given setting
- The sensitivity and specificity of syndromic management has been found to be 68% and 52% respectively, in a study based in Pune, India.

SUGGESTED READING

1. Dicarlo RP, Martin DH. The clinical diagnosis of genital ulcer diseases in men. Clin Infect Dis. 1997;25:292-98.
2. Eggleston SI, Turner AJL. Serological testing for syphilis. Commun Dis Public Health. PHLS Syphilis Serology Working Group. 2000;3:158-62.
3. Morshed MG. Current trend on syphilis diagnosis: issues and challenges. Adv Exp Med Biol. 2014;808:51-64.
4. National Guidelines on Prevention, Management and Control of Reproductive Tract Infections including Sexually Transmitted Infections. Natioanal AIDS Control Organization, Ministry of Health and Family Welfare, Govt. of India, New Delhi; 2007.
5. Roett MA, Mayor MT, Uduhiri KA. Diagnosis and management of genital ulcers. aM Fam Physician. 2012;85(3):254-62.
6. Schmid GP. Approach to the patient with genital ulcer disease. Med Clin North Am. 1990;74(6):1559-72.
7. Vyulsteke B. Current status of syndromic management of sexually transmitted infections in developing countries. Sex Transm Infect. 2004;80:333-4.

CHAPTER 3

Generalized Pruritus

Debabrata Bandyopadhyay

INTRODUCTION

Pruritus is defined as a cutaneous sensation that provokes the desire to scratch. Pruritus is the dominant symptom of dermatological diseases. Commonly limited to the skin lesions and over particular areas, it may involve the entire skin [generalized pruritus (GP)]. GP, particularly when chronic, has the potential to cause markedly reduced quality of life. Chronic itch may be as debilitating as chronic pain with respect to impaired quality of life. Derangement of sleep pattern and associated anxiety and depression occur commonly and may worsen the itching. GP may not only occur in several skin diseases (e.g. atopic dermatitis, scabies, erythroderma from any cause and urticaria) but also occurs in a variety of systemic disorders. In some cases, the underlying cause remains unclear (pruritus of undetermined origin). The mechanisms underlying the various types of GP are complex. A number of mediators and their receptors are involved in the itch sensation. Several local and systemic treatments target these mechanisms. Management of GP is focused on exclusion of dermatological disorders as the primary cause of pruritus, and in their absence, measures to detect and treat any underlying systemic disease. General measures, emollients, and other local agents, and a variety of systemic drugs are employed to treat this disabling symptom.

CASE 1

A 63-year-old retired college teacher presented with generalized itching for the duration of 3 months. He was a known diabetic of 20 years' duration. He was on intermittent hemodialysis for the last 1 year for chronic kidney disease and was scheduled for renal transplantation. The patient described the itching as occurring throughout the day with exacerbation during the night. The itch caused sleep disturbance and waked him several times during the night. The intensity of the itch peaked before dialysis with moderate relief after the procedure. He had no skin lesions prior to the onset of itching. His past medical history was unremarkable and there was no significant family history. He was an ex-smoker and nonalcoholic. His long-term medications included insulin, calcitriol, calcium acetate, erythropoietin and frusemide. There was no history of fever, weight loss, fatigue, night sweats, jaundice or malaise. He had received courses of antiscabetics, emollients, topical steroids and loratadine without any significant benefit.

Cutaneous examination revealed generalized dryness, multiple linear excoriation marks over his limbs and abdomen and areas of lichenified skin over bilateral lower legs. There were no lesions over his finger or toe web spaces. The oral cavity, genitalia, hair and nails were normal. His vitals were within normal limits. He had mild pallor but no icterus or pedal edema. Review of systems was unremarkable and was notable for the absence of organomegaly or enlarged lymph nodes.

Investigations: Laboratory works revealed—hemoglobin: 9.7 mg/dL, blood urea nitrogen: 74 mg/dL (normal range 8–18 mg/dL); serum creatinine: 6.6 mg/dL, fasting blood glucose: 135 mg/dL. Serum electrolytes, liver function tests and thyroid stimulating hormone were within normal limits.

Treatment: A diagnosis of renal pruritus (chronic kidney disease-associated pruritus) was made and the patient was advised frequent liberal application of emollients, cool bath, avoidance of irritants and hot and spicy foods, topical mometasone for application over the excoriated and lichenified areas, and gabapentin 100 mg every alternate nights.

Outcome: There was significant reduction in the intensity of pruritus with the above measures although the patient had occasional bouts of severe pruritus lasting a few hours. There was complete relief from pruritus after renal transplantation done 4 months later. However, the patient was advised to continue application of emollients.

Case Review in a Nutshell

The patient has chronic GP that significantly impaired the quality of his life. The diagnosis of renal pruritus in this case was rather straightforward as he was a known patient of diabetic nephropathy and he had no history of any skin disease prior to the onset of pruritus. However, a thorough mucocutaneous examination was needed to eliminate any dermatological cause for the symptom. Associated xerosis and secondary lesions of excoriations and lichenification as found in this patient are common in many systemic causes of pruritus.

Investigations in this patient revealed changes associated with the underlying renal pathology and absence of any other systemic disease. As seen in the present case, antihistamines are ineffective in the management of renal pruritus. Although, general nonpharmacological measures, liberal application of emollients and gabapentin resulted in moderate relief of the distressful symptom, kidney transplantation ultimately provided complete relief of pruritus in this patient.

INTERACTIVE TOPIC REVIEW

Q.1 What is the pathophysiology of pruritus?

Ans: Pruritus like pain, has evolved as a sensation having a protective role. It may act as an alarm system for quickly removing any potentially harmful substances from the skin by triggering the scratch reflex. However, generalized itch, particularly when chronic, has no protective role and is a distressful symptom. The mechanisms underlying different causes of GP are complex. Various mediators of itch and their receptors, peripheral and central nerve fibers and specific brain regions are involved in the elicitation, transmission and perception of the sensation. Apart from histamine, several mediators and receptors have been identified for having a role in the pathophysiology of itch. These include among others, acetylcholine, proteases, the neurotrophins (nerve growth factor), gastrin-releasing peptide, neurokinins/neuropeptides (e.g. substance P), cytokines (IL-2 and IL-31), and the histamine H4 receptor. Keratinocytes, mast cells, and cell in inflammatory infiltrate such as lymphocytes and eosinophils may also modulate itch by interacting with neuronal cells.

Pruritus originating in the skin is transmitted via free nerve endings of slow conducting itch-specific unmyelinated C fibers and thinly myelinated Aδ fibers located at the dermoepidermal junction and within the epidermis. The afferent nerve fibers enter the dorsal horn of the ipsilateral side of the spinal cord to synapse with itch-specific neurons. The secondary neurons cross to the contralateral side and ascend along the spinothalamic tract to reach the thalamus which relays the signal to various areas of the somatosensory cortex of the brain. Opioid receptors modulate the perception of pruritus in the central nervous system. When activated, μ-opioid receptors incite itch perception, whereas κ-receptors suppresses perception of itch.

Q.2 What are the causes of generalized pruritus?

Ans: The potential underlying causes of GP is categorized into:
- Dermatological diseases (Box 1)

BOX 1 — Dermatologic diseases causing generalized pruritus.

Inflammatory diseases
- Atopic dermatitis
- Allergic/irritant contact dermatitis
- Psoriasis
- Erythroderma
- Bullous diseases (e.g. dermatitis herpetiformis/bullous pemphigoid)
- Eosinophilic folliculitis
- Urticaria
- Drug eruption (e.g. morbilliform)
- Papular urticaria
- Prurigo nodularis
- Mastocytosis

Infection/Infestations
- Scabies
- Pediculosis corporis
- Extensive dermatophytosis

Neoplastic
- Cutaneous T-cell lymphoma
- Sézary syndrome

Other
- Xerosis
- Aquagenic pruritus

BOX 2	Systemic causes of generalized pruritus.
Chronic kidney disease **Endocrine and metabolic disease** • Carcinoid syndrome • Diabetes mellitus • Hyper/hypothyroidism • Hyperparathyroidism **Hematologic** • Hemochromatosis • Iron deficiency anemia • Mastocytosis • Polycythemia vera • Myelofibrosis **Hepatobiliary** • Primary biliary cirrhosis • Viral hepatitis • Biliary occlusion • Sclerosing cholangitis • Cholestasis of pregnancy • Drugs causing cholestasis	**Infections** • Human immunodeficiency virus infection • Parasitic disease (ascariasis, onchocerciasis) **Malignancy** • Leukemia • Lymphoma • Myeloma • Solid tumors **Neurologic** • Cerebral tumor • Cerebral abscess • Multiple sclerosis • Stroke • Creutzfeldt–Jakob disease **Rheumatic diseases** • Dermatomyositis • Sjögren syndrome • Systemic sclerosis

- Systemic diseases (Box 2)
- Psychosomatic/psychogenic diseases
- Drug reaction
- Mixed (any combination of above)
- Idiopathic (pruritus of unknown origin).

Q.2 How would you evaluate a case of generalized pruritus?

Ans: The first step in the evaluation of a patient with GP is to identify any primary cutaneous disease that may be responsible for the symptom. A comprehensive personal, family, travel and psychiatric history may provide important clue to the etiology. A thorough drug history should be obtained from the oral history as well from a review of available prescriptions. An acute onset of GP is less suggestive of a systemic etiology than a chronic itch. While similar symptoms in the patient's cohabitants may suggest a cutaneous disease such as scabies, a history of weight changes, fever, fatigue, night sweats, jaundice, or other constitutional symptoms are important pointers to systemic etiologies.

Meticulous examination of the skin, hair, nails and mucous membrane should be performed. A careful search and assessment should be made of the primary lesions and secondary changes. The primary lesions are often obscured by secondary lesions such as excoriations or nonspecific eczematous lesions. It must be kept in mind that such secondary lesions can accompany systemic cause of persistent pruritus also. Finger webs, intertriginous areas and the genitalia should receive particular attention to exclude scabies.

In absence of any definite lesions, only xerosis and mild scaling may be evident. A general physical examination including the lymph nodes, liver and spleen may disclose a systemic cause. Determining the systemic etiology of generalized itch can be quite challenging since pruritus can antedate other symptoms and signs of a systemic disease such as lymphoma for months. Therefore, detailed review of the case should be repeated at periodic follow-up visits if the diagnosis remains elusive.

In addition to history taking and physical examination, laboratory tests are undertaken either to confirm the dermatologic disease or to screen for an underlying systemic cause. Histopathology and immunofluorescence of a skin biopsy specimen is often required to diagnose a dermatological condition. An initial screening for systemic cause should include complete blood count, fasting glucose, thyroid-stimulating hormone, liver function test, creatinine, blood urea nitrogen levels and human immunodeficiency virus (HIV) antibody assay. Imaging studies such chest X-ray, ultrasonography or computed tomography may be helpful in the diagnosis of an underlying occult malignancy. Further testing for confirmation and assessment of systemic disease is tailored to the individual cases.

Q.3 How is generalized pruritus treated?

Ans: When a definite cause of GP is identified, treatment is tailored to the causative factors such as scabicidals for scabies or thyroxine for hypothyroidism. However, symptomatic relief from generalized itch is required for every patient. Treatment modalities can be categorized into: (i) General nonpharmacologic interventions, (ii) topical therapy, (iii) systemic agents and (iv) physical therapy in the form of ultraviolet exposure.

Q.4 What nonpharmacologic/general measures are used in the management of generalized pruritus?

Ans: Nonpharmacologic interventions might benefit every patient irrespective of the etiology of GP. Frequent bathing with soaps or cleansers and excessive drying of the skin should be avoided. As warmer temperatures lower the threshold of receptors to pruritic stimuli, patients should use lighter clothing and seek cooler surroundings. Hot and spicy foods, and alcoholic and hot drinks should be avoided. Contact with irritants such as woolens should be avoided. Nails should be trimmed regularly to prevent excoriations and infection as well as to break the itch-scratch cycle.

Q.5 Describe the topical therapy of generalized pruritus.

Ans: Emollients are recommended for most patients suffering from GP. Emollients prevent and treat dryness of skin and reduces skin irritation. Emollients are available as ointment, cream, or lotion and contain occlusives mainly in the forms of oils of mineral, vegetable, or animal origin with or without humectants (agents that increase the water-holding capacity of the stratum corneum) such as urea, glycerin, or α-hydroxy acids. Emollients should be applied liberally immediately after bath and as frequently as needed by the patient.

Additional topical antipruritic agents are used when emollients are not adequate, there are contraindications to systemic treatment, or as an adjunct to systemic/etiological treatments. The choice of topical agent (antiscabetics or antifungals) is straightforward when the generalized itch is caused by infection or infestation such as scabies or dermatophytosis. Other agents can be used irrespective of the etiology. These agents act by: (i) Substituting pruritus with some other sensation (cooling, heating, counter irritation), (b) acting on sensory nerve endings or receptors and (c) reducing skin inflammation.

Substitution of pruritus by some other sensation can be achieved by physical methods that include cooling with ice cubes or cold compresses, colloid bath with oat meal or starch, bath oil containing vegetable or mineral oils, calamine lotions and sodium bicarbonate. Chemical methods causing cooling may act on the cold receptors, or by their anesthetic or counterirritant properties. Some of the agents in this category include 0.5–2% phenol, 1% menthol, 0.1–3% camphor, 0.5–1% thymol, 3–10% tars, 2–5% resorcinol, 5–10% urea, 6–20% ammonium lactate and 5–10% precipitated sulfur.

Anesthesia of sensory nerves leading to reduced itch sensation may be achieved by local anesthetics such as pramoxine hydrochloride (0.5–2.5%). Doxepin, a tricyclic antidepressant, is also a histamine H1 and H2 blocker and as a 5% cream or lotion can be used as a local antipruritic.

When cutaneous inflammation is a significant cause of pruritus such as in atopic dermatitis, judicious use of topical anti-inflammatory agents in the form of various topical steroids or calcineurin inhibitors (tacrolimus or pimecrolimus) can be of considerable help in relieving pruritus.

Q. 6 **Which systemic drugs can be used to treat different causes of generalized itch?**

Ans: Several groups of drugs have been used with variable success rates in GP of different etiologies (Table 1). However, for many drugs their efficacy has not been proven by rigorous clinical trials. The following classes of drugs are mainly used.

TABLE 1: Systemic drugs for generalized pruritus.

Class of drug	Medication and adult dosage	Major Indication	Main side effects
Antihistaminics	First generation: • Hydroxyzine (25–75 mg/day) • Chlorpheniramine maleate (4 mg BID/TID) Second generation: • Cetirizine (10 mg/OD) • Loratadine (10 mg/OD) • Fexofenadine (180 mg/OD)	• Nocturnal pruritus • Urticaria • Mastocytosis	• Sedation • Dry mouth • Drowsiness

Continued

Continued

TABLE 1: Systemic drugs for generalized pruritus.

Class of drug	Medication and adult dosage	Major Indication	Main side effects
Antidepressants	Tricyclic antidepressants: • Amitriptyline (25–75 mg at night) • Doxepin (25–100 mg at night) Selective serotonin reuptake inhibitors: • Sertraline (25–100 mg OD) • Paroxetine (10–40 mg OD) • Fluvoxamine (50–150 mg OD) Mirtazapine (7.5–30 mg at night)	• Paraneoplastic pruritus • Pruritus in depression, anxiety • Chronic urticarial • Neuropathic itch • Cholestatic pruritus	• Drowsiness • Dry eyes and mouth • Urinary retention • Drowsiness • Insomnia • Sexual dysfunction • Dry mouth • Sedation • Weight gain
Anticonvulsants	• Gabapentin (300–3600 mg/day in divided dosage, in renal pruritus: 100 mg on alternate days/300 mg before dialysis) • Pregabalin (150–450 mg/day, low dose in renal pruritus)	• Neuropathic pruritus • Renal pruritus • Prurigo nodularis	• Drowsiness • Leg swelling • Ataxia • Constipation
μ-opioid receptor antagonist	Naltrexone (25–50 mg OD)	• Cholestatic pruritus • Atopic dermatitis • Chronic urticaria	• Nausea and vomiting • Insomnia
κ-opioid receptor agonist	Nalfurafine (2.5–5 μg OD)	• Renal pruritus	• Insomnia
Thalidomide	100–200 mg OD	• Renal pruritus • Prurigo nodularis	• Teratogenicity • Drowsiness • Peripheral neuropathy
Neurokinin-1 receptor antagonist	Aprepitant (80 mg OD)	• Paraneoplastic pruritus	• Dizziness • Nausea
Rifampicin	300–450 mg/day	• Cholestatic pruritus	• Flu-like syndrome • Nausea/vomiting • Hepatitis

Antihistaminics

H1-histamine receptor blockers are the most frequently prescribed first line systemic medication in clinical practice owing to their safety, low cost and, wide availability. However, their role is in conditions in which histamine is not the main mediator of itch is questionable. They are drugs of choice in urticaria and mastocytosis. First generation antihistamines, such as hydroxyzine, owing to their soporific effects, may have a role in management of nocturnal itch to improve sleep.

Antidepressants

Selective Serotonin Reuptake Inhibitors

Sertraline has been shown to be effective in cholestatic itch, renal pruritus in hemodialysis patients, polycythemia vera and somatoform pruritus. Paroxetine and fluvoxamine are alternative selective serotonin reuptake inhibitors (SSRIs). Compared to tricyclic antidepressants, SSRIs are better tolerated and have lower cardiovascular adverse effects. Common adverse effects are nausea, dry mouth, dizziness, agitation, sexual dysfunction, insomnia and weight gain or loss.

Serotonin–Norepinephrine Reuptake Inhibitors

Mirtazapine is a tetracyclic antidepressant with additional H1 antihistaminic action. Mirtazapine has been shown to be effective in renal pruritus, cholestatic pruritus and paraneoplastic pruritus (PP). It is especially suitable for relief of nocturnal itch. Mirtazapine does not have any serious adverse effects or drug interaction. The most frequently reported side effects are dry mouth, sedation and weight gain. The most commonly used dosage for adults is 15 mg at night.

Tricyclic Antidepressants

Amitriptyline, nortriptyline and trimipramine are useful in the management of pruritus of neuropathic origin. Doxepin has additional activity both with H1 and H2 receptor. Doxepin may be useful in the treatment of chronic urticaria, renal pruritus and HIV-induced pruritus. The main side effects of tricyclics are drowsiness, hypotension, dry mouth, urinary retention and palpitation. These drugs have anticholinergic actions and should be avoided in patients with prostatic hypertrophy and glaucoma. They are not used as a first-line treatment of chronic itch because of their side effects.

Anticonvulsants

Gabapentin and pregabalin are structural analogs of the neurotransmitter γ-aminobutyric acid (GABA). These drugs are effective for several types of pruritus including neuropathic itch (such as prurigo nodularis), renal pruritus, pruritus associated with lymphoma and pruritus of unknown origin. They are ineffective in cholestatic pruritus. The mechanism of action is uncertain. The most common adverse effects are constipation, drowsiness, ataxia, leg swelling and blurred vision. Compared to gabapentin, pregabalin has a more rapid onset of beneficial effects.

Thalidomide

Thalidomide has been shown to be of benefit in refractory renal pruritus, PP, and prurigo nodularis. The antipruritic effect of this drug may be related to their action against tumor necrosis factor. The most significant toxicity of thalidomide is teratogenicity. Other adverse effects are peripheral neuropathy, sedation, constipation and dizziness. Thalidomide is used when the pruritus is disabling and unresponsive to other treatments.

Opioid Agonists and Antagonists

µ-Opioid Receptor Antagonists

Naltrexone is an orally administered, long-acting, µ-opioid receptor antagonist. Antipruritic effect of naltrexone in GP due to atopic dermatitis and cholestatic itch has been documented by randomized controlled trials (RCTs). Variable results have been obtained in the treatment of itch due to psoriasis, prurigo nodularis and cutaneous lymphoma.

Naloxone is short-acting and must be administered intravenously. A few RCTs have shown their action in intractable cholestatic pruritus. The main adverse effects of these drugs are insomnia, dizziness, headache, nausea vomiting and abdominal cramps. They are not associated with physical dependence and have no abuse potential.

κ-Opioid Receptor Agonists

Nalfurafine is a selective κ-opioid receptor agonist which is useful in intractable renal pruritus in patients on hemodialysis refractory to other treatments. The main adverse effects are insomnia, vertigo, headache, nausea and vomiting. Opioid addiction or withdrawal symptoms were not observed in clinical trials. Nalfurafine is not currently available in most countries.

µ-Receptor Antagonist and κ-Receptors Agonist

Butorphanol modulates opioid system by both its antagonistic and agonistic effects on µ-opioid receptors and κ-opioid receptors respectively. It is administered intranasally and is mainly used in the treatment of migraine. It has been shown to reduce intractable pruritus associated with lymphoma, cholestasis and opioid use.

Neurokinin-1 Receptor Antagonist

Aprepitant is a highly selective neurokinin-1 receptor antagonist. It could reduce pruritus by inhibiting the receptor of substance P, a mediator of itch and a member of the neurokinin group of small peptide neurotransmitters present in the central and peripheral nervous systems. Mainly used as an antiemetic in cancer chemotherapy, aprepitant has given significant benefit in acute and chronic intractable pruritus, particularly in PP. Aprepitant is orally administered in a dose of 80 mg once a day. Adverse effects are generally not serious and include drowsiness, vertigo and gastrointestinal problems. The drug's high cost is a major limitation for its use.

Other Medicines

Various other systemic drugs for GP have been studied, particularly for the management of renal pruritus. These include ondansetron, montelukast, cromolyn sodium, activated charcoal, zinc sulfate, omega-3 fatty acids and erythropoietin. However, the effectiveness of these agents remains uncertain and needs to be confirmed by RCTs.

Q.7 **What is the role of phototherapy in the treatment of generalized pruritus?**

Ans: Pruritus of various etiologies have been successfully managed with whole-body phototherapies with ultraviolet A or ultraviolet B (UVA or UVB) light, either alone or in combination. Both broad-band and narrow-band UVB can be used and their action is comparable to that of UVA therapy. The exact mechanism of action of UV light in relieving pruritus is not known, some studies have suggested their action on opiodergic system.

The UV light can be beneficial in GP associated with chronic kidney disease and skin diseases like atopic dermatitis, psoriasis or cutaneous T-cell lymphoma. Ultraviolet therapy can be particularly useful when systemic agents cannot be used, for example during pregnancy, in old age, in those with serious comorbidities. The UV therapy is also a therapeutic option in those cases in whom topical or systemic drugs have failed. Ultraviolet therapy should not be co-prescribed with topical calcineurin inhibitors.

Q.8 How frequent is renal pruritus? What is the pathogenesis?

Ans: Renal pruritus occurs in patients with advanced or end-stage kidney disease. It is also called nephrogenic pruritus or chronic kidney disease-associated pruritus. The popular term "uremic pruritus" is a misnomer as the pruritus has no relation with raised blood urea or creatinine levels and it does not occur in acute renal failure. More than 40% of patients undergoing hemodialysis suffer from chronic itch, in half of them the pruritus is generalized. The pathogenesis of renal pruritus is unclear. Parathormone, histamine, calcium and magnesium salts, opioid-receptor derangements and microinflammation are thought to be some of the possible etiological factors.

Q.9 Describe the clinical characteristics of renal pruritus. How is it treated?

Ans: The clinical features of pruritus in patients with chronic kidney disease are variable. Some patients may experience intermittent bouts of pruritus lasting for hours or days, while others may be bothered by continuous intractable itch. Pruritus is generally more severe at night. The back is the most frequent body site affected, other common sites of affection being head, arms and abdomen. The itch is exacerbated by dry skin, heat, sweat, stress and rest. Pruritus generally increase just before the hemodialysis and relieved after the procedure. Physical activity and cold ambient temperature also diminish the intensity of the symptom. Uremic pruritus usually resolves completely after renal transplantation.

Renal pruritus may be extremely difficult to control, as therapeutic options are limited in uremic patients. Approaches to treatment include: General nonpharmacological measures, topical treatment with emollients and anti-inflammatory compounds, or systemic treatment with gabapentin, opioid receptor antagonists and agonists and phototherapy. When indicated, successful kidney transplantation will relieve patients from renal pruritus.

Q.10 What causes cholestatic pruritus?

Ans: Cholestatic pruritus may occur in intrahepatic and/or extrahepatic biliary disruption from any cause including primary biliary cirrhosis, chronic viral hepatitis, cirrhosis, sclerosing cholangitis, intrahepatic cholestasis of pregnancy, bile duct obstruction, malignant tumors and prolonged drug-induced hepatitis.

The pathogenesis of pruritus in cholestasis is poorly understood. Some hypotheses include accumulation of pruritogenic substances resulting from impaired bile secretion, derangements of bile salt production and excretion, histamine imbalance, dysregulation of substance P, alterations in progesterone metabolites, and involvement of central pathways mediated via endogenous opioids, serotonin and lysophosphatidic acid.

Q.11 What are the clinical characteristics of cholestatic pruritus? What drugs can be used to treat it?

Ans: Pruritus is a very common and troublesome symptom of cholestasis and can range in severity from mild itch to intolerable pruritus which may cause severe disruption of the patient's quality of life. Cholestatic pruritus may be localized or generalized particularly involving the palms and soles. It is often exacerbated during the night, before menstruation and with psychological stress. Cool temperatures often reduce the pruritus. Long-standing scratching may lead to excoriations, prurigo nodularis and lichenification. The intensity of pruritus has no relation with the severity of the underlying liver pathology.

Antihistamines are largely ineffective in the treatment of cholestatic pruritus. The recommended first line therapy of cholestatic pruritus include rifampicin (300–450 mg/day orally) as a cytochrome P450 enzyme inducer, the bile acid sequestrant cholestyramine (4–16 mg/day orally) and the opioid receptor antagonist naltrexone (25–50 mg/day orally). In the next step, SSRIs (paroxetine 20 mg/day, sertraline 50–100 mg/day) and UVB phototherapy may be used. Ursodeoxycholic acid (10–20 mg/kg/day), butorphanol intranasal spray (1–2 mg/day) are additional options. Finally, liver transplantation may induce complete relief of pruritus.

Q.12 What is senile pruritus? What is the pathogenesis and treatment of this condition?

Ans: Senile pruritus or pruritus of senescence is persistent and widespread itching experienced by elderly people. The main pathogenetic factor involved is xerosis associated with aging. Aging skin has poor water-retaining capacity partly owing to reduced sebum secretion which leads to impaired barrier function, dry skin and pruritus. In some cases, xerotic eczema may ensue which further aggravates the condition. Pruritus is often multifactorial and before a diagnosis of senile pruritus is made, dermatological conditions such as scabies and systemic causes including renal, hepatic, endocrine or malignant disease need to be excluded. Elderly people often have several comorbidities requiring polypharmacy, thus the possibility of drug reaction should always be kept in mind. Pruritus in the elderly may also be a symptom of underlying psychological factors, like depression which may also aggravate pruritus from other causes.

The cornerstone of management of senile pruritus is frequent and liberal application of emollients in association of the general measures outlined above. A nightly dose of antidepressants such as amitriptyline, paroxetine or mirtazapine may help individuals with a significant elementof depression.

Q.13 Can drugs cause generalized pruritus without a rash?

Ans: Drug-induced pruritus is usually associated with morbilliform or urticarial rash; however, a large number of drugs (Table 2) can cause pruritus without any skin rash. The temporal relationship between the initiation of drug therapy and onset of pruritus, resolution after drug withdrawal, and recurrence after rechallenge are useful diagnostic pointers. Drug-induced pruritus is commonly observed in patients taking multiple drugs, as a result of impaired metabolism and/or drug interactions.

TABLE 2: Drugs that may cause pruritus without skin lesions.		
Antihypertensives	• Angiotensin-converting enzyme inhibitors • Angiotensin II inhibitors • Beta-blockers • Calcium channel blockers	
Antidiabetics	• Biguanides • Sulfonylureas	
Antibacterials and chemotherapeutics	• Antimalarials • Penicillins • Cephalosporins • Macrolides • Quinolones	• Tetracyclines • Metronidazole • Rifampicin • Sulfonamides
Psychotropics	• Tricyclic antidepressant • Antipsychotics • Selective serotonin reuptake inhibitors	
Antiepileptics	• Carbamazepine • Phenytoin	
Anti-cancers	• Chlorambucil • Paclitaxel	
Others drugs	• Antithyroid • Opioids • Nonsteroidal anti-inflammatory drugs • Sex hormones • Xanthine oxidase inhibitors	

Q.14 What is paraneoplastic pruritus? How is it treated?

Ans: Paraneoplastic pruritus is a sensation of itch occurring as a systemic reaction to the presence of a tumor or a hematological malignancy which is induced neither by the local presence of cancer cells nor by tumor therapy. Paraneoplastic itch usually disappears after remission of the malignancy and its reappearance may herald tumor recurrence. Paraneoplastic pruritus occurs more commonly in hematological malignancies, although it may occur in association of solid tumors including those of lung, colon, brain, breast, stomach and prostate. The prevalence of PP in Hodgkin's lymphoma is between 15% and 50%, in non-Hodgkin's lymphoma around 30%, and in polycythemia vera about 50%. It may also occur in leukemia (more in lymphocytic type) and myeloma. GP may be a clue for the diagnosis of occult Hodgkin's disease in previously healthy patient as it may occur several months before the diagnosis of Hodgkin disease. The skin in PP may appear normal or secondary lesions such as excoriation, prurigo, lichenification and dyspigmentation may be present. Paraneoplastic pruritus may present as aquagenic pruritus.

The primary management is the treatment of the underlying malignancy which generally leads to amelioration of the symptom. A number of systemic agents can be used to treat PP. H1 antihistaminics are usually ineffective, but first-generation drugs such as hydroxyzine (25–50 mg at night) may be used for their soporific effect. Selective serotonin reuptake inhibitor drugs such as paroxetine (10–20 mg/day), sertraline (25–50 mg/day), of fluvoxamine (25–100 mg/day) have been used with success in PP. Amitriptyline (25–100 mg) or doxepin (50 mg) can be used at night time. Opioid receptor antagonist naloxone (up to 2 mg intravenous) or naltrexone (50–100 mg/day) may provide significant benefit. Gabapentin (300 mg up to 3600 mg in three divided doses), pregabalin (75–300 mg/day in up to three doses) and aprepitant (80–125 mg/day) have been used with variable success rate.

Q.15 What are the causes of generalized pruritus in human immunodeficiency virus infected patients?

Ans: Persistent and distressful GP is a common complaint in many HIV infected patients; it may be the presenting symptom in some. The causes of pruritus in HIV disease is frequently multifactorial and include many ordinary skin disorders, some of which are more common and more severe in presence of HIV infection. These include papulosquamous disorders (psoriasis, seborrheic dermatitis), infestations (scabies, pediculosis), infections (folliculitis), drug eruptions and cutaneous T-cell lymphoma. Xerosis is a frequent association of HIV infection and a common cause of pruritus. Photosensitivity may also be a cause of pruritus and can be due to drugs, porphyria cutanea tarda or an idiopathic photosensitivity associated with advanced HIV infection. In addition, a variety of pruritic skin conditions are peculiar to patients with HIV infection. These include atopic-like dermatitis (eczematous eruption strongly resembling atopic dermatitis), atypical cutaneous lymphoproliferative disorder (widespread pruritic lesions with hyperpigmentation and atypical lymphocytic infiltrate), pruritic papular eruption, and eosinophilic folliculitis.

Pruritus due to drug eruptions occur commonly in the setting of HIV infection and are frequently caused by sulphonamides and antiretroviral drugs. Systemic diseases may also be responsible for GP in HIV infection. These may include HIV nephropathy, cholestatic pruritus (from hepatitis B or C or HAART-induced hepatotoxicity), hypothyroidism and systemic lymphoma.

■ CONCLUSION

There are many dermatological diseases that may cause GP. The GP may also provide a clue to an underlying serious systemic disease. Every patient needs thorough clinical evaluation followed by appropriate investigations to ascertain the underlying etiology. Management of GP is aimed at detection and treatment of the underlying cause and alleviation of symptoms by various measures.

KEY POINTS

- Generalized pruritus is a common problem that can severely impair the quality of life of affected patients
- The pathophysiology of GP is complex and interaction of various cellular and molecular mechanisms in the skin and nervous system are responsible for induction, transmission, perception, and modulation of itch
- Beside many primary dermatological diseases, a large number of systemic diseases can cause GP. It can also be neurogenic or psychogenic in origin
- Renal and cholestatic pruritus are among the more common systemic causes of pruritus and can be extremely distressful
- Generalized pruritus may be an early sign of lymphoma or other malignancies
- Taking a thorough drug history is mandatory as drugs may cause GP without any rash
- General nonpharmacologic measures and emollients could be beneficial in the treatment of all causes of GP
- Several groups of systemic agents that may target various aspects of the pathophysiology of itch are employed in the management of GP. However, robust evidence of their efficacy as confirmed by double-blind RCTs are generally lacking.

SUGGESTED READING

1. Cassano N, Tessari G, Vena GA, Girolomoni G. Chronic pruritus in the absence of specific skin disease: an update on pathophysiology, diagnosis, and therapy. Am J Clin Dermatol. 2010; 11(6):399-411.
2. Hercogova J. Topical anti-itch therapy. Dermatol Therapy. 2005;18:341-3.
3. Metz M, Sander S. Chronic pruritus – pathogenesis, clinical aspects and treatment. J Eur Acad Dermatol Venereol. 2010;24:1249-60.
4. Pongcharoen P, Fleischer AB Jr. Itch management: Systemic agents. Curr Probl Dermatol. 2016; 50:46-53.
5. Raap U, Stnder S, Metz M. Pathophysiology of itch and new treatments. Curr Opin Allergy Clin Immunol. 2011;11:420-27.
6. Singh F, and Rudikoff D. HIV-associated pruritus etiology and management. Am J Clin Dermatol. 2003;4:177-88.
7. Weisshaar E, Weiss M, Mettang T, Yosipovitch G, Zylicz Z et al. Paraneoplastic itch: aan expert position statement from the special interest group (SIG) of the International Forum on the Study of Itch (IFCI). Acta Derm Venereol. 2015;95:261-5.
8. Yosipovitch G, Bernhard JD. Clinical practice. Chronic pruritus. N Engl J Med. 2013;368(17): 1625-34.
9. Yosipovitch G, David M. The diagnostic and therapeutic approach to idiopathic generalized pruritus. Int J Dermatol. 1999;38:881-7.

CHAPTER 4

Diffuse Hyperpigmentation

Komal Agarwal, Anupam Das, Rashmi Sarkar

INTRODUCTION

The prevalence of hyperpigmentary disorders are increasing each day and it is particularly common in skin of color, like our Indian population. The cause of hyperpigmentation is usually traced to the presence and activity of melanocytes, offending drugs or systemic illnesses. Diffuse hyperpigmentation (DHP) does not only cause psychosocial stress but may also be a sign of a life threatening underlying disease. Therefore it is important to take a thorough history and trace the etiology, so as to enable proper treatment of the cause.

CASE 1

A 62-year-old, male presented to the Dermatology outpatient department with complaints of asymptomatic and progressive darkening of skin for past 3–4 years. The hyperpigmentation began as small macules from the face and neck and gradually spread to involve the upper chest, upper back and upper limbs. There was no history of preceding erythema, scaling or pruritus. There was no history of any other major illness or drug intake or of application of any topical preparation. He was a tea garden worker by profession. His family history was insignificant.

Examination: the patient had ill-defined but diffuse brownish-black pigmentation on temporal and preauricular area of face, almost all sides of neck, upper back, chest, upper limbs. The lesions had irregular, poorly defined borders. The hyperpigmentation was symmetrically distributed and was more on the extensors and sun-exposed areas, though entire body was involved (Figs. 1 and 2). There was no sign of inflammation. Palms, soles, scalp, oral mucosa and nails were normal. Systemic examination was within normal limits.

Investigation: no abnormality was detected on routine blood investigations. Skin biopsy of the lesion showed diffuse vacuolar degeneration of basal layer in epidermis. Dermis predominantly showed patchy lymphohistiocytic infiltrate, perivascular inflammation, pigment incontinence and melanophages. There was melanin deposition in superficial dermis. All these were consistent with lichen planus pigmentosus (LPP).

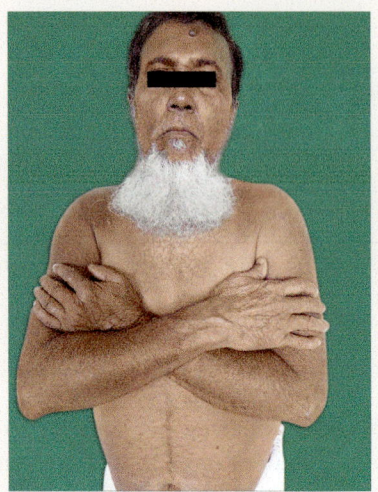

Fig. 1: Ill-defined diffuse brownish-black pigmentation on the face, neck, chest and abdomen (anterior view).

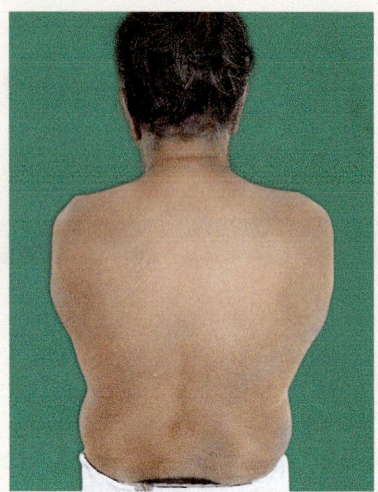

Fig. 2: Ill-defined diffuse brownish-black pigmentation on the back.

Thus, on the basis of the clinical and histopathological examination (HPE), a diagnosis of LPP was made.

Case Review In Nutshell

Any case of DHP is a source of dilemma, not only for the patient but also for the treating doctor. Since, it is not only a cosmetic problem, but may often be a sign of some underlying disorder. Therefore, while dealing with any case of DHP it is imperative to know about all the possible differential diagnosis, so as to make a proper diagnosis and treat the cause.

In the above case the following differentials were considered:
- Lichen planus pigmentosus
- Erythema dyschromicum perstans (EDP) or ashy dermatosis
- Phytophotodermatitis (PPD)
- Riehl's melanosis (pigmented cosmetic dermatitis)
- Postinflammatory hyperpigmentation.

Lichen planus pigmentosus was considered as the first differential. The presence of brownish-black macules mainly on sun exposed areas with no sign of inflammation or pruritus goes in favor of LPP. Moreover, the presence of excessive vacuolar degeneration of basal layer with melanin deposition in superficial dermis was consistent with LPP. EDP was a close differential. However, in EDP the color of the skin appears gray or "ashy", and the hyperpigmentation is not only confined to the sun exposed areas. The lesions may have erythematous and elevated margins. There may be presence of hypo- or hypermelanotic macules simultaneously giving it a polymorphic appearance. Also, on HPE there is focal vacuolar degeneration of basal layer and melanin deposition is seen in deep dermis.

Given the profession of the patient PPD was considered as a differential. However, hyperpigmented lesions, delayed erythema, vesicular and bullous lesions are considered hallmark of PPD which was absent in the present patient. Also, there was no pruritus.

Riehl's melanosis has to have a definite history of application of cosmetic or skin care products. It appears as brownish-gray macules mainly distributed over forehead and temples, may involve other areas like neck, chest, etc. and may have some scaling or horny plugs. It is quite rapid in onset. However, in the above patient the lesions spread gradually, and there was no history of using any kind of cosmetics or other skin care products.

Postinflammatory hyperpigmentation though appears brown to black in color, but as the name suggests there has to be a definite history of allergy or infection at that site. This was not the case in the present patient.

Thus on the basis of history, clinical examination and HPE reports and after ruling out the close possible differentials, a diagnosis of LPP was established.

The patient was counseled regarding the nature of the disease and prognosis. He was advised liberal sun protection, oral and topical steroid and topical tacrolimus. There was significant improvement after 4 months of treatment.

■ INTERACTIVE TOPIC REVIEW

Q.1 What is the normal skin color dependent on?

Ans: There are various factors on which the normal skin color depends, they are:
- Pigments in the epidermis and dermis
- Ethnicity
- Metabolism
- Degree of skin vascularity
- Thickness of stratum corneum
- Environmental influence
- Subjective visual evaluation.

Q.2 What are the pigments present in epidermis and dermis?

Ans: There are mainly four pigments in epidermis and dermis that influence the skin color. They are:
1. Oxygenated hemoglobin (red)—in arterioles and capillaries
2. Deoxygenated or reduced hemoglobin (blue)—in venules
3. Carotenoids (yellow)
4. Melanin—the most important pigment that determines skin color.

Q.3 What is the chemical composition of melanin?

Ans: Melanin is an indole derivative of 3,4-dihydroxyphenylalanine derived from tyrosine.

Q.4 What are the types of melanin?

Ans: Melanin is of two types:
1. Eumelanin
2. Pheomelanin

Q.5 What is the difference between the two types of melanin?

Ans: The differences are enumerated in Table 1.

TABLE 1: Difference between eumelanin and pheomelanin.

	Eumelanin	Pheomelanin
Color	Brown to black	Yellow to reddish-brown
Shape of granules	Elliptical eumelanosomes	Rounded contour
Solubility	Insoluble	Alkali soluble
Composed of	Nitrogen	Nitrogen and sulphur (it is a cysteine rich compound)

Q.6 What do you understand by hyperpigmentation?

Ans: Hyperpigmentation clinically appears as increase in pigmentation of skin which may be due to:
- Increased melanin production (increased melanocyte and tyrosinase activity) or
- Decreased breakdown and removal of melanin.

Q.7 How to clinically differentiate dermal and epidermal hyperpigmentation?

Ans: Refer to Table 2.

TABLE 2: Difference between epidermal and dermal hyperpigmentation.

	Epidermal hyperpigmentation	Dermal hyperpigmentation
Color	Brownish	Bluish-gray (due to Tyndall effect)
Wood's lamp	Enhanced	Not enhanced

Q.8 What are the differential diagnosis of DHP?

Ans: The differentials for DHP will vary depending on the age of the patient (Table 3). Important points to differentiate the above causes:
- Addison's disease—the hyperpigmentation is because of decreased cortisol which in turn causes increased secretion of adrenocorticotropic hormone (ACTH) and melanocyte-stimulating hormone (MSH). There is DHP of mainly sun exposed areas, areas prone to trauma, palmar creases and flexures. Dark longitudinal lines may be seen on the nails. Pre-existing nevi may darken in color. Menstrual abnormalities may be present with systemic features like dehydration, weight loss, hypotension, diarrhea. There is pigmentation of oral mucosa

TABLE 3: Causes of diffuse hyperpigmentation on the basis of age.

Adults	Children
<ul><li>Dermatological causes:<ul><li>Lichen planus pigmentosus</li><li>Erythema dyschromicum perstans or ashy dermatosis</li><li>Postinflammatory hyperpigmentation</li><li>Riehl's melanosis</li><li>Phytophotodermatitis</li></ul></li><li>Endocrine causes:<ul><li>Addison's disease</li><li>Hyperthyroidism</li><li>Cushing syndrome</li><li>Pheochromocytoma</li><li>Carcinoid syndrome</li><li>Acromegaly</li><li>Nelson syndrome</li></ul></li><li>Nutritional causes:<ul><li>Vitamin B12 deficiency</li><li>Malabsorption syndrome</li><li>Folic acid deficiency</li><li>Vitamin A deficiency</li><li>Pellagra</li></ul></li><li>Infections:<ul><li>Tuberculosis</li><li>Malaria</li><li>Kala Azar</li><li>HIV</li><li>Vagabond disease</li></ul></li><li>Malignancies:<ul><li>Metastatic melanomas</li><li>Lymphoma</li><li>Mycosis fungoides</li><li>Cancer cachexia</li><li>Leukemia cutis</li></ul></li><li>Rheumatological:<ul><li>Scleroderma</li><li>Generalized morphea</li><li>Felty's syndrome</li></ul></li><li>Syndromes:<ul><li>Peutz–Jegher syndrome</li><li>Laugier–Hunziker syndrome</li></ul></li><li>Drugs and toxins:<ul><li>Physiological</li><li>Pregnancy</li></ul></li><li>Physical agents:<ul><li>Ultraviolet radiation</li><li>Trauma/friction</li></ul></li><li>Idiopathic</li></ul>	<ul><li>Giant congenital melanocytic nevus</li><li>Bronze baby syndrome</li><li>Postinflammatory hyperpigmentation</li><li>Hyperpigmented stage of incontinentia pigmenti</li><li>Frictional melanosis</li><li>Due to medications</li><li>Systemic causes—nephropathy, malnutrition</li><li>Hemochromatosis</li><li>Porphyria</li><li>Metastasizing melanoma</li><li>Carbon baby or universal acquired melanosis or familial progressive hyperpigmentation</li></ul>

- Acromegaly, Cushing syndrome and Nelson syndrome (corticotropic adenoma of hypophysis)—can all lead to Addisonian type of hyperpigmentation. In addition Nelson syndrome also has features of neuro-ophthalmic symptoms.
- Thyrotoxicosis—it is associated with both vitiligo and DHP. Only 2% patients develop DHP. Oral mucosa is usually spared and there is deposition of hemosiderin in the dermis
- Vitamin B12 deficiency—due to decreased vitamin B12 there is increased tyrosinase activity since glutathione cannot be maintained in its reduced form. The pigmentation may be symmetric and diffuse, scattered or Addisonian type. Face, knuckles and flexures are involved. There is involvement of nails too. Along with it there may be depigmentation of hair, angular cheilitis and glossitis. Vitamin A deficiency—there is DHP of face and limbs with xerosis. There may be pigmentation of lower fornix and bulbar conjunctiva
- Malabsorption syndromes (Whipple or tropical sprue)—Addisonian type of hyperpigmentation but mucous membranes are spared
- Hemochromatosis (Bronze diabetes)—occurs more in males, fifth decade onwards. Its due to excess iron absorption and its deposition in tissues. Brownish or metallic gray pigmentation appears mainly on sun-exposed areas. Other systemic features like hepatomegaly, diabetes mellitus, hypogonadism and heart disease may be present. Diagnostic signs include high ferritin level, Hemosiderin granules are seen on HPE of skin with excessive melanin in basal layer
- Primary biliary cirrhosis—seen more in females than males, sun-exposed areas are involved and there is associated pruritus. On investigation antimitochondrial antibodies are seen
- Chronic renal failure—diffuse brown pigmentation of sun-exposed areas. It is due to increase of beta-MSH due to lack of clearance by kidneys
- Wilson's disease—hepatolenticular degeneration due to disruption of copper metabolism, leading to deposition of copper in basal ganglia. DHP is mainly seen on lower limbs, with greenish pigmentation of face, blue lunula and cirrhosis of liver. On slit lamp examination, Kayser–Fleischer ring is seen around cornea
- Multiple organ failure—there may be diffuse green pigmentation of skin due to dyes in liquid feeding tubes and multiple drugs
- Vagabond disease—commonly seen in old patients, with lack of hygiene and poor diet with pediculosis humanus infestation. Addisonian type of hyperpigmentation with involvement of mucosa. The hypermelanosis is probably postinflammatory due to scratching. Adrenal function is normal
- Peutz–Jegher syndrome—it presents with Addisonian type of hyperpigmentation with hamartomatous polyps in gastrointestinal tract. Occurs due to mutation of serine/threonine kinase 11 gene

- Laugier–Hunziker syndrome—almost similar to Peutz–Jegher syndrome but there are no intestinal polyps
- Porphyrias—there is DPH of sun-exposed skin with erythema, vesicles, bullae, erosions and ulcerations. It is accompanied by photosensitivity and discoloration of urine. Diagnosis is confirmed by analysis of porphyrin metabolites in urine, blood and stool
- Niemann–Pick disease—there is diffuse gray-brown to brown-yellow pigmentation of sun-exposed areas. There may be waxy induration of the face. On skin biopsy melanin is seen in dermis and characteristic lamellar inclusion in the histiocytes are seen
- Scleroderma—diffuse brown pigmentation of face and limbs is seen in advanced cases even without renal involvement. Mucosa is spared. There is increased production of endothelin 1 by keratinocytes and increased soluble L-selectin, and it has been postulated that this is responsible for increased melanogenesis
- Malignancy associated DHP:
  o Diffuse dermal melanosis or diffuse melanosis cutis is characterized by slate bluish-gray to brownish pigmentation. Mucosa is also involved. There are no melanoma cells in the skin and tumor lysis is believed to be the cause of this DHP
  o In mycosis fungoides sometimes DHP may be the only manifestation of the disease and is mostly seen in dark complexioned individuals
  o In lymphomas Addisonian type of hyperpigmentation is seen but mucosa is spared.
- Ultraviolet radiation—also known as tanning. It is seen in sun-exposed areas. It has three distinct phases—immediate pigment darkening, persistent pigment darkening and delayed tanning.

Q.9 What are the drugs and toxins/metals that may cause DHP?

Ans: Drugs that may lead to DHP are as follows:
- Phenothiazines like chlorpromazine, imipramine, trifluoperazine
  o Blue-gray pigmentation of sun-exposed areas due to deposition of drug-pigment complex
  o Chlorpromazine—high dose if used for long term can lead to diffuse purplish pigmentation of skin
  o On HPE golden brown granules are seen in upper dermis.
- Antimalarials like chloroquine or hydroxychloroquine
  o When used for more than 4 months, they cause bluish-gray pigmentation of face, neck, shins and hard palate.
- Mepacrine
  o Yellowish pigmentation due to deposition of complex of melanin, mepacrine, hemosiderin and sulphur.
- Quinine, quinidine
  o Generalized pigmentation.

- Minocycline-induced type 3 pigmentation
  - The pigmentation caused by minocycline has been classified into four types:
    - Type 1—bluish-black pigmentation of acne lesions
    - Type 2—blue-gray pigmentation of shin and arms
    - Type 3—generalized muddy brown hyperpigmentation
    - Type 4—pigmentation of vermillion border of lower lip.
- Busulfan
  - Diffuse brown pigmentation of skin and mucosa. May be associated with drug induced pulmonary fibrosis.
- Clofazimine
  - Red-brown discoloration.
- Dactinomycin
  - Generalized hyperpigmentation which is more prominent on the face.
- Amiodarone
  - If used at daily dose of more than or equal to 800 mg for prolonged duration, leads to slate-gray or purple discoloration of sun-exposed areas.
- Methotrexate
  - Uniform hyperpigmentation in sun exposed areas.
- Adrenocorticotropic hormone/MSH
  - Diffuse brown or bronze pigmentation, more in sun exposed sites.
- Imatinib
  - Diffuse hyperpigmentation of skin and melanonychia, repigmentation of gray hair and pigmentation of teeth and gingiva.
- Cyclophosphamide
  - Generalized pigmentation of trunk, face extremities and black pigmentation of nails.
- Topical agents like carmustine, fluorouracil, mechlorethamine.

Toxins/metals that may lead to DHP:
- Arsenic: Diffuse bronze hyperpigmentation of trunk with macular depigmented areas, giving a "raindrop' appearance". Main source is through drinking water
- Gold (chrysiasis): Blue-gray pigmentation of sun-exposed areas
- Silver (argyria): Generalized blue-gray pigmentation of skin, also involving the nails and sclera
- Lead: Gray discoloration of skin with a blue-black line on the gingiva
- Iron: Hemosiderosis, hemochromatosis.

Q.10 What are the important points while assessing a patient of DHP?

Ans:
- History of any drug intake or use of topical (over the counter or herbal) preparations.
- Family history of similar disease
- Menstrual history (this may give clue to underlying endocrine pathologies like thyrotoxicosis and Addison's disease which may be the cause of DHP

- Any exacerbation of lesions on sun exposure
- Any other systemic complains or chronic illness
- Occupational history (exposure to heavy metals or other allergens)
- Always examine the oral mucosa, hair and nails.

Some important points to reach the etiology of DHP on the basis of HPE findings:
- DHP may be due to melanin or some nonmelanin compounds (Table 4).

Therefore on HPE it's important to first identify, if it's because of melanin or other compounds.

TABLE 4: Diffuse hyperpigmentation due to melanin and nonmelanin compounds.

DHP due to increase in epidermal melanin	DHP due to increase in dermal melanin with/without increased epidermal melanin
• Ultraviolet radiation • Hyperthyroidism • Pregnancy (In case of ultraviolet radiation there is increase in melanocyte count, whereas the other two causes have normal melanocyte count)	• Endocrine causes like Addison's disease, Nelson syndrome • Vitamin B12 deficiency • LPP (superficial dermis) • EDP (deep dermis) • Postinflammatory melanosis • Drugs like minocycline and busulfan • Scleroderma associated DHP • Primary biliary cirrhosis • Tuberculosis • Porphyria cutanea tarda
Due to nonmelanin compounds like	

• Heavy metals like:
  ○ Gold, bismuth—with normal epidermal melanin
  ○ Arsenic, silver—associated with increased epidermal melanin
• Iron
• Deposition of drug compounds like drug-melanin complex as in case of chlorpromazine
• Lipofuscin synthesis—clofazimine	

Note: Some histologically undetectable nonmelanin compounds that may cause DHP are biliverdin (bronze baby), carotenoids, etc.

(DHP: diffuse hyperpigmentation)

Q.11 How would you approach a patient with DHP? Describe briefly.

Ans: Please refer to Flowcharts 1, 2 and 3.

Q.12 What are the differences between EDP and LPP?

Ans: The differences between EDP and LPP can be understood with the help of Table 5.

Q.13 What are the predisposing factors of LPP?

Ans: The etiology of LPP is yet unknown, but some factors that may predispose to LPP are as follows:
- Sunlight
- Hepatitis C virus

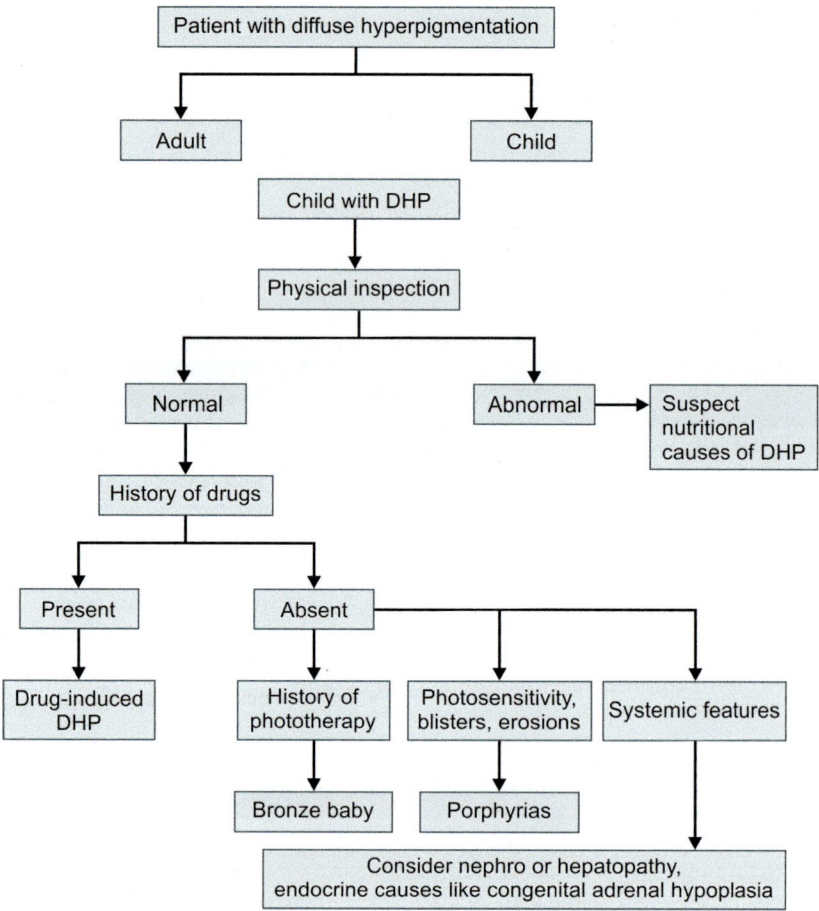

(DHP: diffuse hyperpigmentation)
Flowchart 1: Approach to a patient with diffuse hyperpigmentation.

- Mustard oil (due to allyl thiocyanate—a photosensitizer)
- Various cosmetics like kumkum, hair dye, etc.
- Influence of hormones as it presents in women around the time of menopause.

Q.14 What are the variants of LPP?

Ans:
- Lichen planus pigmentosus inversus
- Localized LPP
- Linear LPP
- Segmental LPP
- Zosteriform LPP
- Lichen planus pigmentosus along Blaschko lines
- Lichen planus pigmentosus of oral mucosa.

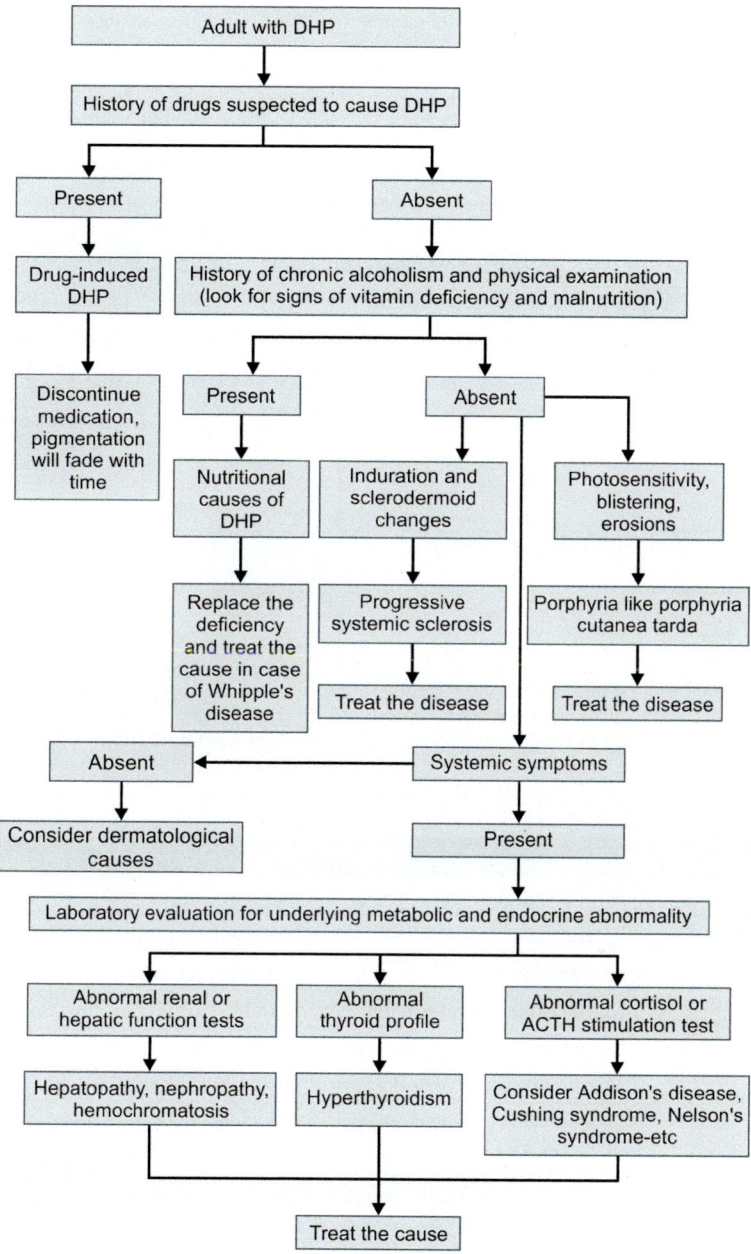

(ACTH: adrenocorticotropic hormone; DHP: diffuse hyperpigmentation)

Flowchart 2: Approach to an adult with diffuse hyperpigmentation.

Q.15 What is LPP inversus?

Ans: Lichen planus pigmentosus inversus is one of the most important variants of LPP. It is similar to LPP both in terms of histological examination and treatment response. The only difference lies in the clinical presentation as given in Table 6.

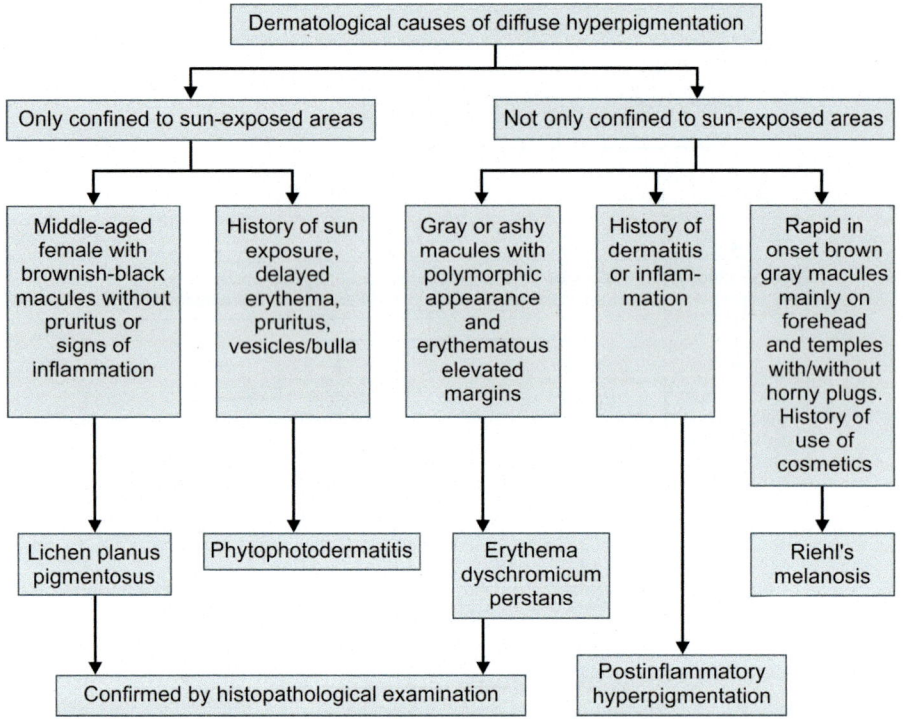

Flowchart 3: Common dermatological causes of diffuse hyperpigmentation.

TABLE 5: Differences between LPP and EDP.

	LPP	EDP (ashy dermatosis of Ramirez)
First reported by	Bhutani et al.	Ramirez
Epidemiology	Worldwide	More in Latin America
Age	Any age	Any age
Sex	More common in females	Equal in both males and females
Color of lesion	Slate-gray to brownish-black	Ash colored
Site	Mainly on sun exposed areas	Not restricted to sun exposed areas
Borders	Discrete macules with diffuse/ill-defined borders	Polycyclic macules with elevated, erythematous border like piece of string
Histopathological examination		
Basal cell degeneration	Diffuse	Focal
Infiltration of dermis	Patchy or band like	Perivascular
Colloid bodies	Plenty	Few
Melanin deposition	Superficial dermis	Deep dermis
Treatment	Partial response to steroids (oral or topical) and immunomodulators	Absent or low response to steroids. Partial response to immunomodulators like tacrolimus and clofazimine

TABLE 6: Difference between LPP and LPP inversus.

	LPP	LPP inversus
Skin type	More in dark skinned	More in fair skinned
Sites	More on sun-exposed areas	More on non-sun-exposed and intertriginous areas especially the axilla (90% cases)

Q.16 What are the other possible associated disorders with LPP?

Ans:
- Frontal fibrosing alopecia (FFA)–LPP on an average occurs 14 months before FFA
- Lichen planopilaris
- Hepatitis C infection
- Endocrinopathies like type 2 diabetes, dyslipidemia and thyroid disease
- Autoimmune disease—lupus erythematosus and vitiligo
- Malignancies—head and neck carcinoma (paraneoplastic LPP)
- Atopic dermatitis
- Nephrotic syndrome.

Q.17 What are the investigations required for LPP?

Ans: Lichen planus pigmentosus is mostly a clinical diagnosis but routine blood investigations may be done as the patient often requires systemic steroids. Also investigations are required to rule out any associated diseases like—hepatitis C serology, fasting lipid profile, fasting and postprandial blood sugar, thyroid profile etc. HPE is confirmatory.

On HPE, we find diffuse vacuolar degeneration of basal cell layer with lymphohistiocytic infiltration of dermis, superficial pigmentary incontinence and melanophages.

Q.18 What is the treatment of LPP?

Ans: **General**
- Avoid triggering factors like mustard oil, amla oil, nickel containing cosmetics, sun exposure
- Broad spectrum sunscreen and other photoprotective measures like use of full sleeve clothing, hats, umbrellas, sunglasses etc.

Topical
- Mid-to-high potency topical steroids may be used as once or twice daily application
- Steroid sparing agents like tacrolimus (0.03% or 0.1%)
- Adjuvant treatment with depigmenting agents like kojic acid.

Oral
- Oral corticosteroids–dexamethasone 2.5 mg as pulse therapy for two days/week for 12 weeks.
- Dapsone—100 mg daily for 16 weeks
- Isotretinoin.

Lasers
- Q switch laser (1064 nm NdYAG).

CONCLUSION

There are various causes of DHP, both dermatological as well as nondermatological. DHP is usually cosmetically very distressing for the patient and it may be a clue to underlying pathology. Therefore proper history taking, clinical examination and appropriate investigations are imperative in each case of DHP. The management of DHP depends on the diagnosis and treatment of the underlying cause.

KEY POINTS

- Diffuse hyperpigmentation may be benign and nonspecific or it may be a sign of some underlying systemic disease
- They cause great psychosocial distress and affect the quality of life of the patient
- Melanin is the most important pigment. It is an indole derivative of 3,4-dihydroxyphenylalanine derived from tyrosine. It is of two types – eumelanin and pheomelanin.
- Diffuse hyperpigmentation can be broadly divided into epidermal (brown) or dermal (bluish) hyperpigmentation
- Causes of DHP can be divided on the basis of age of the patient. LPP and EDP are the common dermatological causes of DHP that we come across in everyday practice
- Erythema dyschromicum perstans is also known as ashy dermatosis of Ramirez or dermatosis cenicienta
- Menstrual history is important in cases of DHP as it may give clue to underlying endocrine pathologies like thyrotoxicosis and Addison's disease
- Some nonmelanin compounds may also cause DHP like heavy metals (gold, bismuth), deposition of drug-melanin complex (chlorpromazine) or due to lipofuscin synthesis (clofazimine)
- Lichen planus pigmentosus—mainly over sun exposed areas, discrete macules with ill-defined borders
- Erythema dyschromicum perstans—involves both sun exposed and sun protected areas, polycyclic macules with elevated erythematous border like a piece of string
- Lichen planus pigmentosus inversus is one of the most important variants of LPP. It is similar to LPP both in terms of histological examination and treatment response. The only difference lies in the clinical presentation
- The treatment of DHP depends on the management of the underlying cause.

SUGGESTED READING

1. Akarsu S, Ilknur T, Özer E, Fetil E. Lichen planus pigmentosus distributed along the lines of Blaschko. Int J Dermatol. 2013;52:253-4.
2. Al-Mutairi N, El-Khalawany M. Clinicopathological characteristics of lichen planus pigmentosus and its response to tacrolimus ointment: an open label, non-randomized, prospective study. J Eur Acad Dermatol Venereol. 2010;24:535-40.
3. Bhutani LK, Bedi TR, Pandhi RK, et al. Lichen planus pigmentosus. Dermatologica. 1974;149:43-50.
4. Cho S, Whang KK. Lichen planus pigmentosus presenting in zosteriform pattern. J Dermatol. 1997;24:193-7.

5. Dlova NC. Frontal fibrosing alopecia and lichen planus pigmentosus: Is there a link? Br J Dermatol. 2013;168:439-42.
6. Feingold ML, Koss LG. Effects of long-term administration of busulfan. Arch Intern Med. 1969;124:66-71.
7. Fistarol SK, Itin PH. Disorders of pigmentation. J Dtsch Dermatol Ges. 2010;8(3):187-201;quiz 201-2.
8. Ghosh A, Coondoo A. Lichen planus pigmentosus: The controversial consensus. Indian J Dermatol. 2016;61:482-6.
9. Gupta D, Thappa DM. Dermatoses due to Indian cultural practices. Indian J Dermatol. 2015;60:3-12.
10. Hashimoto K, Joselow SA, Mauray JT. Imipramine hyperpigmentation: A slate gray discoloration caused by a long-term imipramine administration. J Am Acad Dermatol. 1991;25:357-61.
11. Hong S, Shin JH, Kang HY. Two cases of lichen planus pigmentosus presenting with a linear pattern. J Korean Med Sci. 2004;19:152-4.
12. Kanwar AJ, Dogra S, Handa S, et al. A study of 124 Indian patients with lichen planus pigmentosus. Clin Exp Dermatol. 2003;28:481-5.
13. Kim JE, Won CH, Chang S, et al. Linear lichen planus pigmentosus of the forehead treated by neodymium: Yttrium aluminum-garnet laser and topical tacrolimus. J Dermatol. 2012;39:189-91.
14. Kim KJ, Bae GY, Choi JH, et al. A case of localized lichen planus pigmentosus on the thigh. J Dermatol. 2002;29:242-3.
15. Kumar YH, Babu AR. Segmental lichen planus pigmentosus: An unusual presentation. Indian Dermatol Online J. 2014;5:157-9.
16. Mancuso G, Berdondini RM. Coexistence of lichen planus pigmentosus and minimal change nephrotic syndrome. Eur J Dermatol. 2009;19:389-90.
17. Murzaku EC, Bronsnick T, Rao BK. Axillary lichen planus pigmentosus-inversus: Dermoscopic clues of a rare entity. Diagnosis: Lichen planus pigmentosus (LPP). J Am Acad Dermatol. 2014;71:e119-20.
18. Muthu SK, Narang T, Saikia UN, et al. Low-dose oral isotretinoin therapy in lichen planus pigmentosus: An open-label non-randomized prospective pilot study. Int J Dermatol. 2016;55:1048-54.
19. Rieder E, Kaplan J, Kamino H, et al. Lichen planus pigmentosus. Dermatol Online J. 2013;19:20713.
20. Sassolas B, Zagnoli A, Leroy JP, et al. Lichen planus pigmentosus associated with acrokeratosis of Bazex. Clin Exp Dermatol 1994;19:70-3.
21. Satanove A. Pigmentation due to phenothiazines in high and prolonged dosage. JAMA. 1965;191(4):263-8.
22. Sehgal VN, Verma P, Bhattacharya SN, et al. Lichen planus pigmentosus. Skinmed. 2013;11:96-103.
23. Seidel A. Lichen planus pigmentosus (LPP) and lichen planus pigmentosus: 35 cases in Armenia, Colombia. J Am Acad Dermatol. 2015;72:AB114.
24. Sindhura KB, Vinay K, Kumaran MS, et al. Lichen planus pigmentosus: A retrospective clinico-epidemiologic study with emphasis on the rare follicular variant. J Eur Acad Dermatol Venereol. 2015;30:e142-4.
25. Torres J, Peña Romero AG, Reyes E, et al. Lichen planus pigmentosus in patients with endocrinopathies and hepatitis C. J Am Acad Dermatol. 2013;68:AB139.
26. Vachiramon V, Suchonwanit P, Thadanipon K. Bilateral linear lichen planus pigmentosus associated with hepatitis C virus infection. Case Rep Dermatol. 2010;2:169-72.
27. Vega ME, Waxtein L, Arenas R, et al. Ashy dermatosis and lichen planus pigmentosus: A clinicopathologic study of 31 cases. Int J Dermatol. 1992;31:90-4.
28. Verma P, Pandhi D. Topical tacrolimus and oral dapsone combination regimen in lichen planus pigmentosus. Skinmed. 2015;13:351-4.
29. Vineet R, Sumit S, Garg VK, et al. Lichen planus pigmentosus in linear and zosteriform pattern along the lines of Blaschko. Dermatol Online J. 2015;21(10).

CHAPTER 5

Fever with Rash in a Child

Nitin Nadkarni, Aayushi Mehta

■ INTRODUCTION

Fever with rash in children is a common case scenario encountered both in the dermatology and pediatric departments. This is a diagnostic challenge and the major consideration is to distinguish benign from serious clinical presentations, with the common sequence of a history, physical examination and investigations, it is mostly possible to make a correct diagnosis and choose a proper treatment.

It is seen that the pattern of rash is more important than the type of the fever. Hence, the dermatologist's role in the management of fever with rash is extremely vital, while the pediatrician comes into the picture once a diagnosis is made, from the view of treatment.

CASE REPORT

A 5-year-old child was brought by his mother to dermatology outpatient department with history of fever since 5 days, redness of eyes, running nose, irritability and generalized rash since 2 days. The rash started from the face, neck and progressed downwards to trunk. Mother reported loss of appetite and irritability. There was no history of contact or similar rash in family members.

Clinical Features: On examination, the child was febrile with a toxic look. There was a generalized erythematous maculopapular rash involving face, neck, postauricular region, chest, back, and arms, extending on lower legs up to the knees. Congestion was seen in the eyes (Figs. 1 and 2).

Treatment: The child was advised rest, isolation and adequate hydration. Antipyretics were given along with oral antihistamines. Soothing emollients were given for local application.

Outcome: The child had recovered completely on follow-up after 10 days.

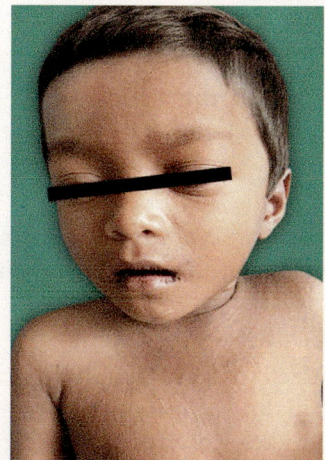

Fig. 1: Maculopapular rash on face with mucosal congestion and oral involvement.
Courtesy: Nitin J Nadkarni, , Professor, Department of Dermatology, DY Patil School of Medicine, Nerul, Navi Mumbai, Maharashtra .

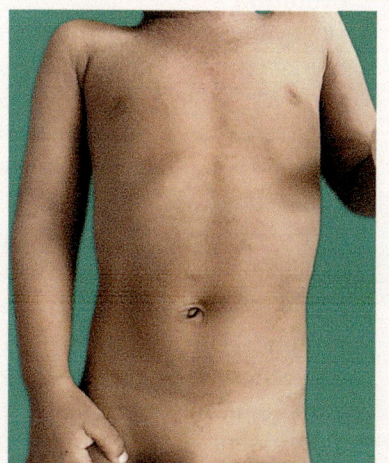

Fig. 2: Maculopapular rash progressively involving trunk and limbs (cephalocaudal progression).
Courtesy: Nitin J Nadkarni, , Professor, Department of Dermatology, DY Patil School of Medicine, Nerul, Navi Mumbai, Maharashtra.

INTERACTIVE TOPIC REVIEW

Q.1 What are the important points in history taking of a child presenting with fever and rash?

Ans: Box 1 includes the important points to be covered in history taking of a child with fever and rash.

Age

The age of the child gives us important clues about the possible etiology. Infants and small children having a rash with fever would make one think of viral exanthems. Kawasaki disease is often found in slightly older children, while varicella can be found at 3–10 years of age. Meningococcal septicemia is also found in <5 years of age. Collagen vascular conditions, though rare in children, usually affect an older child. Henoch–Schönlein purpura (HSP) occurs between 3 and 8 years.

Dengue and chikungunya can occur at any age.

BOX 1	History taking.
• Age of the child	• History of recent intake of drugs
• Mode of onset	• Nature of fever
• Initial site of rash	• Recent travel abroad
• Evolution of the rash	• History of similar rash in family members
• Type of rash	• Immunization status
• Symptoms of severe systemic involvement	

Evolution

The evolution of a rash gives important clues, e.g. measles start in a cephalo-caudal pattern. Varicella starts on the trunk and spreads outwards (centripetal pattern), while meningococcemia often starts on the hands and feet and progresses to the trunk (centrifugal pattern). HSP starts on the lower legs and buttocks and progresses upward.

Systemic Involvement

It is very important to diagnose presence of systemic involvement since it indicates a worse prognosis and warrants urgent referral to a pediatrician. Thus, the following systemic features herald a serious course (Table 1).

Temporal Onset of Rash with Fever

A prodrome of upper respiratory tract infection (URTI) indicates a viral exanthem. However, it can also occur in certain drug reactions.

A mnemonic given in Box 2 can predict the likely etiology depending on the time of the rash after the onset of fever.

Drug History

A recent intake of drugs confuses the issue, since patients are often given antipyretics by a primary care physician or by the parents themselves. In the personal experience of most physicians, paracetamol is relatively safe, however, agents like diclofenac can cause erythema multiforme major or Stevens–Johnson syndrome.

Ampicillin, given for fever can cause the rash of infectious mononucleosis to appear after 1 week. Many other drugs can precipitate Stevens-Johnson syndrome or even toxic epidermal necrolysis.

TABLE 1: Signs indicative of systemic involvement in a child with fever and rash (and the possible associations).

Polyarthritis	Dengue, chikungunya, juvenile arthritis, systemic lupus erythematosus, dermatomyositis
Hepatosplenomegaly	Leptospirosis, Epstein–Barr virus infection
Lymphadenopathy	Tuberculosis, leukemias, lymphomas
Bleeding from gums/nose	Henoch–Schönlein purpura, dengue, chikungunya, meningococcemia
Multiorgan failure	Dengue, meningococcemia, toxic shock syndrome

BOX 2: Mnemonic to predict the likely etiology depending on the time of the rash after the onset of fever.

- **V**ery
- **S**ick
- **P**atients
- **M**ust
- **T**ake
- **D**ouble
- **T**reatment

Varicella—Rash on 1st day of fever
Scarlet Fever—Rash on 2nd day of fever
Small **P**ox—Rash on 3rd day of fever
Measles—Rash on 4th day
Typhus—Rash on 5th day
Dengue—Rash on 6th day
Typhoid—Rash on 7th day

Q.2 What are the causes of acute onset of fever and rash in a child?

Ans: When the fever with rash is of acute onset, the following causes have to be taken into consideration (Box 3).

BOX 3	Causes of acute onset of fever with rash.
• Viral exanthems • Drug reactions • Pyogenic infections (staphylococcal scalded skin syndrome)	• Kawasaki disease • Rheumatic fever

Q.3 What are the causes of a subacute onset of fever with rash in a child?

Ans: The causes of a subacute onset of fever with rash in a child are shown in Box 4.

BOX 4	Causes of subacute onset of fever with rash.
• Henoch-Schönlein purpura • Autoimmune diseases • Polyarteritis nodosa	• Wegener's granulomatosis • Juvenile rheumatoid arthritis

Q.4 What are the causes of fever with rash in a neonate?

Ans: The causes of fever with rash in a neonate are shown in Box 5.

BOX 5	Causes of fever with rash in a neonate.
• Neonatal herpes simplex • Neonatal varicella • Septicemia • Severe bullous impetigo/staphylococcal scalded skin syndrome	• Neonatal erythroderma (secondary to severe congenital ichthyosis) • Neonatal candidiasis • Neonatal lupus erythematosus

Q.5 What are the common infectious and noninfectious causes of fever with rash in a pediatric age group?

Ans: Common infectious and noninfectious causes of fever with rash in pediatric population are shown in Table 2.

TABLE 2: Common infectious and noninfectious causes of fever with rash in pediatric population.

Infectious Causes	Noninfectious Causes
Rubella	Erythema multiforme
Rubeola	Stevens–Johnson syndrome
Human herpesvirus 6	Toxic epidermal necrolysis
Fifth disease	Systemic lupus erythematosus
Epstein–Barr virus	Juvenile dermatomyositis
Typhoid	Systemic onset juvenile rheumatoid arthritis
Meningococcemia	Sweet's syndrome

Q.6 How to classify causes of fever with rash on basis of morphology?

Ans: The classification is shown in Table 3.

TABLE 3: Classification of fever with rash on basis of morphology (common causes).		
Morphology of Rash	**Infectious Causes**	**Noninfectious Causes**
Macular/ Maculopapular/ Erythematous/ Desquamative/ Scarlatiniform	• Measles • Rubella • Other viral infections • Chikungunya fever • Infectious mononucleosis • Scarlet fever	• Serum sickness syndrome • Drug hypersensitivity • Neonatal and systemic lupus erythematosus • Juvenile rheumatoid arthritis • Rheumatic fever (erythema marginatum) • Kawasaki disease • Juvenile dermatomyositis
Vesicular/ vesiculopustular rash	• Neonatal varicella • Neonatal herpes • Varicella zoster virus • Hand, foot, and mouth disease • Rickettsialpox • *Candida* infections	• Steven–Johnson syndrome • Acute generalized exanthematous pustulosis • Pustular psoriasis • Autoimmune bullous dermatosis • Bullous erythema multiforme
Petechial/purpuric rash	• Dengue Fever • Chikungunya fever • Meningococcemia • Rickettsial infections • Gonococcemia • Typhoid • Hepatitis B • Epstein–Barr Virus • RMSF	• Rheumatic fever • Systemic lupus erythematosus • Henoch–Schönlein purpura • Childhood polyarteritis nodosa • Purpura fulminans
Urticarial rash	Infectious mononucleosis	• Urticarial vasculitis • Malignancies • Serum sickness
Nodular	–	• Erythema nodosum • Nodular vasculitis
Rash with skin failure	• Staphylococcal scalded skin syndrome • Toxic shock syndrome	• Steven–Johnson syndrome/toxic epidermal necrolysis

Q.7 What are the salient initial steps in management of a child with fever and rash?

Ans:
- Note whether patient is toxic or not. If so, referral to a pediatrician and/or admission is advisable
  - Note the type of the rash. A petechial or purpuric rash indicates a more serious prognosis, and at least a few basic investigations

Fever with Rash in a Child | 77

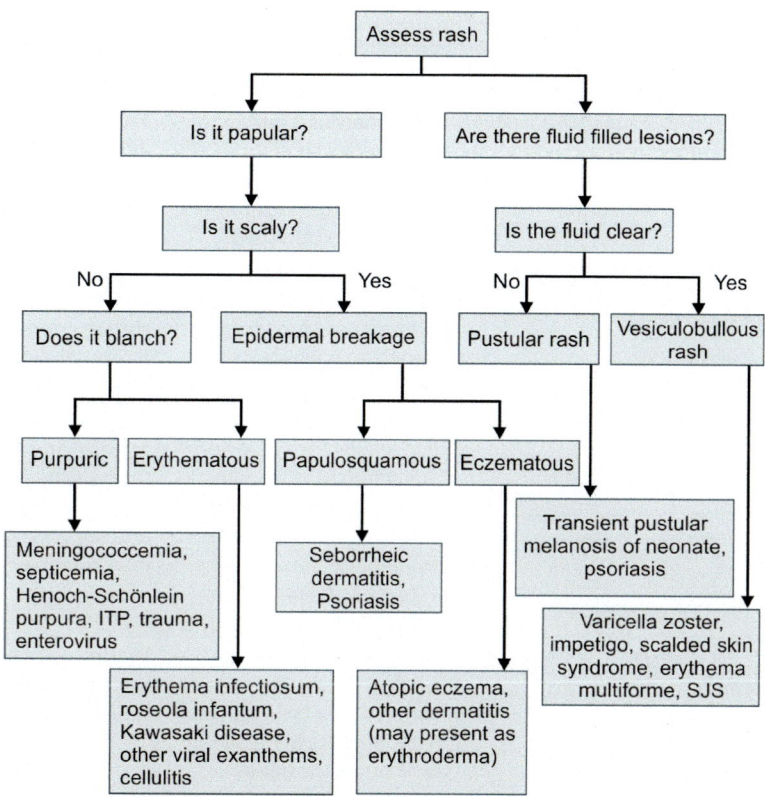

(ITP: idiopathic thrombocytopenic purpura; SJS: Stevens–Johnson syndrome).

Flowchart 1: Approach to patient presenting with fever and generalized rash.

Adapted with permission from: Algorithm for Common Childhood Rashes (2015) by Dr. Mary Harding at Patient UK Website. Available at: https://patient.info/doctor/common-childhood-rashes.

- Supportive and symptomatic management remains the mainstay in most cases
- Counseling and isolation when indicated.

The algorithm presented in Flowchart 1 indicates a good approach to patient presenting in outpatient department with fever and generalized rash.

Q.8 What are the typical clinical features of common viral exanthems of childhood?

Ans: The typical clinical features of common viral exanthems of childhood are shown in Table 4.

Q.9 What are the features of commonly occurring hemorrhagic fevers in childhood?

Ans: The features of commonly occurring hemorrhagic fevers in childhood are shown in Table 5.

TABLE 4: Important clinical features of common viral exanthems of childhood.

Disease	Infectious agent	Incubation period	Characteristics of rash	Other features
Measles	Measles virus (Paramyxovirus)	10–11 days	Erythematous, blanching, maculopapular rash, begins behind ears and anterior hairline. Progresses to neck, trunk and extremities	Prodrome of coryza, conjunctivitis, cough and fever. Fever rises when rash appears. Koplik's spot
Rubella	Rubella virus	17 days	Cephalocaudal spread. Light pink macules and papules spreading from face downwards. Forchheimer spots	Prodrome of fever, headache, malaise, sore throat; suboccipital lymphadenopathy
Varicella	Varicella zoster virus	16 days	Polymorphous rash with successive crops of lesions. Characteristic: Clear vesicle on an erythematous base "dew drops on rose petal appearance". Rash begins on trunk and spreads to neck, face and limbs	Prodrome of malaise and fever. Complications such as varicella pneumonia and secondary infection may occur
Erythema infectiosum (Fifth disease)	Parvovirus B19	7 days	Characteristic "slapped cheek appearance", followed by a lacy, reticular, generalized rash involving trunk and extremities	Prodrome of fever, malaise, pharyngitis, nausea, diarrhea

TABLE 5: Clinical features of common viral hemorrhagic fevers seen in pediatric population.

Name	Causative agent	Incubations period	Clinical features	Cutaneous manifestations
Dengue Fever	Dengue virus (DEN–1, 2, 3, 4)	4–10 days after bite of infected mosquito	Biphasic fever, myalgia, arthralgia, headache, retrobulbar pain, rash	• Cutaneous lesions occur in 50–82% patients • Maculopapular eruption with islands of sparing (white islands in a sea of red); possible petechiae and purpura • The rash starts peripherally and spreads to trunk
Chikungunya fever	Chikungunya virus (family Togaviridae)	1–12 days	Biphasic/saddleback fever, polyarticular and migratory arthralgias	• Generalized pigmentation, flagellate or streaky pigmentation, mucosal and nail pigmentation • Generalized maculopapular eruption may occur • Rarely vesiculobullous lesions

CONCLUSION

It is necessary to be constantly vigilant, and investigate further whenever indicated, when assessing cases of fever with rash in children. Although the most common causes remain self-limiting infections, every case needs to be carefully assessed to rule out other plausible causes; keeping in mind the wide spectrum of diseases which can present with this clinical picture.

KEY POINTS

- History taking and clinical assessment are keys to making the diagnosis
- Causes can be broadly classified as infectious and noninfectious
- Investigate when underlying systemic diseases suspected
- Management remains supportive.

SUGGESTED READING

1. Drago F, Ciccarese G, Gasparini G, et al. Contemporary infectious exanthems: An update. Future Microbiol. 2017;12:171-93.
2. Kang JH. Febrile illness with skin rashes. Infect Chemother. 2015;47(3):155-66.
3. Manoharan KS, Ramasamy K, Heinz P. Rash with fever in children: A clinical approach. Paediatrics and Child Health. 2017;27(4):196-201.
4. Sanders CV, Lopez FA. Cutaneous manifestations of infectious diseases: Approach to the patient with fever and rash. Trans Am Clin Climatol Assoc. 2001;112:235-51.
5. Sarkar R, Mishra K, Garg VK. Fever with rash in a child in India. Indian J Dermatol Venereol Leprol. 2012;78:251-62.

CHAPTER 6

Nerve Thickening with or without Hypoesthetic Patch

Mala Bhalla, Kavita Poonia

■ INTRODUCTION

Nerve thickening may involve a single nerve or multiple nerves; it may occur in isolation or in association with skin lesions and may lead to sensory and/or motor impairment. Peripheral nerve thickening may be due to various underlying causes like diabetes, amyloidosis, etc., but the most common cause in dermatology for nerve thickening is leprosy as *Mycobacterium leprae* infects and damages the Schwann cells in the peripheral nervous system, leading first to sensory and then to motor deficits. Involvement of peripheral nerves as demonstrated by thickening or loss of sensation over the area supplied is one of the three cardinal features of leprosy in addition to a hypopigmented or erythematous cutaneous lesion with loss of sensation and skin smear positivity for acid fast bacilli (AFB). Leprosy patients are usually susceptible to the development of neuropathy during the course of the disease, which may lead to nerve thickening, asymmetry and dysfunction. Regularly palpating peripheral nerves helps a clinician in detecting nerve thickening and is an essential part of the cutaneous examination of a patient suspected to have leprosy. Rarely in the pure neuritic form of leprosy, only the peripheral nerves are involved without any cutaneous lesions. Pure neural leprosy (PNL) affects only 3–10% of patients and its clinical diagnosis is challenging as the characteristic skin lesions are absent and the identification of the leprosy bacillus is not easily achieved even when a nerve biopsy is performed. Hence, other causes of peripheral nerve thickening need to be excluded in such cases.

Leprosy is the most common treatable cause of peripheral neuropathy. Early detection and management of leprosy neuropathy is important for preventing deformities and disabilities which may otherwise lead to severe disability and long term morbidity.

CASE 1

A 10-year-old male resident of Uttar Pradesh, presented with complaints of paresthesia of left forearm since 15 months. He initially had decreased sensation on medial aspect of the left hand and slowly developed progressive weakness of the hand over the last

6 months. He was unable to lift heavy objects and there was partial flexion of the left little finger. There was no history of trauma, fever or any severe illness preceding the complaints. There was no history of epistaxis and slippage of footwear. Immunization and developmental history was unremarkable. There was no history of any neurological disease in family members. There were no cutaneous lesions. Sensory examination revealed decreased sensation to touch, temperature, and pain in the distribution of left ulnar nerve. On palpation, left ulnar nerve was moderately enlarged (grade 2) up to 4 cm above the elbow joint without any nodularity and tenderness. The left radial cutaneous nerve was also moderately enlarged. Rest of the peripheral nerves, i.e. supraorbital, supratrochlear, greater auricular, clavicular, median, lateral popliteal and dorsal tibial were normal. Cranial nerve examination was normal. There was no muscle weakness identified by voluntary muscle testing (VMT) using the 0–5 modified Medical Research Council scale except inability to adduct the little finger. Deep tendon reflexes were present. There was no evidence of lagophthalmos. Examination of eyelashes, eyebrows were normal and corneal reflexes were present.

Investigations: The hemogram, blood sugar, serum electrolytes, hepatic and renal function tests were within normal limits. Slit skin smear examination revealed no lepra bacilli. Nerve biopsy which is gold standard for definitive diagnosis was taken from the left radial cutaneous nerve. It showed thickening and infiltration of the perineurium and extension of the granuloma to the endoneurium along with a partial loss of fibers but no bacilli were seen.

Treatment: A diagnosis of PNL was made and the patient was started on paucibacillary multidrug therapy (PB-MDT) child dose along with oral prednisolone in a dose of 30 mg/day.

Outcome: The PB-MDT was continued for 6 months. Oral prednisolone was slowly tapered every 2 weeks as per the World Health Organization (WHO) guidelines. The progressive weakening of the left hand stopped and there was improvement in the flexion deformity of the little finger and anesthesia though some amount of anesthesia persisted.

Case Review in a Nutshell

The patient, a young boy, presented with unilateral limb involvement with nerve thickening, sensory and motor impairment in the absence of cutaneous features. In view of the young age of presentation, hereditary causes of nerve involvement should be excluded. Hereditary neuropathy usually affects nerves in a bilateral, symmetrical pattern and is unlikely to cause an asymmetrical localized presentation. Moreover, long standing hereditary motor sensory polyneuropathy patients usually have significant muscle atrophy which was absent in the present patient. The insidious onset and slow progression of the weakness excluded traumatic and postural causes of neuropathy which usually have a sudden onset.

Neural leprosy is difficult to diagnose as skin lesions are absent and it needs histological confirmation. Though neural involvement can occur in any spectrum of the disease, but the earliest and most common form is sensory mononeuropathy followed by multiple mononeuropathy and polyneuropathy. Hence, causes of polyneuropathy like diabetic and amyloid neuropathy also need to be excluded depending on the clinical presentation. For diabetic and amyloid neuropathy associated features can be a clue. However, deep tendon reflexes are usually well preserved in leprosy in contrast with these two conditions. Chronic inflammatory demyelinating polyneuropathy usually presents with symmetrical presentation and absent reflexes.

In view of the insidious onset of sensory neuropathy which later progressed to motor impairment in a resident of an area endemic for leprosy and the histopathological features consistent with tuberculoid leprosy despite the inability to demonstrate AFB, a diagnosis of PNL was made. The PB-MDT was started along with systemic steroids to halt the progression of the disease. It was the correct decision to start systemic steroids along with multidrug therapy (MDT) to decrease the chances of developing ulnar claw hand which would have led to long term disability and deformity.

■ INTERACTIVE TOPIC REVIEW

Q.1 What are the causes of peripheral nerve thickening?

Ans: Detecting enlargement of accessible nerves is very helpful in assessing these patients, as only a few types of neuropathy lead to nerve thickening. Most distal nerves can be palpated clinically, but proximal segments are less easily accessible. It is imperative to know all the common differentials of nerve thickening to reach a correct diagnosis (Table 1).

TABLE 1: Important conditions causing thickened nerves.	
Hereditary	• Hereditary motor and sensory neuropathy types 1 and 3 • Charcot–Marie–Tooth neuropathy • Refsum's disease
Acquired immune mediated	• Chronic inflammatory demyelinating polyradiculoneuropathy (CIDP) • Chronic inflammatory sensory polyradiculopathy (CISP) • Multifocal acquired demyelinating sensorimotor neuropathy (MADSAM)
Tumours of nerves or sheath	• Perineuroma (localized hypertrophic neuropathy) • Neurofibroma • Schwannoma • Malignant peripheral nerve sheath tumor • Neurofibromatosis 1 and 2 • Intraneural synovial tumor
Amyloidosis	–
Infection	Leprosy
Nerve infiltration	Neurolymphomatosis

Q.2. What should be the clinical approach to a patient suspected to have neuropathic disorders?

Ans: When a person presents with features of sensory loss like trophic ulcers, spontaneous blistering, etc. or motor impairment, a detailed history and complete physical examination is imperative to reach the correct diagnosis.

The following causes of neuropathy should be kept in mind while taking the history:
- Systemic diseases that are associated with neuropathy like diabetes, hypothyroidism, etc.
- Medicines that are known to cause neuropathy like thalidomide, vincristine, cisplatin, paclitaxel, colchicines, etc. and also indigenous medication
- Nutritional disorder: Alcohol, thiamine deficiency, vitamin B12 deficiency, folate deficiency, etc.
- Heavy metal exposure such as arsenic, mercury, organophosphorus poisoning, carbon monoxide which may be occupational or through complementary and alternative systems of medicine
- Human immunodeficiency virus risk factors
- History of tick bite (Lyme disease) or history of travel
- In case of a person suspected to have leprosy: History of anesthesia/hypoesthesia, epistaxis, pedal edema, episodes of reaction, any deformity or disability and family history.

A complete physical examination should include:
- All peripheral and cranial nerves examination
- Testing of muscle power enervated by cranial nerves such as V, VII, IX/X, XI and XII
- Peripheral sensations, i.e. temperature, touch, pain, vibration should be checked in the cutaneous lesions as well as in the glove and stocking distribution
- Motor examination: Testing for bulk, power, tone, pattern of weakness, symmetric or asymmetric, distal or proximal
- Palpation of all peripheral nerves for nerve thickening
- Deep tendon reflexes should always be elicited
- Radiographic examination for trophic changes such as loss of bone density, thinning of phalanges, phalanges resorption, pathological fractures, arthropathy etc.
- Complete spine examination for spina bifida.

Q.3 What are the nerves to be examined in leprosy and how to do examination of nerves?

Ans: A peripheral nerve is palpated with the pulp of index, middle and ring fingers and not by the tip of digits. The nerve should be rolled to and fro over the surface of the underlying bone in a direction perpendicular to the long axis of the nerve. It is necessary to compare nerves bilaterally for nerve enlargement and to detect any abnormality. The clinician should note the consistency, thickness, regularity and tenderness of nerves (Table 2).

TABLE 2: Grading of nerve thickness.

Grade	Degree	Description
0	Not thickened	Nerve normal and not thickened
1	Mild thickening	Thickened compared to contralateral side
2	Moderate	Thickened, rope like
3	Severe	Thickened, feels nodular or beaded

Peripheral nerves to be examined in leprosy:
- Supraorbital
- Supratrochlear
- Infraorbital
- Greater auricular
- Supraclavicular
- Ulnar
- Median
- Superficial radial cutaneous nerve
- Common peroneal nerve
- Anterior and posterior tibial
- Sural nerve
- All cranial nerves should be examined, but most important are:
    - Trigeminal nerve (for corneal reflex)
    - Facial nerve (for facial palsy).

Q.4 Which are the commonest nerve trunks to be affected in leprosy?

Ans: The commonest peripheral nerve trunks to be affected is the ulnar nerve followed by the lateral popliteal and radial cutaneous nerve. Temperature and pain sensation are the first to be affected. Neural involvement includes damage to nerve trunks and cutaneous nerve endings resulting in sensory and/or motor impairment. The earliest and most common disease forms are sensory with mainly mononeuropathy (60%) followed by multiple mononeuropathy and polyneuropathy.

Q.5 How to assess nerve damage clinically in leprosy?

Ans: Clinical method of assessing nerve damage includes:
- Palpation of nerve
- Testing motor integrity
- Testing sensory integrity
- Testing autonomic integrity.

Palpation of Nerve
- Done at predetermined sites of the body along the course of the nerves commonly involved
- Look for enlargement, bilateral or unilateral, extent, pain, nodularity, and compressibility.

Testing Motor Integrity
- Voluntary muscle testing

Graded as:
- Grade 5: Normal power
- Grade 4: Full range but less than normal
- Grade 3: Full range against gravity but not against resistance
- Grade 2: Range of movement is incomplete and effective neither against gravity nor against resistance
- Grade 1: Perceptible contraction not resulting in joint movement
- Grade 0: No movement.

- Individual nerve involvement
  - Ulnar nerve: Card test, Froment's sign, Egawa's test
  - Median nerve: Pen test, Oschner's clasp showing Benediction sign.

Testing Sensory Integrity
- Pain
  - Pin prick
  - 23 gauge disposable needle.
- Touch
  - Ball point pen (in field conditions)
  - Wisp of cotton
  - Feather
  - Nylon monofilament testing [graded Semmes-Weinstein (SW) mono filaments]: Most effective.
- Temperature
  - For hot and cold sensation.

Testing Autonomic Integrity
- Histamine test
- Sweat test
- Starch iodine test.

Q.6 What are the other methods to examine the nerve damage?

Ans:
- Electrophysiological testing
  - Nerve conduction study (NCS): It is a bedside procedure for the assessment of various peripheral neuropathies and considered as an important tool for the early detection of nerve function impairment (NFI). Abnormalities in nerve conduction include:
    - Prolonged distal latencies and reduced sensory or motor nerve conduction velocity
    - Absent or low amplitude sensory nerve action potential (SNAP), reduced amplitude of compound muscle action potentials
    - Both axonal and demyelination patterns seen.
- Electromyography (EMG): It detects and records the electrical activity from a portion of a muscle by recording motor action potential. In case of myopathy, it demonstrates a motor unit potential that is lower in amplitude and shorter duration than normal
- Imaging of the nerve: Imaging of peripheral nerves help to observe and record structural changes in nerves

- Ultrasonography (USG): Normal peripheral nerves have been described as echogenic tubular structure with multiple hypoechoic, but discontinuous linear areas separated by hyperechoic bands in the longitudinal plane and multiple rounded hypoechoic areas in a homogenous background in the transverse plane (honeycomb pattern). Nerve sonography can demonstrate five main pathologic changes: (i) Nerve enlargement; (ii) increased hypoechogenicity or hyperechogenicity; (iii) enlarged fascicles; (iv) increased thickness of the epineurium; and (v) increased endoneural or epineural blood flow (Color Doppler)
- Magnetic resonance imaging (MRI): It can detect nerve abnormalities and also depict soft tissues with excellent resolution, but it is expensive compared to USG and it is difficult to follow the superficial course of peripheral nerves to identify any pathology.

- Nerve biopsy: Two important characters, i.e. cellular infiltrates and bacillary load helps in histological classification of nerve biopsy specimen to either tuberculoid or lepromatous pole. Most common clinical pattern of nerve damage seen in leprosy is mononeuropathy or "mononeuritis multiplex" that histologically shows tuberculoid pattern and less commonly polyneuritic form which shows lepromatous pattern histologically. Neural leprosy is difficult to diagnose in absence of skin lesions and needs histological confirmation
  - Tuberculoid pole: There is thickening and infiltration of the perineurium with extension of the granuloma to the endoneurium. There may be partial or total loss of nerve fibers. Usually no bacilli are seen. In long standing cases, there is complete hyalinization, granuloma subsides, and the nerve structure is altered by fibrosis
  - Lepromatous pole: There is moderate to intense inflammatory infiltrate consisting of macrophages, plasma cells, and lymphocytes mainly in the endoneural space, with absence of true granuloma. Vacuolated "foamy cells" may be present. Mild fibrosis of endoneurium, perineurium and epineurium, axonal degeneration and asymmetrical partial or total loss of fibers are also present. The fascicular structures of the nerve remain noticeable. Large numbers of bacilli are seen in Schwann cells, endothelial cells, and macrophages. These may form the globi.

Q.7 What are the various ways in which nerve involvement in leprosy may present?

Ans: Nerve involvement in leprosy may present at different time durations during the course of disease and with a variable clinical picture.
- Acute neuritis: There is an acute onset of pain, tenderness and/or swelling due to nerve abscess and/or recent onset neurological deficit less than 6 months in duration, mostly seen in type 1 or 2 reaction
- Chronic neuritis: There is long standing (>6 months) gradually progressive neurological deficit with nerve tenderness or pain

- Recurrent neuritis: There are recurring episodes of pain after a symptom free period of at least 3 months
- Silent neuritis/quiet nerve paralysis: Progressive sensory or motor impairment in the absence of symptoms such as pain, paraesthesia or tenderness of the nerve develops with no obvious sign of reaction
- Catastrophic paralysis: The patient develops sudden paralysis
- Complete destruction: There is complete destruction of nerve with no residual nerve function
- Chronic neuropathic pain: It is a late complication which presents with pain in absence of reaction and NFI, after completion of MDT. The pain is predominantly continuous burning type with glove and stocking distribution.

Q.8 What is segmental necrotizing granulomatous neuritis?

Ans: Segmental necrotizing granulomatous neuritis (SNGN) is an uncommon presentation affecting the peripheral nerves of leprosy patients. It can be the initial presentation of pure neuritic leprosy or may develop in association with a cutaneous lesion. It is usually associated with tuberculoid and borderline tuberculoid leprosy with higher immunological spectrum. It can present as a single or multiple nodules along the course of a thickened peripheral nerve and has been reported most commonly in the ulnar nerve. It may be confused with nerve abscess because of similar clinical presentation, but has a different histopathological presentation. Histopathologically, it is characterized by central area of caseous necrosis surrounded by multiple epitheloid granulomas, which is different from true nerve abscess that shows dense mixed inflammatory infiltrates of neutrophils, few eosinophils, lymphocytes, macrophages, few well defined granulomas and areas of necrosis. Management requires surgical drainage along with multidrug therapy.

Q.9 Other than slit skin smear and histopathology what are the other diagnostic tests for leprosy?

Ans: Diagnosis of leprosy is based on classical cardinal signs and characteristic histopathology of skin or nerve lesions. However, this standard method for assessing leprosy has limited value in diagnosing new suspicious cases, indeterminate leprosy and for monitoring treatment. So, specific serodiagnostic and molecular methods may help in early diagnosis and provide valuable information.
- Serodiagnostic test: Using specific *M. leprae* antigens and their epitope specific antibodies
    - *M. leprae* specific lipid antigen: Phenolic glycolipid-1 (PGL-1) present on *M. leprae* cell wall. About 90–90% of BL/LL and 25–60% of TT/BT patient found to be positive for PGL-1 antigen
    - The 35 kDa antigen serology: Monoclonal antibody, MLO4 which specifically reacts with 35 kDa epitope of *M. leprae*. Using radio-immunoassay, almost 100% of active BL/LL and 40% of TT/BT patient were found to be positive. These antibody levels gradually fall with treatment

- *M. leprae* recombinant proteins such as early secretory antigenic target 6 and culture filtrate protein 10: Using enzyme-linked immunosorbent assay, antibody to this specific antigen is helpful in evaluation of leprosy patient.
- Molecular methods: For early diagnosis, monitoring of treatment and detection of drug resistance.
  - Probes targeting deoxyribonucleic acid: Probes for detection of specific sequences of *M. leprae*
  - Gene amplification (polymerase chain reaction) techniques.

CASE 2

A 9-year-old, male presented with an asymptomatic, single, erythematous, well-defined, raised plaque 4 × 4 cm with dry looking surface over the right side of cheek since 5 years (Fig. 1). The parents had noticed that the lesion had slowly increased in size though the child had no complaints. There was no history of epistaxis, slippage of footwear, no history of spontaneous blister formation, difficulty in chewing. On cutaneous examination, no similar lesion was present over rest of the body. No definite loss of sensation could be demonstrated over the lesion but a nerve to the patch was palpable. Peripheral nerve examination revealed no thickening. Examination of cranial nerves was normal. There were no gloves and stocking anesthesia. There was no history of difficulty in chewing or deviation of angle of mouth and no evidence of lagophthalmos. Examinations of eyelashes, eyebrows were normal and corneal reflexes were present.

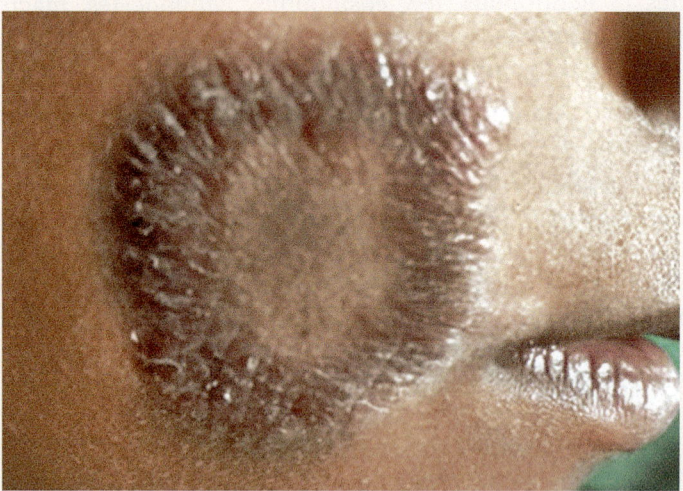

Fig. 1: Erythematous, well defined, plaque with raised border with dry looking surface over the right side of cheek.

Investigations: The hemogram, blood sugar, serum electrolytes, hepatic and renal function tests were within normal limits. In slit skin smear, no lepra bacilli were seen.

Skin biopsy from the lesion showed numerous noncaseating epitheloid cell granulomas with few langerhans giant cells. The granulomas were just abutting the epidermis but not destroying it.

Treatment: The patient was diagnosed as borderline tuberculoid leprosy, using the Ridley-Jopling classification or paucibacillary leprosy as per the WHO classification. He was started on PB-MDT (child pack) for 6 months.

Outcome: The PB-MDT was continued for 6 months. At the end of therapy, the lesion became slightly hypopigmented with a partial regression in size.

Case Review in a Nutshell

The patient presented with an asymptomatic, single, well defined erythematous plaque over right cheek with a palpable feeding nerve. Due to the rich and overlapping nerve supply over the face, sensory loss is usually difficult to demonstrate over the facial lesions and the slit skin smear may show no AFB in the paucibacillary spectrum of the disease. So, a definitive diagnosis of leprosy requires histological confirmation though the enlargement of intradermal nerve near the lesion known as "feeding nerve to the lesion" is typically seen in leprosy.

This patient was at risk of developing facial nerve involvement because of the site of the skin lesion which may get inflamed during the type 1 reaction. The possibility for nerve damage and deformities increase when there are coexisting skin lesions with type 1 reaction. The incidence of type 1 reaction in borderline tuberculoid leprosy varies from 8–36% and usually occurs during first 6 months of therapy. Early recognition of nerve damage and treatment with steroids may result in full restoration of nerve function. Follow-up of the patient should be done for next three years as per WHO guidelines to look for reversal reaction (RR) and relapse.

■ INTERACTIVE TOPIC REVIEW

Q.1 In what way are facial lesions of leprosy different from the classical lesion of leprosy?

Ans:
- Lesions on the face usually do not show the expected degree of hypoesthesia due to the rich and overlapping nerve supply over the face and sensory loss is usually difficult to demonstrate over these lesions
  - Lesions on the face tend to be more erythematous compared to other body lesions due to extensive blood supply and photosensitivity
  - Leprosy lesion over face may present with diverse clinical manifestation and may be more infiltrated which may mimic other infectious and non-infectious diseases such as lupus vulgaris, leishmaniasis, sarcoidosis. So facial lesions of leprosy require cautious physical examination and histopathological confirmation to rule out other causes.

Q.2 What are the causes of facial nerve palsy?

Ans: The causes of facial nerve palsy is summarized in Table 3.

TABLE 3: Causes of facial palsy.

Idiopathic	Bell's palsy
Infection	• Ramsay Hunt syndrome • Leprosy • Lyme disease
Trauma	Temporal bone fracture
Tumors	• Cerebellopontine angle tumors: Acoustic neuromas, meningioma • Parotid cancer: Pleomorphic adenoma, squamous cell carcinoma, adenoid cystic carcinoma, adenocarcinoma, mucoepidermoid carcinoma • Head and neck tumors
Metabolic	• Diabetes mellitus • Hyperthyroidism
Toxic	• Thalidomide • Arsenic intoxication • Ethylene glycol • Tetanus • Alcoholism • Diphtheria
Neurologic	• Guillain-Barré syndrome
Congenital	• Möbius syndrome • Hemifacial microsomia • Myotonic dystrophica

Q.3 What are the risk factors for nerve function impairment?

Ans: The various risk factors for developing NFI in leprosy are:
- Extensive clinical or multibacillary disease
- Borderline leprosy
- Pregnancy and puerperium
- Stress
- Facial patch
- Thickened nerves
- Bacterial index (BI) positivity
- Anti-PGL-1 positivity
- Lepromin test positive
- Male sex
- Bacillus Calmette-Guérin vaccination status positive.

Q.4 What are the consequences and complications due to neurological deficit?

Ans: The consequences of neurological deficit are:
- Impairment: It is defined as loss or abnormality in physiological, psychological, and anatomical structure and function because of some disorder, e.g. sensory loss, trophic ulcers

- Deformity: Visible alteration in the form, shape or appearance of body due to impairment produced by the disease
- Disability: It is defined as lack of ability to perform activity that is considered normal for a person of the same age, gender and culture resulting from deformity
- Handicap: The social disadvantages experienced by disabled persons.

The various complications of neurological deficit are:
- Due to sensory loss:
  - Trophic ulcer
  - Mutilation of fingers and toes
  - Charcot' joints (also due to loss of proprioception)
  - Corneal ulcers (due to involvement of trigeminal nerve).
- Due to motor loss:
  - Facial palsy
  - Exposure keratitis
  - Wrist and foot drop, claw hand and foot, etc.
  - Wasting of muscles and contracture.
- Due to autonomic loss:
  - Anhidrosis
  - Ichthyosis and xerosis
  - Loss of appendages.

Q.5 What are the differential diagnoses of trophic ulcer?

Ans: Any disorder that causes sensory loss can result in trophic ulcers. Following causes should be ruled out:
- Diabetes: Same site as leprosy, no thickened nerve
- Tabes dorsalis
- Syringomyelia, spina bifida, hereditary sensory neuropathy can all lead to trophic ulcer.

Q.6 How to manage a patient who presents with nerve function impairment?

Ans:
- Nerve examination and functional assessment should be done at first visit and then at every visit to monitor the onset and progress of nerve damage
- Aim is to prevent or limit irreversible nerve damage through early detection and treatment
- If NFI is less than 6 months then recovery is possible
- Principles of management
  - Continue or start MDT
  - Early treatment of reactions
  - Effective and prolonged anti-inflammatory therapy
  - Analgesia
  - Physical therapy and rest
  - Surgery when indicated
  - Physiotherapy during recovery phase.

CASE 3

A 35-year-old male resident of Bihar, farmer by occupation presented with multiple, well-defined, hypopigmented plaques with sloping edges, dry looking surface, localized predominantly on the face, upper limbs, lower limbs, buttocks and back for 18 months. The lesions ranged from 3 to 7 cm in diameter, with largest lesion on the back. Few lesions over back and thigh were annular with sharp inner border and sloping outer border. There was no loss of eyebrows, ear lobe infiltration or saddling of nose. On sensory examination, there was mild-to-moderate sensory loss to temperature, touch and pain over hands and feet that extended up to the elbows and knees with complete sensory loss over hypopigmented plaques. Palpation along the course of nerves found thickened bilateral ulnar nerves, superficial radial cutaneous nerves, lateral popliteal and posterior tibial nerves with uniform consistency without nerve tenderness and nodularity. Right side nerves were more thickened than left side. The other peripheral nerves and cranial nerves were normal. There was no muscle weakness identified by VMT using the 0–5 modified Medical Research Council scale. Nasal mucosa was normal. No history of redness or grittiness of eyes, epistaxis, hoarseness of voice, slippage of footwear, difficulty in chewing or deviation of angle of mouth. Eyelid closure was tested and there was no evidence of lagophthalmos, eyelashes were normal, corneal reflexes normal.

Investigation: A skin smear demonstrated a BI of 3 with a morphological index (MI) of 33%. Skin biopsy demonstrated a diffuse lymphocytic infiltrate with few epitheloid cell granulomas with multiple foamy macrophages. Stain for AFB showed few bacilli.

Treatment: Based on the morphology of the lesions, slit skin smear finding and skin biopsy report, diagnosis of mid-borderline or borderline-borderline (BB) leprosy without any reaction with no deformity was made, using the Ridley–Jopling classification or multibacillary leprosy as per the WHO classification. He was started on multibacillary multidrug therapy (MB-MDT) for 12 months.

Outcome: After 3 months of therapy, he noticed that previously hypopigmented plaques became red and swollen. He also complained of weakness in both hands and feet. Cutaneous examination revealed no new lesions but the previous lesions had become inflamed, swollen and tender. There was increased sensory loss in the distribution of ulnar and popliteal nerve. Peripheral nerve examination showed tenderness of the thickened ulnar, popliteal and posterior tibial nerves. A diagnosis of mid-borderline leprosy with type 1 reaction was made. Along with continuation of MB-MDT, he was started on oral corticosteroids dose of 0.5–1 mg/kg which was continued till the erythema, pain in skin lesions and nerve tenderness subsided and then the dose was tapered off according to the WHO regimen. He completed 12 months of MB-MDT and tapering course of corticosteroids.

Case Review in a Nutshell

A 35-year-old farmer presented with multiple, hypopigmented, hypoesthetic plaques with peripheral nerve thickening and AFB demonstrable on slit skin smear examination, which is a classical presentation of leprosy. According to Ridley–Jopling classification i.e. on the basis of clinical, bacteriological, histological, and immunological features, he was classified as mid borderline type of leprosy. After 3 months of MB-MDT therapy patient developed type 1 reaction/RR, as existing skin lesions became inflamed and swollen. Leprosy reactions are immunologically mediated episodes divided into two forms, type 1 and type 2. Type 1, RR, is a type IV hypersensitivity reaction, whereas type 2 reaction known as erythema nodosum leprosum (ENL) is a type 3 hypersensitivity reaction. Reactions can occur at any time, either during the natural course of the disease, during treatment or even after the completion of treatment with MDT. Most of the deformities and disabilities in leprosy results from these leprosy reactions. Timely initiation of treatment for reaction can reduce morbidity as well as prevent deformities. However, leprosy reaction does not indicate the failure of treatment rather it indicates killing of bacteria and clearance of antigen. Treatment should include MDT that has to be started or continued, if already started and specific treatment for reaction that includes nonsteroidal anti-inflammatory drugs in case of mild reaction and immunosuppressants, i.e. corticosteroid in case of severe reaction.

▍INTERACTIVE TOPIC REVIEW

Q.1 What are the cardinal signs of leprosy?

Ans: Presence of any one out of three cardinal signs is essential to diagnose leprosy. The three cardinal signs of leprosy are:
1. Hypopigmented or erythematous skin lesions with definite sensory deficit
2. A thickened or enlarged peripheral nerve with loss of sensation and/or weakness of the muscles supplied by that nerve
3. The presence of AFB in slit skin smears or histopathology.

Q.2 What all is required to be done in the clinical assessment of persons affected by leprosy?

Ans: After confirming the diagnosis of leprosy by the presence of one or more of the cardinal signs, the persons affected by leprosy must be clinically assessed in detail (as outlined below), to determine extent of involvement and management decisions:
- Elicit detailed history
- Carry out general physical examination
- Examine complete skin for presence of skin lesions
- Note the number of skin patches
- Test for loss of sensation in the skin patch(es)
- Palpate nerves for thickening/tenderness/consistency, and number affected
- Test sensation in the palm and soles
- Look for normal blinking and redness of the eyes and visual acuity
- Observe for presence of any deformity/disability due to leprosy
- Perform VMT

- Grade the disability and record the eyes, hands and feet (EHF) score
- Record the findings
- Decide the needs of the person
- Register the person for treatment and counsel the persons affected by leprosy.

Q.3 What is the WHO grading of disability for leprosy?

Ans: The WHO grading of disability for leprosy is summarized in Table 4.

TABLE 4: World Health Organization disability grading.		
Grade	Hands and feet	Eyes
Grade 0	No disability found	No disability found
Grade 1	No visible deformity and damage Anesthesia present	No grade 1 for eye
Grade 2	Visible damage [disability, wound, ulcer, deformity due to muscle weakness (foot drop, claw hand, resorption of fingers and toes)]	Inability to close eyes, redness, lagophthalmos, iridocyclitis, corneal opacities and blindness

CONCLUSION

Peripheral nerve thickening is associated with various causes. Most common infective etiology for nerve thickening is leprosy and it is one of the cardinal features for its diagnosis. Nerve assessment in leprosy mainly depends on clinical examination by palpating the nerve and testing the nerve function, but other noninvasive imaging tools such as nerve USG and MRI are also available these days which may give better information regarding degree of nerve enlargement and early morphological alteration. These may be of help in the early diagnosis of nerve damage, an important factor for deformities and disability, especially in pure neuritic leprosy where the cutaneous lesions are absent.

KEY POINTS

- Leprosy has a variable presentation depending on the spectrum of the disease and the presence of reaction, but the presence of the cardinal features, i.e. typical cutaneous lesions, features of nerve involvement and demonstration of bacilli help in making the diagnosis
- Pure neuritic leprosy is a rare clinical entity in which leprosy involves the peripheral nerves in the absence of cutaneous features. It is peculiar to India and is seen in 3–10% of patients affected with leprosy
- The clinical diagnosis of PNL remains a challenge, because the cardinal features of leprosy may be absent and it requires histological confirmation
- Leprosy is an important treatable cause of peripheral neuropathy which presents with nerve thickening. The most common clinical pattern seen is mononeuritis multiplex and less commonly diffuse peripheral nerve involvement.

SUGGESTED READING

1. Jain S, Visser LH, Suneetha S. Imaging techniques in leprosy clinics. Clinics in Dermatology. 2016;34:70-8
2. Kar HK, Kumar B. IAL Textbook of Leprosy. New Delhi: JPB; 2010.
3. Khadilkar SV, Yadav RS, Soni G. A practical approach to enlargement of nerves, plexuses and roots. Pract Neurol. 2015;2:105-15.
4. Marcos RG, Freitas D, Said G. Leprous neuropathy. In: Said G, Krarup C (Eds). Handbook of Clinical Neurology. 2013; p. 115.
5. Wilder Smith EP, Van Brakel WH. Nerve damage in leprosy and its management. Nature Clinical Practice Neurology. 2008;4:656-63.

CHAPTER 7

Papulonodular Lesions of Face

Anupam Das, Anand Toshniwal

∎ INTRODUCTION

Papulonodular lesions of the face always pose an enigma to a dermatologists as various infectious, benign and malignant etiologies can manifest in this form. The final diagnosis is achieved by an accurate cutaneous and systemic examination and noting the age, mode of onset and morphology of the predominant lesions as well as by, dermoscopy. The final confirmative clincher is the histopathological examination.

CASE 1

A 23-year-old female presented with multiple asymptomatic skin colored papulonodules on face since 5 years of age (Fig. 1). Patient was otherwise healthy without any systemic complaints. Family history was insignificant. On cutaneous examination multiple dome shaped yellowish waxy appearing nodules predominantly affecting the T-area (pericentral) area of face were seen. Radiological examination was normal. Biopsy was done and the histopathological examination revealed keratinized stratified squamous epithelium overlying proliferating packets of basaloid cells with hyperchromatic nuclei, along with several keratin horn cysts and moderate stroma infiltrate of chronic inflammatory cells. Based on clinical and histopathological examination a diagnosis of trichoepithelioma was made.

Case Review in Nutshell

Papulonodular lesions on face pose a diagnostic dilemma as it could be an underlying long standing infectious disease or a genodermatosis. Based on the age of onset and clinical examination the following differentials were considered:
- Trichoepithelioma
- Trichilemmoma
- Steatocystoma.

Trichoepithelioma was considered the first differential considering the age of onset and waxy yellowish hue nodules involving pericentral areas of face with basaloid cells and keratin horn cysts supporting the same.

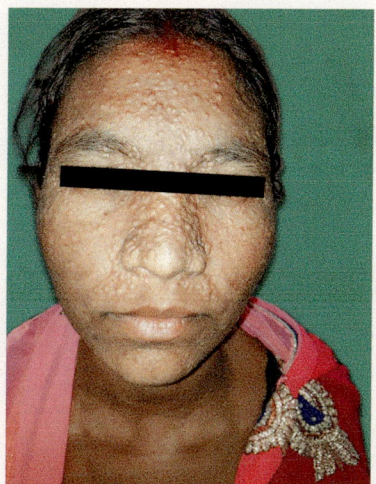

Fig. 1: Multiple trichoepitheliomas affecting the face.

Trichilemmomas are solitary or multiple skin colored papules seen on face. Multiple are seen in Cowden syndrome, wherein they are associated with oral papillomatosis and acral keratosis. On histopathological examination, plate like growth of pale pink glassy cells with palisading at the periphery is observed.

Steatocystomas are yellowish papulonodules seen mainly at puberty with trunk and face predominantly involved. On histopathological examination it shows empty cyst lined by squamous epithelium and minimal granular cell layer. Sebaceous glands are found adjacent to cyst.

Thus, on the basis of clinical and histopathological findings, a diagnosis of trichoepithelioma was made. The benign nature of the disease was explained and surgical excision was advised for cosmetic concern.

CASE 2

A 36-year-old female patient came with complaints of asymptomatic nodules around eyes for 5 years (Fig. 2). She had a similar lesion 8 years back which she got excised. Lesions were gradually progressive in nature. Family history was nil significant with no other systemic complaints. Cutaneous examination revealed soft to firm nontender yellowish brown nodules involving the infraorbital area, not fixed to underlying tissues. There was no hepatosplenomegaly and lymphadenopathy. On investigations she was found to have a normal lipid profile, raised lactate dehydrogenase and immunoglobulin G1 (IgG1) spike on electrophoresis. Radiological examination revealed no abnormalities. Biopsy was done. Histopathological examination revealed unremarkable epidermis with dermis showing unencapsulated lesion comprising sheets of nodular collections of large foamy histiocytes admixed with lymphoplasmacytic infiltrate with extensive areas of hyaline necrobiosis. Touton and foreign body giant cells were also seen. Based on the clinical and histopathological correlation, diagnosis of necrobiotic xanthogranuloma was made.

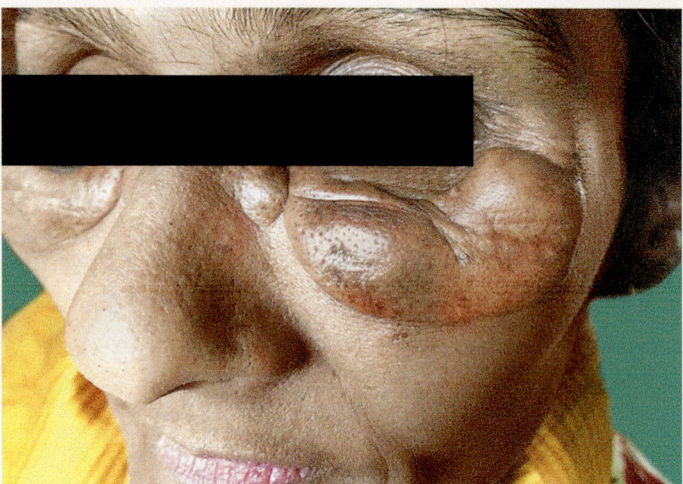

Fig. 2: Necrobiotic xanthogranuloma.

Case Review in Nutshell

Papulonodular lesions around the eye are usually misdiagnosed and treated as xanthelasma and may not receive proper investigations and follow-up. In the above case the following differentials were considered:
- Necrobiotic xanthogranuloma
- Necrobiosis lipoidica
- Diffuse xanthoma.

Necrobiotic xanthogranuloma was considered as a differential based on the clinical appearance of nodules, slow progression and IgG spike on electrophoresis which can be seen in necrobiotic xanthogranuloma associated with monoclonal gammopathy. The histopathological examination also showed necrobiosis with Touton giant cells and lymphoplasmacytic infiltrate with foamy cells.

Necrobiosis lipoidica in its atypical presentation involves the periorbital area. On histopathological examination it shows predominant involvement of septa and cholesterol clefts. Atypical giant cells, foam cells and dense infiltrate is absent.

Diffuse xanthoma usually presents as yellowish plaques and nodules. On histopathological examination it would reveal large sheets of foamy cells present throughout dermis and absence of Touton giant cells.

On the basis of clinical and histopathological correlation a diagnosis of necrobiotic xanthogranuloma was made and a complete surgical excision was done with regular follow-up every 6 months. No recurrence has been reported yet.

▮ INTERACTIVE TOPIC REVIEW

Q.1 How to classify the causes of papulonodular lesions of face?

Ans: **Infections**

Molluscum contagiosum, tinea faciei, demodicosis, lupus vulgaris, Hansen's diseases, leishmaniasis, verruca vulgaris.

Inflammatory Disorders

Acne vulgaris, Acne rosacea, lupus miliaris disseminatus faciei, sarcoidosis, facial Afro-Caribbean childhood eruption, perioral dermatitis, follicular mucinosis, Peli incarniti.

Differentials for normal surfaced eythematous papules is described in Flowchart 1.

Tumors

- Benign epidermal tumors and cysts: Milia, dermatosis papulosa nigra, keratoacanthoma, seborrheic keratosis
- Premalignant: Actinic keratosis, cutaneous horn
- Malignant: Basal cell carcinoma, squamous cell carcinoma, lymphoma, metastasis.

Tumors of Skin Appendages

- Eccrine gland: Syringoma, eccrine hidrocystoma
- Apocrine gland: Syringocystadenoma papilliferum
- Sebaceous gland: Sebaceous hyperplasia, sebaceoma, sebaceous adenoma
- Hair follicle mesenchyme: Trichodiscoma
- Hair follicle: Dilated pore of winer, trichoadenoma
- External root sheath: Trichilemmoma
- Hamartomas: Trichofolliculoma, trichoepithelioma
- Soft tissue tumors: Fibrous papule of nose, atypical fibroxanthoma
- Others: Granuloma faciale, angiofibroma, colloid milia, keratosis pilaris, lichen planus, lichen nitidus, dermatofibroma, hemangioma, palisaded encapsulated neuroma, pilomatrixoma, xanthoma.

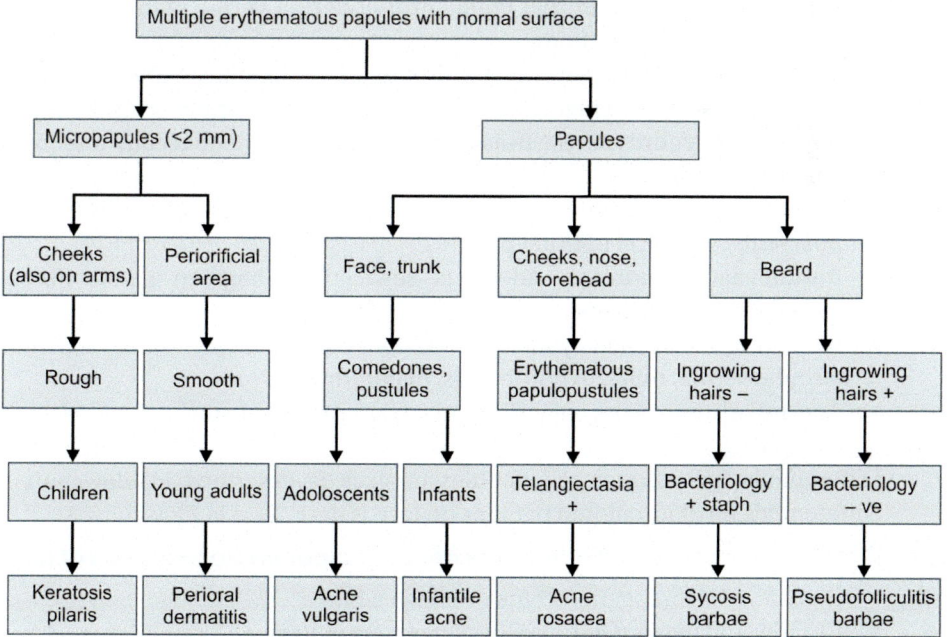

Flowchart 1: Differentials for normal surfaced erythematous papules.

Q.2 What are the differentials for colored papules on face?

Ans:
- White papules: Molluscum contagiosum, cutaneous calculus, milia, closed comedones
- Brown papules: Compound nevus, seborrheic keratosis, pigmented basal cell carcinoma, nodular melanoma, plane warts
- Black papules: Dermatosis papulosa nigra, seborrheic keratosis, melanoma, trichostasis spinulosa
- Purple: Kaposi's sarcoma
- Blue: Blue nevus, apocrine hidrocystoma
- Skin/yellowish papules: Xanthoma, necrobiotic xanthogranuloma, fibrous papule of nose, keratosis pilaris, histoid Hansen's, post-kala-azar dermal leishmaniasis, angiofibromas, syringomas, etc.

Q.3 What is the significance of the surface of papulonodular lesions on face?

Ans:
- Pigmented and hairy: Congenital melanocytic nevus
- Crusted surface: Actinic keratosis, Bowen's disease, basal cell carcinoma, leishmaniasis, lupus vulgaris
- Smooth dome shaped: Intradermal nevus, compound nevus, colloid milia, apocrine hidrocystoma
- Flat topped papules: Plane warts, syringomas, trichilemmomas.

Q.4 What are syndromes associated with papulonodular lesions of face?

Ans:
- Brooke-Spiegler syndrome: Multiple cylindromas with trichoepitheliomas
- Birt–Hogg–Dubé syndrome: Fibrofolliculomas, trichodiscomas, acrochordons
- Cowden syndrome: Trichilemommas, oral papillomas, palmar keratosis, epidermal nevi, macrocephaly
- Rombo syndrome: Multiple milia, atrophoderma vermiculatum, telangiectasias, basal cell carcinoma
- Basaloid follicular hamartoma syndrome: Multiple milia, comedone like or dermatosis papulosa nigra like follicular lesions, hypotrichosis, palmar pits
- Muir-Torre syndrome: Gastrointestinal malignancy, Sebaceous adenoma, keratoacanthoma
- Grzybowski syndrome: Keratoacanthoma like papules, ectropion, hoarseness of voice, perioral papules
- Bourneville's syndrome: Adenoma sebaceum, Shagreen patch, fibrous plaque, Koenen tumors
- Bazex–Dupré-Christol syndrome: Multiple basal cell carcinomas, follicular atrophoderma, milia, hypotrichosis, hypohidrosis
- Apert syndrome: Acne vulgaris, syndactyly, craniosynostosis, crowded teeth, cleft palate.

Differentials for skin-colored nodules on face is described in Flowchart 2. Differentials for skin-colored papules on face is described in Flowchart 3.

Q.5 What are dermoscopic findings of common papulonodular lesions of face?

Ans:
- Blue nevus: Homogenous blue or bluish white
- Intradermal nevus: Globular homogeneous pattern

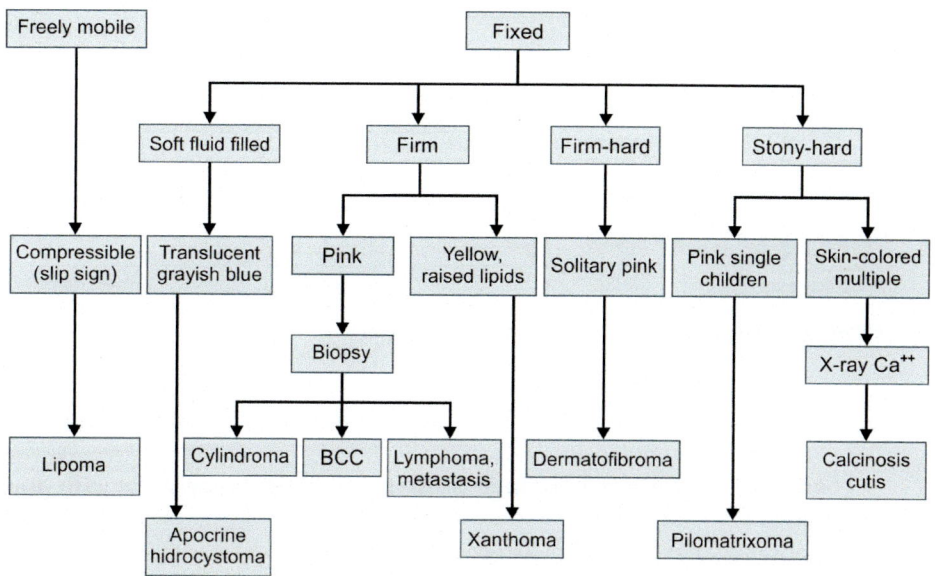

Flowchart 2: Differentials for skin-colored nodules on face.

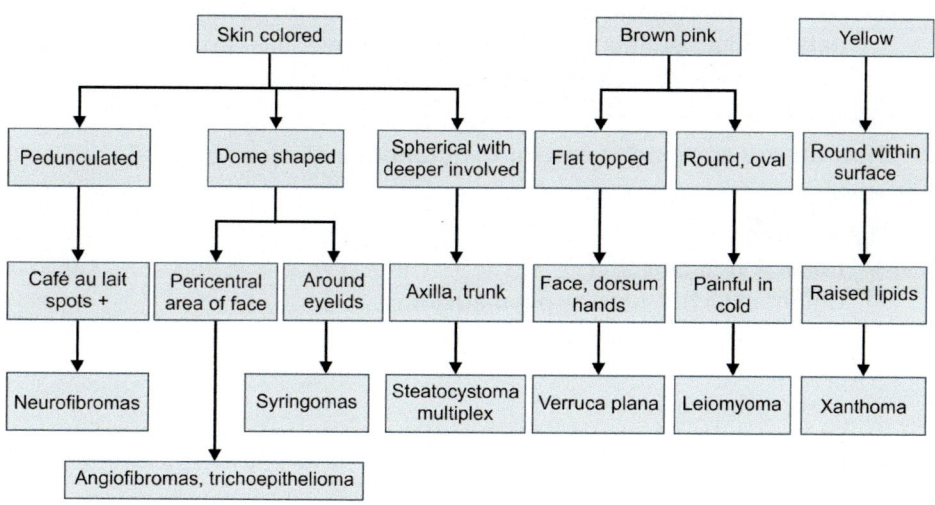

Flowchart 3: Differentials for skin-colored papules on face.

- Seborrheic keratosis: Sharply demarcated borders, milia-like cysts, comedo-like openings, ridges, fissures and hairpin vessels surrounded by a halo
- Sebaceous hyperplasia: Yellow to yellow white lobular structures; crown vessels or linear winding serpentine vessels at the periphery of the lesion that radiate toward the center

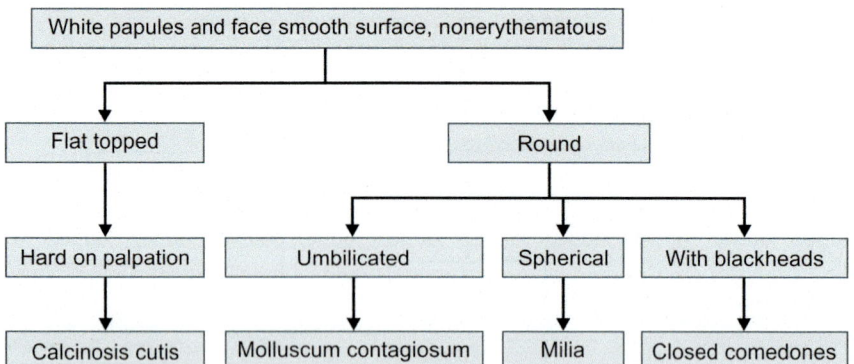

Flowchart 4: Differentials for white-colored papules on face.

- Granuloma faciale: White gray background with whitish streaks and elongated telangiectasia
- Sarcoidosis: Yellowish orange structure less globular area with linear vessels
- Lupus vulgaris: Fine yellowish gold background with telangiectasias and few milia-like cysts
- Actinic keratosis: Erythema with a pink to red pseudonetwork surrounding the hair follicles; fine, linear wavy vessels surrounding the follicular openings; and follicles with yellowish keratotic plugs
- Basal cell carcinoma: Leaf-like structures; multiple nonaggregated blue gray dots or blue globular structures, spoke wheel like structures, serpentine branched vessels, absence of pigmented network.

Differentials for white-colored papules on face as described in Flowchart 4.

Q.6 How do you approach a case of papulonodular lesions of face?

Ans: History

Age of Onset
- Infancy: Hemangioma
- Children: Lichen nitidus, pilomatrixoma
- Adults: Basal cell carcinoma.

Duration
- Acute: Tinea facei
- Chronic: Lupus vulgaris.

Evolution
- Sudden: Eruptive syringomas, acne vulgaris
- Gradual: Acne agminata, pseudolymphoma.

Mucosal Lesions
- Lichen planus, papular xanthoma, Cowden syndrome, Darier's disease.

Triggering Factors
- Sunlight: Polymorphic light eruption, acne rosacea.

Photosensitivity
- Photoallergic contact dermatitis, polymorphic light eruption.

Systemic Complaints
- Joint pains: Acne fulminans, lymphoma
- Lymphadenopathy, pulmonary symptoms: Sarcoidosis.

Cutaneous Examination
Morphology of lesions, color, size, surface, shape, symmetry, distribution of lesions, diascopy, dermoscopy. Biopsy and relevant systemic investigations.

CONCLUSION

Papulonodules on the face require a holistic approach as it could be a manifestation of a spectrum of diseases ranging from infectious etiology to malignancy. A detailed clinical examination to look out for any associated systemic involvement and the use of dermoscope would be useful to obviate the need for biopsy in certain scenarios although histopathology would be the gold standard for confirmation.

KEY POINTS

- Always look for the colour, surface, shape, size and number of lesions along with examination of lymph nodes
- Dermoscopy is an invaluable tool and recognition of vascular, keratin pattern would help to differentiate benign from malignant lesions
- Acute erythematous lesions tend to be benign or infectious etiology and the chronic lesions tend to be towards granulomatous or malignant etiology
- Systemic fungal infections should be borne in mind while dealing with sudden evolution of lesions with associated immunosuppresion.

SUGGESTED READING

1. Ardigo M, Zieff J, Scope A, et al. Dermoscopic and reflectance confocal microscope findings of trichoepithelioma. Dermatology. 2007;215:354-8.
2. Char DH, LeBoit PE, Ljung BM, et al. Radiation therapy for ocular necrobiotic xanthogranuloma. Arch Ophthalmol. 1987;105:174-5.
3. Giacomel J, Zalaudek I. Dermoscopy of superficial basal cell carcinoma. Dermatol Surg 2005;31:1710-3.
4. Harada H, Hashimoto K, Ko MS. The gene for multiple familial trichoepithelioma maps to chromosome 9p21. J Invest Dermatol. 1996;107:41-3.
5. Mehregan DA, Winkelmann RK. Necrobiotic xanthogranuloma. Arch Dermatol. 1992;128:94-100.
6. Mohammadi AA, Jafari SMS. Trichoepithelioma: A rare but crucial dermatological issue. World J Plast Surg. 2014;3:142-5.
7. Rajesh G, Thappa DM, Jaisankar TJ, et al. Spectrum of seborrheic keratoses in south Indians: A clinical and dermoscopic study. Ind Dermatol Venereol Leprol. 2011;77:483-8.
8. Wood AJ, Wagner MV, Abbott JJ, et al. Necrobiotic xanthogranuloma: A review of 17 cases with emphasis on clinical and pathologic correlation. Arch Dermatol. 2009;145:279-84.
9. Zalaudek I, Kreusch J, Giacomel J, et al. How to diagnose nonpigmented skin tumors: A review of vascular structures seen with dermoscopy Part I. Melanocytic skin tumors. J Am Acad Dermatol. 2010;63:361-74.

CHAPTER 8

Vesiculopustular and Bullous Disorders in Children

Indrashis Podder, Rashmi Sarkar

■ INTRODUCTION

Several disorders present clinically with vesicles, pustules and bullae in children. Vesicles are well circumscribed elevated lesions filled with clear fluid, sized <0.5 cm while bullae are >0.5 cm. Pustules can be of any size, containing purulent fluid. Vesicles, pustules and bullae are the primary skin lesions while erosions and ulcerations are the secondary skin lesions. Blister is a collective term for any fluid filled lesion. These disorders are a challenging domain to treat as they may have varied presentations. Accurate and prompt diagnosis is essential to prevent iatrogenic complications, unnecessary expense and parental anguish. Also the etiopathogenesis of these disorders vary widely in children and adults, therefore information pertaining to the adult population cannot be extrapolated to the pediatric age group.

The authors have attempted to discuss the different aspects of pediatric vesiculopustular and bullous disorders to help in their prompt diagnosis and management.

CASE 1

A 6-day-old neonate, born by normal vaginal delivery at term, developed several vesicles all over her body, including the genitalia and flexural areas on an erythematous background. Some of the vesicles gradually transformed into pustules after about 24–72 hours followed by crusting. Fever and lethargy developed subsequently. On enquiry, her mother revealed that she had developed some painful, fluid filled lesions on her introitus 3 days prior to delivery. She also reported the development of similar lesions occasionally in the past. There was no history of seizure and application of any other drug. The child was born out of nonconsanguinous parentage.

Dermatological examination revealed several small vesicles and pustules, ranging from 2–4 mm, on an erythematous background, distributed all over the body and scalp, especially the vertex. Vesicles and shallow ulcerations were also noted within the oral mucosa. Some of these lesions were found to be clustered together. Crusted papules and plaques were observed at the site of older lesions. There was no evidence of neurological or any other organ involvement.

Investigations: An intact vesicle was de-roofed and the fluid was sent for histopathological Tzanck smear examination, which revealed multinucleated giant cells. Swab specimens were collected from the skin vesicles, mouth, nasopharynx, conjunctiva and anus for herpes simplex virus (HSV) cell culture which demonstrated the presence of HSV-2 virus in the skin and oral samples. Polymerase chain reaction and culture analysis of the cerebrospinal fluid (CSF) was within normal limits. Serum alanine transaminase (ALT) level was not raised.

A diagnosis of neonatal (perinatal) HSV infection was made; and intravenous acyclovir was administered.

Case Review in a Nutshell

A full-term neonate presented with acute eruption of clustered vesicles and pustules on an erythematous base by the 6th day of her life. Oral mucosal lesions also developed in the form of shallow ulcerations. The classical clinical picture and maternal history of perinatal herpes 3 days prior to delivery points towards a diagnosis of neonatal/perinatal herpes. This diagnosis was confirmed by Tzanck smear examination and culture, which demonstrated evidence of HSV infiltration. There was no evidence of neurological (no CSF abnormality detected by PCR/culture) or any other organ involvement including eye (normal serum ALT), thus hinting towards a diagnosis of the milder SEM variety (HSV infection involving the skin, eyes or mouth).

Neonatal HSV can manifest in three characteristic forms:

1. Mucocutaneous disease—limited to the skin, eyes or mouth (SEM) [present case]
2. Disseminated disease—multiorgan involvement viz. liver, lungs or disseminated intravascular coagulation
3. Central nervous system disease—CSF or brain abnormalities are present in the absence of other visceral involvement.

Skin lesions may occur in all the types.

The management of this condition essentially comprises of intravenous acyclovir administration, regardless of clinical presentation. The dosage is 60 mg/kg/day in three divided doses for a minimum period of 14 days for our SEM variety (minimum 21 days is required for CNS/disseminated disease). In patients presenting with renal involvement, dosage should be adjusted accordingly. Daily suppressive dose may be used for about 6 months to prevent recurrences, if needed. Oral valacyclovir is also efficacious, but no liquid formulation exists till date.

CASE 2

A 5-day-old infant developed several bizarre shaped erythematous rashes on her face and trunk, which developed within 24–48 hours of her birth, which resembled "flea bite". Some of the rashes presented with superimposed, elevated yellowish fluid filled lesions on their surface. Parents provided a history of waxing and waning of the lesions. The child was born by vaginal delivery at term, birth weight 2750 g. There was no history of any family disorder, drug history or consanguineous marriage. There was no complaint of fever or any systemic illness.

Barely elevated, yellowish papules and pustules on an erythematous background were noted on local examination, measuring roughly 1–3 mm in diameter. The erythematous macules were bizarre shaped, with irregular margins, resembling "flea-bites". All the lesions were restricted to the face and trunk. Palms and soles, mucosa, hair and nails were spared.

Scraping was obtained from one of the pustules and histologically examined after staining with Wright stain. Sheets of eosinophils were observed around the hair follicles, concentrated around the pilosebaceous duct, localized in the upper part of epidermis (subcorneal). Scattered neutrophils were also observed. Peripheral blood examination was within normal limits.

A diagnosis of erythema toxicum neonatorum/toxic erythema of the newborn/flea bite dermatitis was made.

Case Review in a Nutshell

A full-term neonate presented with tiny yellowish papules and pustules, superimposed on erythematous macules and flares, which developed by 24–48 hours of her birth. The erythematous macules were bizarre shaped resembling, flea bites. Lesions initially started on the face and subsequently developed on the trunk. Palms, soles and mucosa were spared. She was born out of nonconsanguineous parentage and had an uneventful vaginal delivery. There was no history of fever or any systemic illness. A history of waxing and waning of the lesions was obtained. The typical morphology, distribution and time of onset prompted the diagnosis of erythema toxicum neonatorum. This diagnosis was confirmed by histological evidence of intra and perifollicular eosinophilic infiltration in the upper layers of epidermis. In the present case differential lymphocyte count was unremarkable, although peripheral blood eosinophilia has been reported in about 15% patients. The diagnosis is essentially clinical, skin biopsy is not warranted.

This is essentially a transient and benign condition, with lesions usually resolving spontaneously by one week following birth; although atypical cases have been reported (late onset, persistence beyond 10 days and neutrophilic predominance on histology). There is usually no residual pigmentation following the resolution of lesions (if residual pigmentation persists transient neonatal pustular melanosis must be considered). No therapy is needed except for parental counseling and reassurance.

CASE 3

A 7-year-old boy presented with multiple tense, fluid filled lesions on his lower trunk, buttocks and thighs, associated with pruritus for the last 3 weeks. He also complained of difficulty in swallowing since last 10 days. Family history and drug history are unremarkable. There was no history of fever or any other systemic illness.

Dermatological examination revealed multiple, tense fluid filled bullae, ranging from 2–3 mm in diameter scattered on erythematous skin affecting the lower trunk, buttocks and thighs. Some of the lesions had ruptured to form subsequent crusts. Some of the bullae were arranged in an annular pattern, to attain the classical "string of pearl" configuration. Genitalia and oral mucosa were involved which showed the presence of shallow erosions.

Clinically, chronic bullous disorder of childhood (CBDC)/childhood linear immunoglobulin A (IgA) disease (childhood LAD) was suspected. Skin biopsy was undertaken which demonstrated subepidermal bullae filled with neutrophils. Direct immunofluorescence (DIF) revealed a linear deposition of IgA along the basement membrane zone. Histopathology and DIF confirmed the diagnosis of CBDC/childhood LAD. Oral dapsone 50 mg twice daily was started in this patient.

Case Review in a Nutshell

A 7-year old boy presented with multiple pruritic and tense bullae arranged in an annular configuration, forming the "string of pearl appearance" which is characteristic of CBDC. Typical sites have been affected in the present case which include the lower part of torso (lower trunk, thighs, perineum and genitalia). Oral mucosa has been involved in the present case, which occurs in almost 75% of all such cases. Histopathology (subepidermal cleft filled with neutrophils) and DIF (linear deposition of IgA along the basement membrane zone) corroborate the diagnosis.

The commonest differential is childhood bullous pemphigoid which can be differentiated by DIF (granular deposition of IgG and IgM along the basement membrane zone).

Dapsone is the drug of choice for this condition, sulfapyridine also shows varying levels of efficacy. Occasional cases have responded to corticosteroids (topical > systemic), mycophenolate mofetil, colchicine, topical calcineurin inhibitors and dicloxacillin.

INTERACTIVE TOPIC REVIEW

Q.1 Classify vesicopustular and bullous disorders in children.

Ans: Vesicopustular and bullous disorders may be classified under the following heads in the pediatric population:
- Infective conditions
- Transient skin lesions
- Genodermatoses
- Immunological disorders/inflammatory disorders
- Drug reactions
- Uncommon and rare causes.

Q.2 What are the infective causes of pediatric vesiculopustular disorders and their salient features?

Ans: There are several infections which may present as vesicles and pustules in the pediatric age group. They can be classified as bacterial, viral, fungal and parasitic according to the etiologic agents. Some of the important causes are tabulated below along with their salient features (Table 1).

TABLE 1: Infective disorders presenting with blisters in children.

Name of disorder	Causative agent	Clinical features	Diagnosis/ Investigations
Bacterial disorders			
Impetigo (bullous and nonbullous)	*Staphylococcus* > *Streptococcus*	• Can occur in any age • Vesicles, pustules, often bulla (bullous impetigo), follicular distribution, furuncles, associated purulent discharge, lesions rupture and result in "honey colored" crusting • Associated sore throat, fever and other systemic symptoms hint towards streptococcal infection • Any site, but usually involves the periorificial, flexural and diaper areas	Skin or tissue Gram stain (gram-positive cocci) and bacterial culture to identify the causative organism
Perianal erythema	Group A *Streptococcus*	• Pustules, erosions and fissures on an erythematous base; perianal area (differential diagnosis: Perianal dermatitis) • Associated fever and other systemic symptoms (more than *Staphylococcus* infection), history of sore throat in family member may be present	Gram stain (gram-positive cocci in chains), bacterial culture, throat swab culture
Blistering distal dactylitis	Group A *Streptococcus*	• Vesicles, pustules and erosion at the distal end of volar fingertips • Associated fever and other systemic symptoms (more than *Staphylococcus* infection), history of sore throat in family member may be present	Gram stain (gram-positive cocci in chains), bacterial culture, throat swab culture
Psudomonas infection	*Pseudomonas* species	• Any age • Erythema, pustules, hemorrhagic bullae and necrotic ulcerations • Diaper and periorificial areas predominantly affected • Usually occurs in immunosuppressed children	Skin or tissue Gram stain (gram-negative rods), bacterial culture; blood culture
Congenital syphilis	*Treponema pallidum*	• Usually appears at birth to first few days • Tense bullae and/or erosions • Periorificial and acral areas show predilection • Other stigmata of congenital syphilis may be present viz. snuffles, Hutchinson's teeth, bulldog jaw etc.	Dark ground illumination microscopy, serological tests (VDRL, RPR), skin biopsy

Continued

Continued

TABLE 1: Infective disorders presenting with blisters in children.

Name of disorder	Causative agent	Clinical features	Diagnosis/ Investigations
Viral disorders			
Intrauterine herpes	HSV-2 > HSV-1	• Usually present at birth or appear within first few days • Vesicles, pustules, erosions, areas of scarring and missing skin • Scalp and upper torso predominantly affected • Other features of TORCH infections may be present viz. low birth weight, microcephaly, chorioretinitis • History maternal genital herpes few days before delivery (in case of vaginal delivery)	Tzanck smear, fluorescence antibody test, PCR, viral culture
Neonatal/ perinatal herpes simplex	HSV-1 > HSV-2	• Usually occurs between 5–14 days • Vesicles, pustules and crusted erosions • Three characteristic presentations- SEM/mucocutaneous, disseminated and CNS type • Usually the upper part of body, mucosae may be involved	Same as above
Herpes simplex in older children	HSV-1 > HSV-2	• Primary gingivostomatitis, recurrent episodes • Painful, grouped vesicles and erosion • Punched out discreet erosions and vesicles in a "honey-comb" pattern showing extensive body surface involvement– eczema hepeticum (disseminated HSV infection); usually occurs in background of atopic dermatitis	Same as above
Congenital/fetal varicella	VZV	• Scarring in a dermatomal distribution, erosions, vesicles and bullae are rare • Limb hypoplasia, chorioretinitis, low birth weight may be associated. • History of maternal primary varicella (chicken pox) in the first trimester	Cord blood examination for IgM, Tzanck smear, viral culture

Continued

Continued

TABLE 1: Infective disorders presenting with blisters in children.

Name of disorder	Causative agent	Clinical features	Diagnosis/ Investigations
Neonatal varicella	VZV	• Widespread vesicles and crusted papules on an erythematous base • Generalized distribution • Lesions usually in same stage of development • History of maternal varicella 7 days before to 2 days after vaginal delivery	Same as above
Primary varicella in older children (Chicken pox)	VZV	• Vesicles on an erythematous base: "Dew drops on rose petal" appearance • Face à trunk à extremities, mucosae may be involved • Palms and soles spared • Moderate to severe pruritus • Lesions heal with scab formation, usually in different stages of development	Same as above
Herpes zoster (Fig. 1)	Reactivation of latent VZV in ganglion	• Painful vesicles on an erythematous base, unilateral and dermatomal distribution • Usually affects older children	Same as above
Hand foot mouth disease	Coxsackievirus A16, Enterovirus 71, etc.	• Small vesicles on palms, soles, oral cavity and buttocks • Oblong shaped vesicles, longitudinal axis parallel to the palmar and plantar creases • Fever, vomiting, diarrhea and upper respiratory tract symptoms may be present	PCR or viral culture, best samples obtained from nasopharynx and intact skin vesicles
Chikungunya	Chikungunya virus (flavivirus family)	• Generalized vesiculobullous eruptions, usually associated with fever • Congenital Chikungunya has characteristic nasal pigmentation	PCR or viral culture
Fungal infection			
Candidiasis	*Candida albicans* and other species	• Beefy red patches, macerated plaques with overlying fine scale • Satellite papules and pustules • Mainly affects the diaper and intertriginous areas	Potassium hydroxide (KOH) examination (hyphae and budding yeast), fungal culture

Continued

Continued

TABLE 1: Infective disorders presenting with blisters in children.			
Name of disorder	Causative agent	Clinical features	Diagnosis/ Investigations
Parasitic infestation			
Scabies (Fig. 2)	Sarcoptes scabiei hominis (mite)	• Generalized pruritus with nocturnal exacerbation • Excoriated papules, vesicles, nodules, crusts, burrows • Head to foot (infants), neck to foot (>1 year), web space of fingers and toes, periumbilical area, genitalia, palms and soles (only in infantile scabies) • History of pruritus in family/contacts	Clinical diagnosis, scrapping from burrows to demonstrate mites

(VDRL: venereal disease research laboratory; RPR: rapid plasma reagin; HSV: herpes simplex virus; PCR: polymerase chain reaction; TORCH: toxoplasmosis, other (syphilis, varicella-zoster, parvovirus B19), rubella, cytomegalovirus, herpes; SEM: skin, eyes, mouth; CNS: central nervous system; VZV: varicella zoster virus)

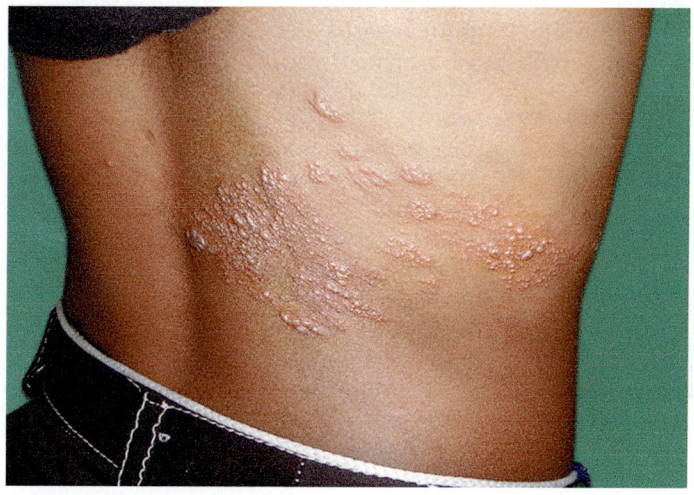

Fig. 1: Herpes Zoster.
Courtesy: Dr Anirban Das, Clinical Tutor, Murshidabad Medical College, West Bengal.

Q.3 Mention briefly about some transient skin disorders presenting with blisters in the pediatric population.

Ans: Some blistering disorders heal spontaneously within days to weeks, thus requiring no active treatment except parental counseling and reassurance. Some of the important transient skin disorders are presented in Table 2.

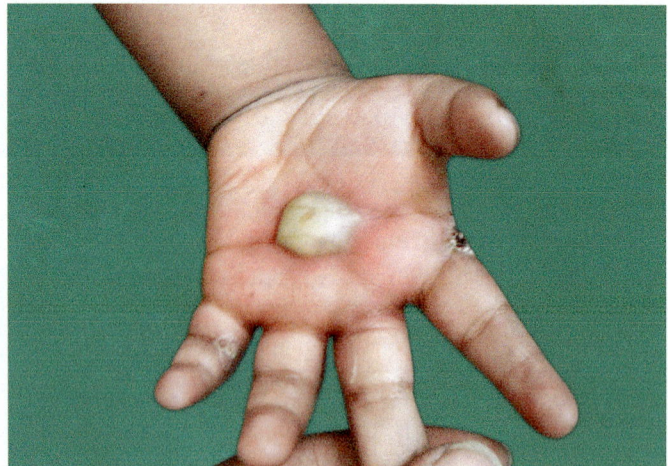

Fig. 2: Secondary pyoderma following scabies.
Courtesy: Dr. Anirban Das, Clinical Tutor, Murshidabad Medical College, West Bengal.

TABLE 2: Transient blistering disorders in children.

Disorder	Usual age of presentation	Clinical features	Associated findings	Diagnosis/ Investigations
Erythema toxicum neonatorum	Within 24–48 hours of birth, absent at birth	• Small papules and pustules on irregular erythematous macules and wheals (flea bite marks) • Usually the lower torso, may affect any site except palms and soles • Usually resolve spontaneously by 7–10 days	Occur in term infants, birth weight >2500 g, first pregnancy, vaginal delivery and summer/autumn season are other predisposing factors	Clinical, Wright's stain shows lesional eosinophilic infiltration
Neonatal pustular melanosis	Birth or shortly thereafter	• Pustules without underlying erythema, collarette of scales, lesions heal with formation of hyperpigmented macules • More commonly affects the forehead, ears, back, fingers and toes	Black term infants have the highest predilection	Clinical, Wright stain shows neutrophils > eosinophils
Miliaria crystallina	May present at birth, neonatal or infantile period	• Fragile, clear fluid filled shiny vesicles on normal skin • Forehead, upper trunk, arms, neck most common sites	History of fever is characteristic in acquired cases	Clinical, Wright, Gram and Tzanck smears are negative

Continued

Continued

TABLE 2: Transient blistering disorders in children.

Disorder	Usual age of presentation	Clinical features	Associated findings	Diagnosis/Investigations
Miliaria rubra	Neonatal or infantile period	• Discreet, pruritic erythematous papulovesicles with superimposed pustules showing localized distribution • Prickling, burning > pruritus • Forehead, upper trunk, arms, neck most common sites	History of overwarming, fever, or use of occlusive garments may be obtained	Clinical, Wright, Gram and Tzanck smears are negative
Neonatal acne/benign cephalic pustulosis	Days to weeks	• Papules and pustules on erythematous base • Face (cheeks, forehead, eyelids), neck, upper trunk	Scaly lesions on scalp (seborrheic capitis)	Clinical diagnosis, no stain is positive for any infective agent
Suction blisters (Fig. 3)	At birth	• Flaccid *bullae* or linear erosions at the site of trauma • Occasionally two symmetric lesions may be seen • Fingers, wrists > feet	Evidence of trauma due to suction, use of vacuum devices or forceps for delivery, monitoring electrodes etc.	Clinical diagnosis, corroborative history
Insect-bite hyper-sensitivity	Any age	• Tense vesicles and bulla (blister beetle dermatitis) on erythematous base • Often pruritus leads to excoriations and crusting • Occasionally arranged in a linear array "breakfast, lunch and dinner sign" • Affects the exposed parts of body, hands, feet, ankles • If skin biopsy shows increased dermal eosinophils, Well's syndrome/eosinophilic cellulitis may be considered	History of exposure to different insects and fleas, overcrowding, lack of adequate hygiene	Clinical diagnosis, skin biopsy (if needed) shows eosinophilic infiltration

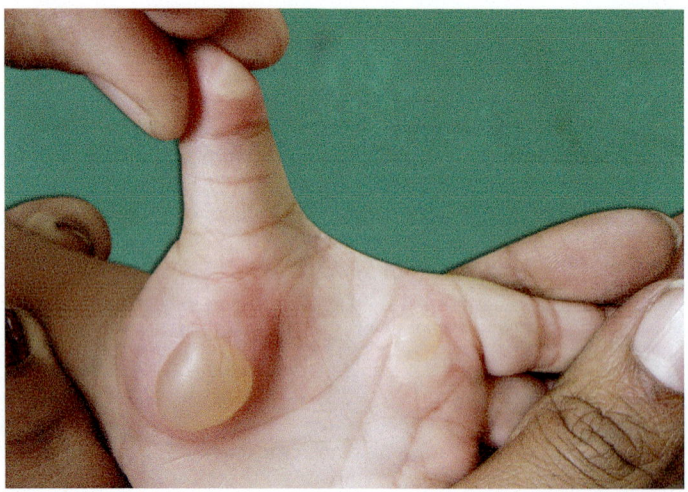

Fig. 3: Friction blister.
Courtesy: Dr. Anirban Das, Clinical Tutor, Murshidabad Medical College, West Bengal.

Q.4 **What are the common genodermatoses presenting with vesicles and bullae in children?**

Ans: Some of the important blistering genodermatoses with their salient features are given below:

Epidermolysis Bullosa
- Autosomal dominant, recessive or X-linked condition
- Usually presents at birth or within first few days
- Extreme skin fragility, exacerbated by trauma and shearing forces, bullous lesions, milia, nail dystrophy and mucosal erosions may be present
- Predominantly affects the trauma prone areas—hands, feet, buttocks
- Three types depending on depth of pathology—superficialis, junctional and dystrophic
- Occasionally muscular dystrophy, pyloric atresia and other systemic pathologies may be present
- Diagnosis is confirmed by skin biopsy, electron microscopy, salt-split examination and genetic profiling
- Treatment is symptomatic, prevention of trauma and genetic engineering.

Incontinentia Pigmenti
- X-linked dominant disease, mutation of *NEMO* gene
- Appears at birth or within first few days
- Four stages in sequence—vesicular, verrucous, hyperpigmented and hypopigmented lesions
- All lesions are arranged linearly along the lines of Blaschko
- Common sites—trunk and extremities
- May be associated with ocular, dental, skeletal and neurological defects

- Skin biopsy shows eosinophilic spongiosis with dyskeratosis, gene testing is confirmatory
- Treatment is symptomatic and parenteral counseling.

Bullous Ichthyosiform Erythroderma
- Autosomal dominant disorder
- Generalized bullous eruption, thickened keratotic skin, may present with erythroderma
- Excessive ridging is seen at the flexural areas
- Biopsy shows characteristic epidermolytic hyperkeratosis
- Treatment is symptomatic.

Q.5 What are the different causes of immunological/inflammatory blistering disorders?

Ans: This is a rare subgroup of vesiculo-bullous disorders in children. Immunological/inflammatory bullous disorders in children may be classified under two heads:
1. Those occurring due to maternal antibodies
2. Autoimmune bullous disease in children.

Blistering Disorders Occurring due to Maternal Antibodies
Some blistering disorders may occur in the neonate born to mothers having IgG mediated immunobullous disorders, as IgG can cross the placenta. Neonatal lupus erythematosus is an exception which occurs due to transplacental anti-SS-A, anti-SS-B and U1-RNP antibodies.

This group contains the following important diseases:
- Pemphigoid gestationis or herpes gestationis
- Pemphigus vulgaris (neonatal pemphigus or pemphigus neonatorum)
- Pemphigus foliaceus
- Epidermolysis bullosa acquisita
- Neonatal lupus erythematosus.

Autoimmune Bullous Disease in Children
These disorders occur rarely in children. This group includes three main disorders:
1. Childhood linear IgA disease (chronic bullous disease of childhood), most common
2. Childhood dermatitis herpetiformis
3. Childhood bullous pemphigoid.

The basic differences between the two groups is presented in Table 3.

Q.6 Name some drug reactions which may present with vesiculobullous lesions in children.

Ans: Some drug reactions which may rarely present with vesiculobullous lesions in children are given below:
- Toxic epidermal necrolysis: Blisters on the face and palatal erosions, confluent and generalized eruption is absent
- Bullous erythema multiforme: Very rare, usually postviral infection more than drugs

TABLE 3: Immune mediated blistering diseases in children—salient features.

Blistering disorders occurring due to maternal antibodies	Autoimmune bullous disease in children
Blistering is virtually always present at birth	Blisters never present at birth, usually appear around 5 years of age
History of autoimmune blistering disease in mother must be present, most mothers have active disease during pregnancy	No such history may be obtained
The extent and type of disease depends on maternal disease	No such correlation
Blisters usually do not occur after neonatal period	Blistering starts around mean age of 5 years
Treatment is supportive with bland emollients, topical corticosteroids may be used if needed; spontaneous resolution occurs as maternal autoantibodies are gradually cleared from the affected neonate	Treatment with corticosteroids and other immunomodulators necessary; there is no spontaneous resolution

N.B. If blistering occurs in a neonate after phototherapy, porphyria must be suspected.

- Acute generalized exanthematous pustulosis: Very rare cause, sudden onset of fever and widespread erythema and minute sterile, discreet and nonfollicular pustules. Most commonly occurs due to beta-lactam antibiotics. (Commonest differential is pustular psoriasis where the pustules coalesce to form "lakes of pus").

Q.7 Name some rare and uncommon disorders which can present with vesiculobullous lesions in children.

Ans: Some of the important rarer conditions which may present as blistering disorders in children are given below:
- Acropustulosis of infancy: Pruritic vesicles and pustules limited to the hands and feet
- Bullous mastocytosis: Thickened, infiltrated skin with superimposed bullae (localized or generalized), usually affects the torso within weeks to months of birth, may be associated with hives, flushing (Darier's sign positive); skin biopsy shows increased dermal mast cells and serology shows serum tryptase level >20 ng/mL
- Acrodermatitis enteropathica: Sharply demarcated vesicles, bullae, erosions and crusted plaques in a periorificial distribution, mostly occurs in breast fed infants of zinc deficient mothers, low serum zinc (<50 µg/dL)
- Langerhans cell histiocytosis: Presents with necrotic and hemorrhagic vesicles and bullae, pustules, erosions and crusting, usually affects the intertriginous areas (groins), three forms—congenital self-healing, Hashimoto-Pritzker, Weber–Christian and eosinophilic granuloma (localized), skin biopsy shows increased number of histiocytes with reniform nucleus and abundant cytoplasm

- Eosinophilic pustular folliculitis: Pustules on an erythematous base mainly affecting the scalp and face, appear in crops, histologic diagnosis
- Neonatal Behcet's disease: Small punched out vesicles, pustules, ulceration and scarring, mucosal affection, history of maternal Behçet's disease
- Erosive pustular dermatosis of the scalp: May be associated scalp edema, areas of alopecia and necrosis; Hay–Wells syndrome and Rapp–Hodgkin syndrome to be suspected if associated with ectodermal dysplasia
- Hyper IgE syndrome: Single or grouped vesicles, pustules and crusting; affects face, scalp and upper torso, blood eosinophilia and elevated serum IgE levels
- Lipoid proteinosis: Erythematous papulovesicles with atrophic scarring, face, ears mainly affected, upper eyelid develops a beaded appearance and histopathological examination shows deposition of periodic acid-Schiff positive hyaline material.

Q.8 What is the difference in approach to blistering disorders in children versus adults?

Ans: There is a conspicuous difference in approach to blistering disorders in children and adults owing to the difference in etiology.

In children the commonest causes of vesiculo-bullous disorders are infection (bacterial, viral, fungal, or parasitic) (Table 2) and genetic disorders (epidermolysis bullosa, incontinentia pigmenti, etc.). Immunobullous disorders are extremely rare and most of them occur due to transplacental passage of maternal antibodies (Table 3). So, in any child with blistering disorders we should rule out infections first, thus early institution of empirical antimicrobials is necessary as any delay may be fatal. Treatment should be continued when the clinical suspicion is high despite negative initial culture results. Even if a genetic disorder is suspected, antimicrobials should be administered as we can't rule out co-existence of an infection.

On the other hand, immunobullous disorders comprise the commonest cause of blistering disorders in an adult, so corticosteroids form the mainstay of treatment in this population.

Q.9 What are the major differences between pediatric bullous pemphigoid and its adult counterpart?

Ans: Bullous pemphigoid (BP) is primarily a disease of the elderly population; however, rare cases of this disorder have been reported in the pediatric population also, although some conspicuous differences exist between these two populations a (Table 4).

Q.10 How does childhood epidermolysis bullosa acquisita (EBA) differ from the adult variant?

Ans: Some of the important diseases are presented in Table 5.

Q.11 Is there any difference between childhood linear IgA disease and adult IgA disease?

Ans: Although the presentation is similar in children and adults (annular configuration of blisters in a "cluster of jewels" or "string of pearls" pattern with

TABLE 4: Difference between childhood bullous pemphigoid and adult bullous pemphigoid.

Childhood bullous pemphigoid	Adult bullous pemphigoid
Females > males	Males > females
Three clinical varieties: Infantile, childhood and localized vulvar disease, acral involvement (palms, soles and head) is more common in infantile bullous pemphigoid	Trunk > extremities, preceded by pruritic urticarial wheals and plaques
Mucosal involvement more common than adults	Mucosal involvement extremely rare
Favorable prognosis, most patients achieving remission in weeks to months	More chronic course with significant mortality and morbidity
Eosinophils and neutrophils seen on histopathology	Mainly eosinophilic infiltration, very sparse neutrophils may be observed
Tetracyclines contraindicated in children <8 years	Tetracyclines form an effective therapeutic tool

TABLE 5: Difference between Childhood and adult epidermolysis bullosa acquisita.

Childhood epidermolysis bullosa acquisita	Adult epidermolysis bullosa acquisita
• Extremely rare condition • Mainly inflammatory variety occurs, mimicking bullous pemphigoid, scarring and milia less common • Mucosal involvement more common (oral > ocular) • Anti-bodies formed against the NC2 or triple helical domain of collagen 7 • Better prognosis	• More common than the childhood variant • Mainly the mechanobullous variety occurs, blisters occurring on extensor surfaces of extremities at trauma prone sites, can be hemorrhagic or filled with serous fluid. Scarring and milia are more common • Mucosal involvement less common • Antibodies formed against the NC1 domain of collagen 7 • Poorer prognosis

new lesions appearing at the periphery of older lesions), the hallmark difference is the site of lesions.

Children: Lesions appear on the abdomen, groin and thighs with a predilection for the anogenital skin.

Adults: Face, extensor surfaces, buttocks and trunk is more commonly involved.

N.B. Drug induced linear IgA disease is more common in adults, the commonest drug being vancomycin.

Q.12 Which blistering diseases may clinically resemble child abuse?

Ans: Some autoimmune diseases have predilection for the genital region, presenting with blisters and erosions. These disorders should be evaluated carefully as they may clinically resemble child abuse. Some the important disorders belonging to this group are given below:
- Linear IgA disease/chronic bullous dermatosis in children (Fig. 4)
- Childhood bullous pemphigoid—localized vulvar variant

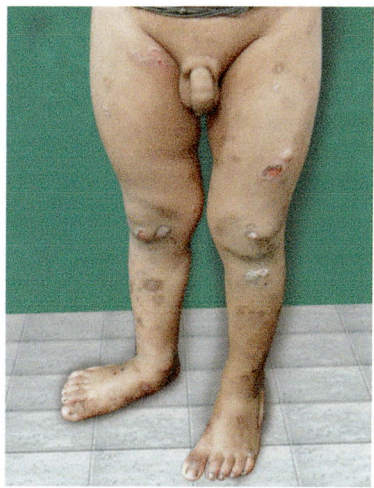

Fig. 4: Chronic bullous dermatosis of childhood (CBDC).
Courtesy: Dr Anirban Das, Clinical Tutor, Murshidabad Medical College, West Bengal.

- Pemphigus
- Epidermolysis bullosa acquisita
- Vulvar-only cicatricial pemphigoid.

CONCLUSION

Vesiculopustular and bullous disorders encompass a wide gamut of conditions in children ranging from infections, inflammatory disorders, some rare genetic disorders and even some child abuse manifestations. A rational approach is needed for proper diagnosis and management of these condition. In this chapter, we have provided a comprehensive list of these conditions in tabular formats and also provided a pragmatic diagnostic approach for their early evaluation and management.

KEY POINTS

- Proper history is the cornerstone for the diagnosis of the different varieties of vesiculopustular disorders in children
- Appropriate investigations are complementary to confirm the clinical diagnosis.

SUGGESTED READING

1. Chi CC, Wang SH, Charles-Holmes R, et al. Pemphigoid gestationis: Early onset and blister formation are associated with adverse pregnancy outcomes. Br J Dermatol. 2009;160:1222-8.
2. Eichenfield LF, Frieden IJ, Zaenglein A, et al. Neonatal and Infant Dermatology. 3rd ed. Elsevier Health Sciences; 2014. P. 111-39.
3. Fortuna G, Salas-Alanis JC, Guidetti E, et al. A critical reappraisal of the current data on drug induced linear immunoglobulin A bullous dermatosis: A real and separate nosological entity? J Am Acad of Dermatol. 2012;66:988-94.
4. Gajic-Veljic M, Nikolic M, Medenica L. Juvenile bullous pemphigoid: The presentation and follow-up of six cases. J EurAcad Dermatol Venereol. 2010;24:69-72.

5. Hogeling M, Nakano T, Dvorak CC, et al. Severe neonatal congenital erythropoietic porphyria. Pediatr Dermatol. 2011;28:416-20.
6. James WD, Berger TG, Elston DM, et al. Andrews' diseases of the skin: Clinical Dermatology. 11th ed. Saunders Elsevier. P. 464-7.
7. Marathe K, Lu J, Morel KD. Bullous diseases: Kids are not just little people. Clin Dermatol. 2015;33:644-56.
8. Srinivas SM, Sheth PK, Hiremagalore R. Vesiculobullous disorders in children. Indian J Pediatr. 2015;82:805-8.
9. Waisbourd-Zinman O, Ben-Amitai D, Cohen AD, et al. Bullous pemphigoid in infancy: Clinical andepidemiologic characteristics. J Am Acad Dermatol. 2008;58:41-8.

CHAPTER 9

Vesiculobullous Disorder in Middle Age

Monica Chahar, Paschal D'Souza, Lalit K Gupta, Sudheer K Arava

■ INTRODUCTION

Vesiculobullous lesions are encountered quite commonly in dermatological practice. Several disorders present with such lesions ranging from mild and benign acute irritant dermatitis to life threatening junctional epidermolysis bullosa, pemphigus and drug induced toxic epidermal necrolysis. While some of these diseases can present at birth (epidermolysis bullosa), most appear at later stages including most of the autoimmune bullous disorders.

One of the common autoimmune blistering disease that occurs in middle age is pemphigus which may have varied presentations. In this chapter the disorder has been taken as a prototype example of vesiculobullous disease in middle age and a management approach has been outlined around it.

CASE 1

A 48-year-old housewife presented with recurrent painful erosions and ulcers in the mouth for 5 months. Two months later she developed multiple, slightly itchy, fluid filled lesions on scalp, face, arms, trunk and thighs. These lesions gradually increased in number and size and ruptured spontaneously in 2–3 days leaving behind painful red eroded areas which did not heal completely.

Further enquiry revealed that the eruptions started de novo as oral ulcerations, followed by skin lesions. There was no history of any drug treatment, excessive exposure to heat, cold, sunlight or any occupational irritants. There was no history suggestive of active infections at any other site, difficulty in swallowing, hoarseness of voice, fever, malaise, joint pains, diarrhea, significant weight loss or similar complaints in her family. She is a vegetarian and nonsmoker and attained menopause 3 years back.

Her physical examination was unremarkable except for the presence of mild pallor. Systemic examination was within normal limits.

Cutaneous examination revealed multiple discrete, clear fluid filled, mostly flaccid bullae ranging in size from 1 cm × 0.5 cm to about 1.5 cm × 1 cm present over trunk

(Fig. 1a) and upper limbs along with multiple reddish oval irregularly shaped erosions over neck (Fig. 1b), upper chest, back and thighs. Crusted lesions were present around her eyes (Fig. 1c), trunk and upper limbs. Few smaller blisters were present over dorsa of hands which appeared tense (Fig. 1d). Palms were spared. Nikolsky's sign (direct and marginal) and bulla spread sign were positive. There were no pigmentary changes, scarring or milia formation at the site of healed lesions.

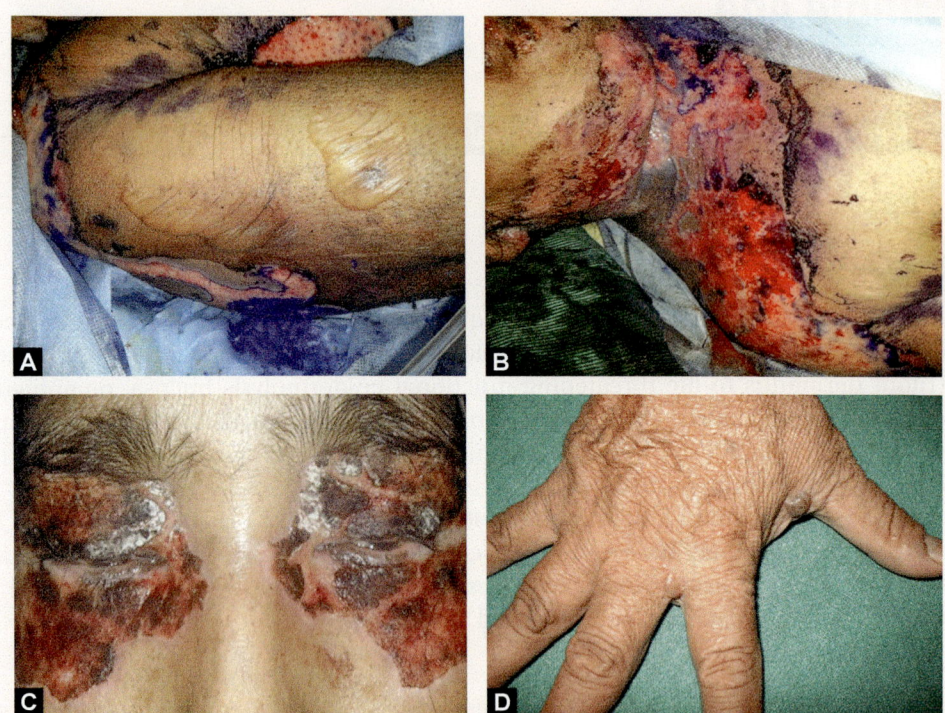

Fig. 1: (A) Flaccid bullae of pemphigus vulgaris; (B) Crusting over neck; (C) Periocular crusting; (D) Smaller tense blisters seen on the hand.
Courtesy: Fig. 1 (A), (B) and (C) Dr Rohini Soni, ESIPGIMSR, New Delhi; Fig. 1 (D) Dr Tapan Dhali, Professor Dermatology, ESIPGIMSR, New Delhi.

Scalp had multiple linear-irregularly shaped erosions with red oozing surface covered by yellowish-brown crusts (Fig. 2a). Oral examination revealed multiple, irregularly shaped erosions and ulcers, a few of which revealed shelving margins with overlying hanging edge (Fig. 2b). Ocular, genitalia and nail examination was within normal limits.

On investigations, Tzanck smear from blister floor on right hand and erosion on left buccal mucosa revealed multiple acantholytic cells (Fig. 3a). Skin biopsy from an intact blister on left forearm revealed mild spongiosis, suprabasal cleft with acantholytic cells simulating a tomb stone appearance (Fig. 3b). Dermis showed mild chronic perivascular lymphocytic infiltration. Direct immunofluorescence from perilesional skin showed intercellular IgG and C3 deposits (Fig. 3c). Indirect immunofluorescence was not done. Enzyme-linked immunosorbent assay (ELISA) test from serum showed IgG antibodies to both desmoglein 1 and 3 in a titer of 30 U/mL and 160 U/mL, respectively. Rest of the routine hematological, biochemical and radiological investigations were within normal range.

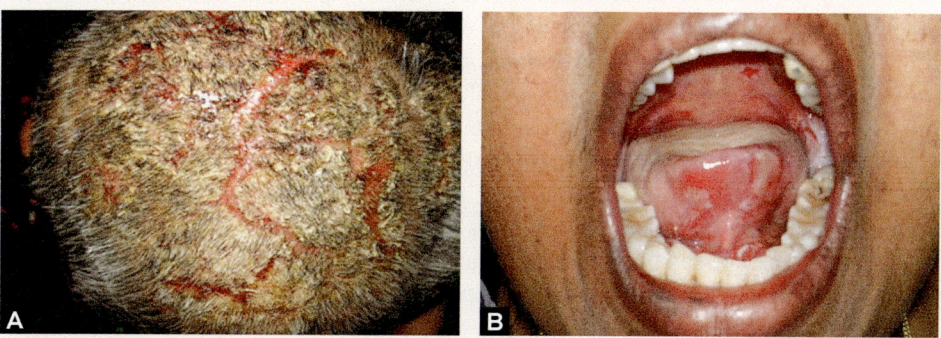

Fig. 2: (A) Fissuring and thick crusting over scalp; (B) Ulcers in oral mucosa with shelving edematous margins.
Courtesy: Fig. 2 (A) Dr Tapan Dhali, Professor Dermatology, ESIPGIMSR, New Delhi.

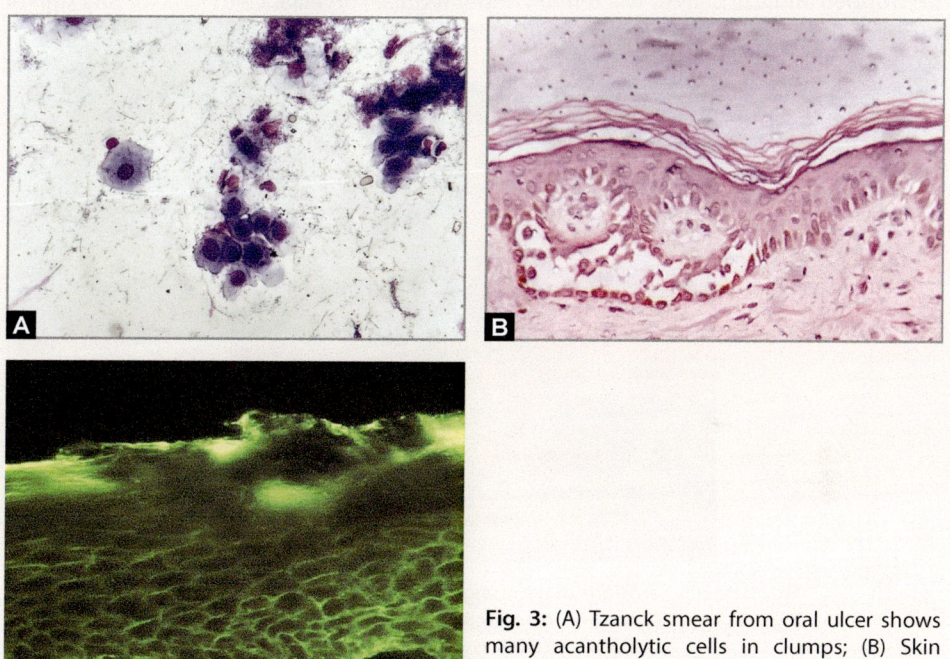

Fig. 3: (A) Tzanck smear from oral ulcer shows many acantholytic cells in clumps; (B) Skin biopsy of intact blister shows suprabasal cleft containing acantholytic cells and single row of basal cells in the floor resembling tombstones; (C) Fishnet appearance of epidermis on direct immunofluorescence due to IgG deposits is diagnostic of pemphigus vulgaris.

On the basis of history, examination and investigations, a final diagnosis of pemphigus vulgaris was made. The patient was started on dexamethasone-cyclophosphamide pulse

(DCP) therapy, phase 1, which comprised of inj. dexamethasone 100 mg in 500 mL of 5% dextrose intravenous, administered for 3 consecutive days, inj cyclophosphamide 500 mg intravenous on day second and oral cyclophosphamide 50 mg daily. In addition she was also given oral prednisolone 20 mg once daily. Symptomatic treatment comprising of fluticasone + mupirocin ointment for eroded skin lesions, betadine mouth rinse, triamcinolone acetonide gel for oral ulcers, ciprofloxacin 500 mg twice daily as antibiotic prophylaxis, ranitidine 150 mg twice daily, fluconazole 150 mg once a week and multivitamin once a day, was also provided.

The patient reported improvement in the eroded areas from day 4 and by 6 weeks, majority of the cutaneous erosions had healed completely with postinflammatory hyperpigmentation (Fig. 4). The old blisters also started to subside by day 10 although few new blisters appeared over limbs during first week of therapy, but they gradually ceased to appear. The oral erosions too improved with reduction in pain by the end of 2 weeks. The patient is under regular follow-up.

The DCP is planned to be repeated every month till disease activity is brought under complete control and then will be continued further for 6–9 months (phase II). The patient will then be kept on oral cyclophosphamide for a year (phase III) after which it will be stopped and the patient will remain under regular surveillance to look for any sign of relapse (phase IV).

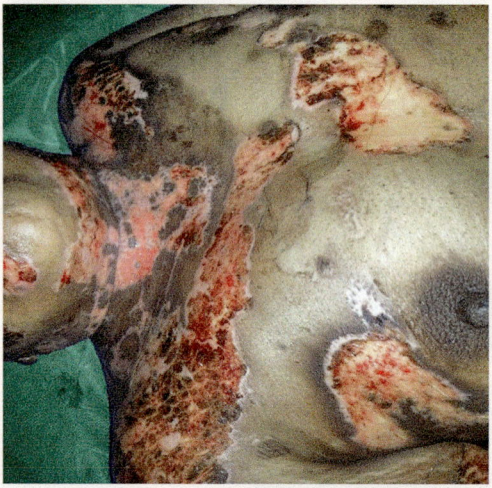

Fig. 4: Healing erosions of pemphigus vulgaris patient on 7th day.
Courtesy: Dr Rohini Soni, ESIPGIMSR, New Delhi.

■ INTERACTIVE TOPIC REVIEW

Q.1 What are the differential diagnosis of vesiculobullous lesions in this age group?

Ans: Box 1 provides a list of the differential diagnosis.

| BOX 1 | **Vesiculobullous disorders in middle age.** |

Infectious
- Viral: Herpes group (herpes simplex/herpes zoster/varicella zoster)
- Bacterial: Impetigo, staphylococcal scalded skin syndrome (SSSS)
- Fungal: Vesicular dermatophytosis

Genetic
- Hailey–Hailey disease

Autoimmune disorders
- Pemphigus group: Pemphigus vulgaris/foliaceus/erythematosus/drug induced/paraneoplastic
- Bullous pemphigoid
- Epidermolysis bullosa acquisita (EBA)
- Dermatitis herpetiformis (DH)
- Pemphigoid gestationis (in pregnant females)
- Bullous lupus erythematosus (LE)

Inflammatory/metabolic diseases
- Transient acantholytic dermatosis
- Polymorphous light eruption (vesicular PMLE)
- Porphyria cutanea tarda (PCT)
- Bullous Sweet's syndrome
- Bullous lichen planus and lichen planus pemphigoides
- Mucha-Habermann disease
- Dyshidrotic dermatitis
- Id reaction
- Allergic contact dermatitis (ACD)
- Irritant contact dermatitis (ICD)

Drug induced
- Erythema multiforme major
- Bullous fixed drug eruption (FDE)
- Stevens–Johnson syndrome: Toxic epidermal necrolysis (SJS-TEN)

Others
- Insect bite
- Friction blisters
- Burns (sunburn/frostbite/electrodessication)

Q.2 How does the history and clinical presentation of this patient help to approach/arrive at/to your diagnosis?

Ans: With the above case scenario, many of the differentials listed below will be eliminated:
- Drug induced disorders like erythema multiforme major (Fig. 5a), bullous fixed drug eruption (Fig. 5b), Stevens-Johnson syndrome/toxic epidermal necrolysis (Fig. 5c) due to absence of any drug history. This has to be carefully excluded as many times patient may not give a correct history or may not consider treatment from alternate system of medicines as drugs. Clinically

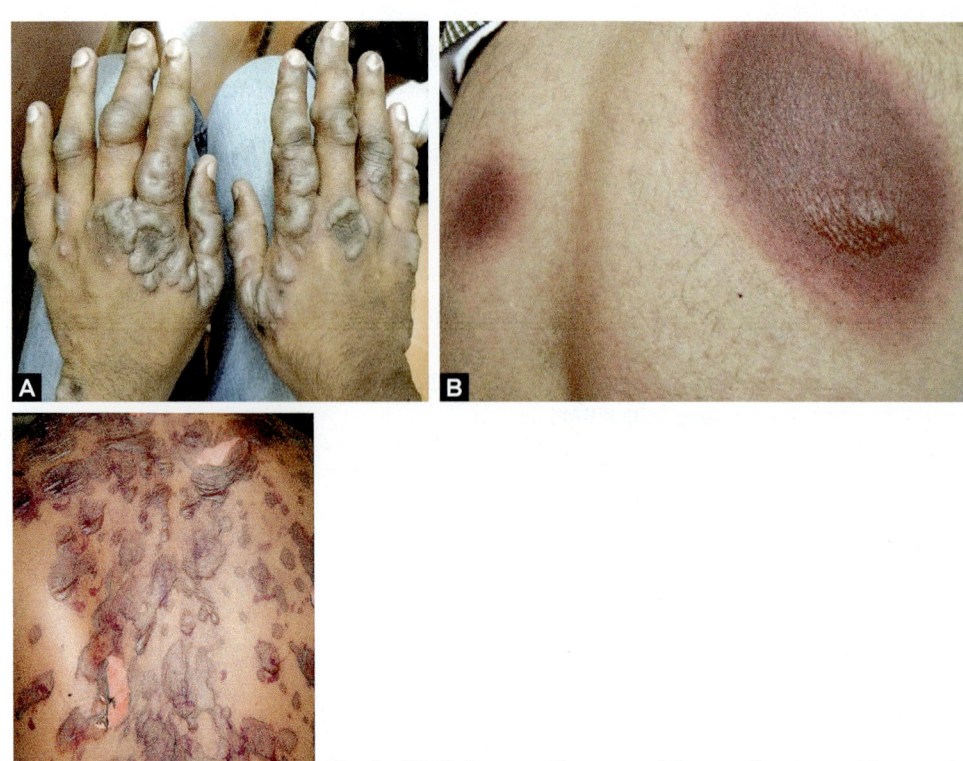

Fig 5: (A) Bullous erythema multiforme due to co-trimoxazole; (B) Multiple bullous fixed drug eruption due to tinidazole; (C) Toxic epidermal necrolysis in a patient due to carbamazepine.
Courtesy: Fig. 5 (B) Dr Raj Kumar Kothiwala, Professor Dermatology, JLN Medical College, Ajmer, Rajasthan.

these disorders are sufficiently characteristic and can be easily recognized in the presence of an appropriate history
- Pemphigoid gestationis (nonpregnant menopausal patient).

Q.3 What are the differential diagnoses still being considered at this stage and how do we go about sorting them out?

Ans: On the basis of the clinical presentation, the possibility that she is suffering from a primary autoimmune vesiculobullous disorder notably pemphigus vulgaris appears strong. On the other hand, some conditions from the list above can be excluded while others require further workup:
- Infectious disorders can manifest with blisters. Herpes zoster commonly is segmental dermatomal (Fig. 6a) while herpes simplex is localized and grouped. Disseminated herpes simplex seen in atopics or immunosuppressed is more like dermatitis than blistering, i.e. eczema herpeticum (Fig. 6b). Staphylococcal scalded skin syndrome (SSSS) may uncommonly present in an adult with renal failure and presents with fever, malaise, toxemia and widespread sloughing of tender skin. Vesicular tinea usually maintains the

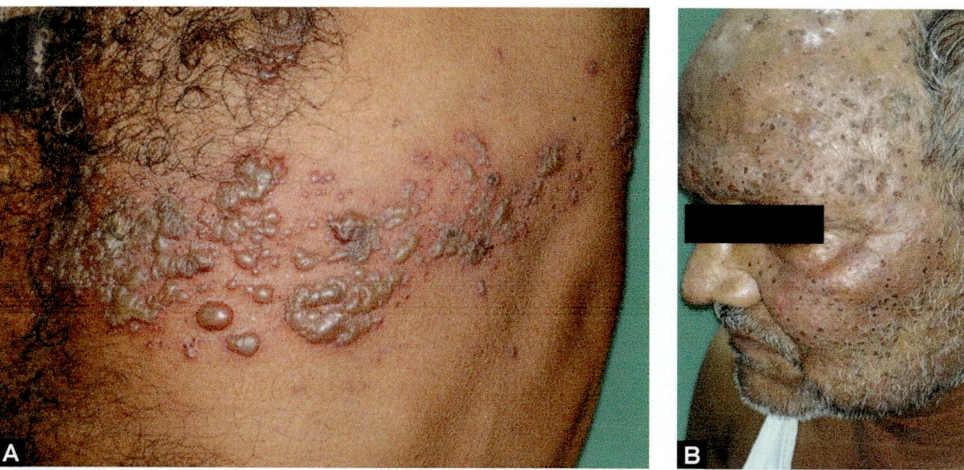

Fig. 6: (A) Herpes zoster over left side of chest; (B) Eczema herpeticum: Scattered deep seated vesicles of herpes simplex with eczematization over face.

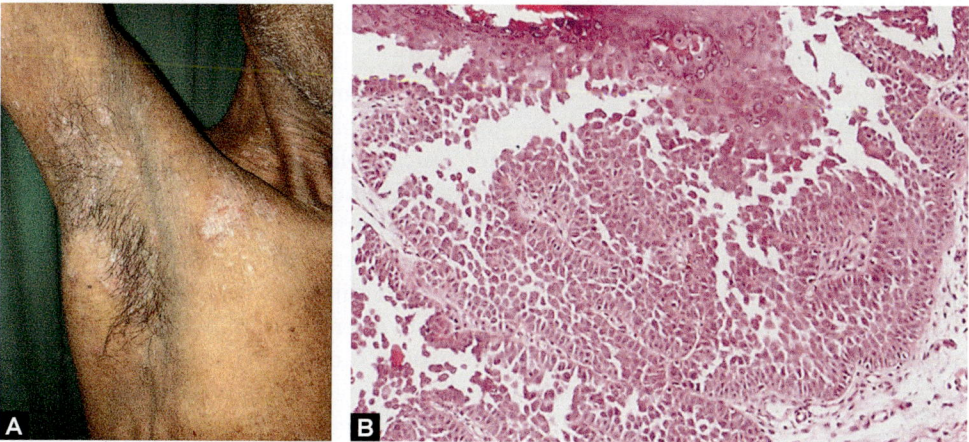

Fig. 7: Hailey-Hailey disease (A) Intertriginous fissures and scale crusts; (B) Prominent supra basal separation in the epidermis with many acantholytic cells causing lacunae, bulla and villi formation. Direct immunofluorescence (DIF) test was negative.
Courtesy: Fig. 7 (A) Dr Rohini Soni, ESIPGIMSR, New Delhi.

characteristics annularity of ringworm with vesicles superimposed on scaly papular margins
- Genetic disorder like Hailey–Hailey disease has a positive family history in around 70% patients. It is characterized by recurrent vesicles and transient flaccid bullae which quickly evolve into irregular erosions and fissures, mainly located in the intertriginous areas (Fig. 7a). Histopathology shows acantholytic dyskeratosis and dilapidated brick wall appearance which is quite characteristic (Fig. 7b)
- Other diseases: Localized nature of bullous insect bites (unless secondary to lymphoreticular malignancies), friction blisters, burns, contact dermatitis

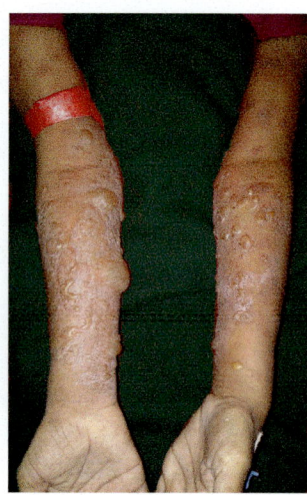

Fig. 8: Irritant contact dermatitis forearms due to alkali spill.

(Fig. 8) is usually obvious. Id reaction generally presents as bilaterally symmetrical acral vesico-pustules with or without an obvious primary dermatoses like inflamed tinea cruris. Polymorphic light eruption occurs in spring-summer season on sun-exposed parts with varying spectrum of lesions like pruritic papules, papulovesicles, plaques or erythema multiforme like lesions on sun-exposed skin; frank bullous lesions are rarely observed. In porphyria cutanea tarda, there is characteristic history of photosensitivity with tense blisters and erosions over mostly sun-exposed areas like dorsa of hands and forearms (Fig. 9a). Scarring and milia may be seen around healed lesions together with hypertrichosis and sclerodermoid changes. Teeth are yellowish brown (Fig. 9b) and urine usually shows red discoloration (Fig. 9c).

Bullous lupus erythematosus has an acute presentation where patients can exhibit features such as fever, arthralgia, arthritis, photosensitivity, etc. Clinically, cutaneous changes are characterized by vesicles and tense bullae (subepidermal blister) on erythematous or urticated base with a predilection for face, upper trunk and proximal extremities. It can clinically mimic toxic epidermal necrolysis. Test for antinuclear antibodies is usually positive calling for further diagnostic workup. Bullous lichen planus and lichen planus pemphigoides will both manifest classical violaceous papules of lichen planus in addition to blisters. In Grover's disease, the characteristic lesions are crusted erythematous papules, pustules, or papulovesicles over chest, back and proximal extremities. Although termed "transient acantholytic dermatosis", the lesions may persist for years, especially in the inframammary regions

- Primary auto immune vesiculobullous disorders: Table 1 lists the features which help to differentiate between various primary autoimmune vesiculobullous disorders, a category to which the present patient probably belongs.

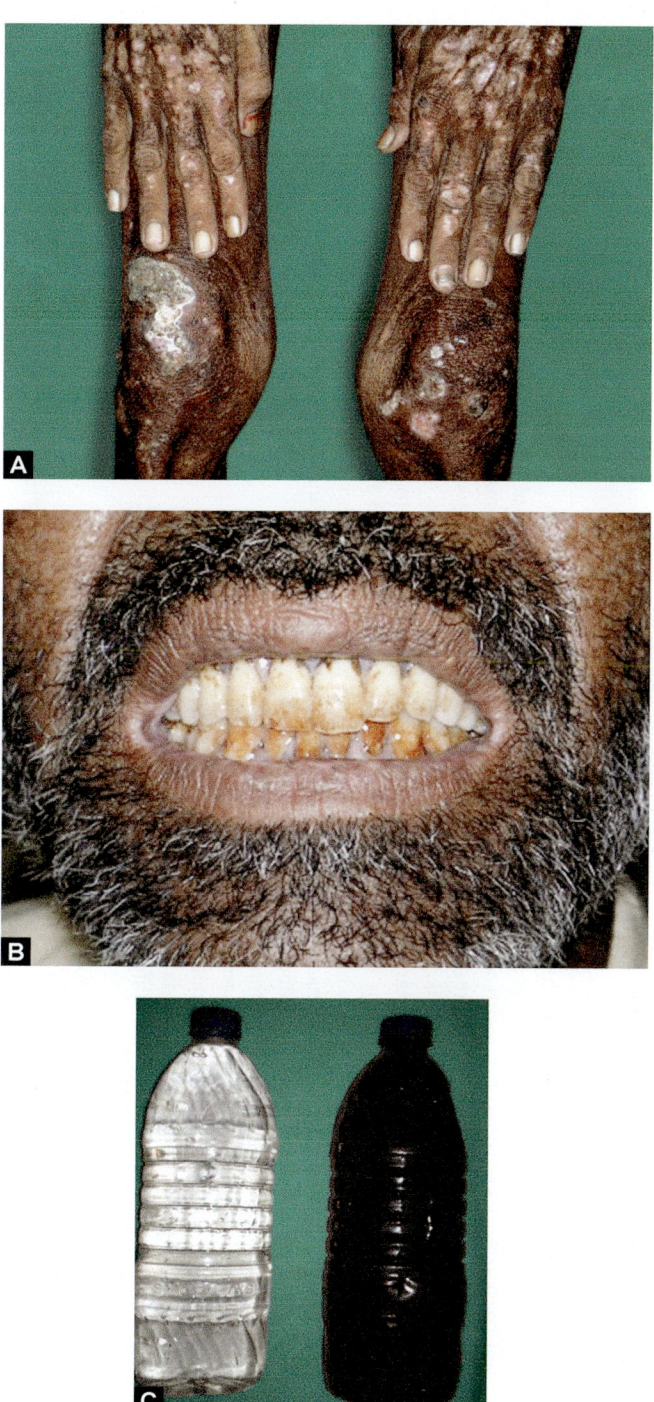

Fig. 9: Porphyria cutanea tarda (A) Hemorrhagic crusts, healing erosions, scarring, milia and hypertrichosis involving dorsa of hands and knees; (B) Yellowish-brown discoloration of teeth; (C) Reddish-black discoloration of urine.

TABLE 1: Differentiating features between various autoimmune vesiculobullous disorders.

Clinical features	Pemphigus Vulgaris	Pemphigus foliaceus	Paraneoplastic pemphigus	Bullous pemphigoid	Dermatitis herpetiformis	Linear IgA dermatosis (Adult)	Epidermolysis bullosa acquisita
Age group	40–60 years	Same as P. Vulgaris	45–70 years	Majority of cases in adults >60 years although may occur earlier	30–50 years	Peak onset in adults >60 years, but may occur any time after puberty	30–60 years
Cutaneous morphology	Flaccid blisters usually on normal skin. Superficial, painful erosions with little tendency to heal. (Fig. 1a) Nikolsky sign positive. Recurrent fresh lesions smaller and tense (Fig. 1d)	Small transient flaccid blisters which rupture very fast and so may not be found. Crusting, scaling and moist erosions predominate. May present as erythroderma (Fig. 10)	Polymorphous lesions. Presents with confluent erythema of the trunk, on which blisters and erosions form. Extremities may have lesions mimicking erythema multiforme. Clinical patterns may be of pemphigus, pemphigoid, exudative erythema multiforme, graft-versus-host disease (GVHD)-like and lichen planus-like	Prodromal nonbullous phase characterized by itching, urticated papules and excoriations may be present commonly. Bullous phase characterized by tense blisters (clear hemorrhagic fluid) on normal erythematous skin with or without urticarial papules, plaques and excoriations (Fig. 12)	Usually group of erythematous papule/small vesicles on erythematous base or areas of excoriations seen (Fig. 13)	The cutaneous bullae often have a distinctive symmetrical and grouped appearance. Vesicles present in an annular distribution that resembles a cluster of jewels (Fig. 14). Some patients may present with tense bullae similar to those in bullous pemphigoid	Tense vesicles, bulla and erosions on trauma-prone sites

Continued

Continued

TABLE 1: Differentiating features between various autoimmune vesiculobullous disorders.

Clinical features	Pemphigus Vulgaris	Pemphigus foliaceus	Paraneoplastic pemphigus	Bullous pemphigoid	Dermatitis herpetiformis	Linear IgA dermatosis (Adult)	Epidermolysis bullosa acquisita
Mucosal involvement	Oral lesions seen in almost all patients (i.e. 50–70%) and may be the first presentation (Fig. 2b). Involvement of pharynx, larynx, conjunctiva, esophagus, anus and genital mucosa have also been reported. Any stratified squamous mucosal surface may be involved	Oral lesions rarely present.	Oral lesions extensive and extremely painful and persistent (recalcitrant stomatitis); conjunctival, bronchial mucosal involvement common (Fig. 11)	Oral cavity involvement may be present in minority of cases but is usually of mild intensity. Other mucosae may also be rarely affected	Mucosal surfaces rarely involved	Oral, ocular, nasal mucosa may be involved	Mucosal lesions common (oral/conjunctival) common
Healing	Nonscarring, pigmentary changes common	Usually heals without scar, pigmentary changes frequent	Pigmentary changes and scarring (mucosal) may be present	Pigmentary changes and milia formation common	Scarring rare, pigmentary changes may be present	Scarring usually not seen, transient pigmentary changes occur	Healing with atrophic scars, milia formation and pigmentary changes

Continued

Continued

TABLE 1: Differentiating features between various autoimmune vesiculobullous disorders.

Clinical features	Pemphigus Vulgaris	Pemphigus foliaceus	Paraneoplastic pemphigus	Bullous pemphigoid	Dermatitis herpetiformis	Linear IgA dermatosis (Adult)	Epidermolysis bullosa acquisita
Common sites	Oral mucosa, scalp, face, axilla, groin, trunk	Seborrheic sites (later may be generalized)	Trunk, extremities, oral, ocular and other mucosal surfaces	Involvement of flexures, lower trunk and abdomen common	Symmetrical distribution over shoulders, lower back, buttocks, elbows, knees and scalp	Similar to dermatitis herpetiformis. In bullous pemphigoid like presentation, flexures and trunk mainly involved	Mucosa, extremities at trauma prone sites like knees, elbows, palms and soles
Associated symptoms	Itching may be associated	Itching may be present	Itching common	Itching of varying intensity may be commonly present	Intense itching with burning	Itching of variable intensity with burning	Some patients may have itching
Associated conditions	Myasthenia gravis, thymoma	None significant	Lymphoproliferative neoplasms, Waldenström's macroglobulinemia, thymoma, retroperitoneal sarcomas	Marginal increased risk of malignancy (gastrointestinal tract, urinary bladder, lymphoproliferative)	Gluten sensitive enteropathy, autoimmune diseases, lymphomas	Lympho-proliferative and autoimmune disorders	SLE, inflammatory bowel disease and other autoimmune disorders

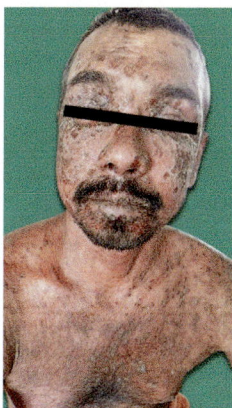

Fig. 10: Pemphigus foliaceus with scale crusts and moist erosions over face and trunk in a seborrheic pattern.

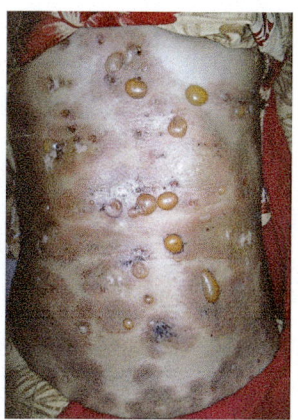

Fig. 11: Paraneoplastic pemphigus showing irregular confluent erythema with tense bullae over trunk.

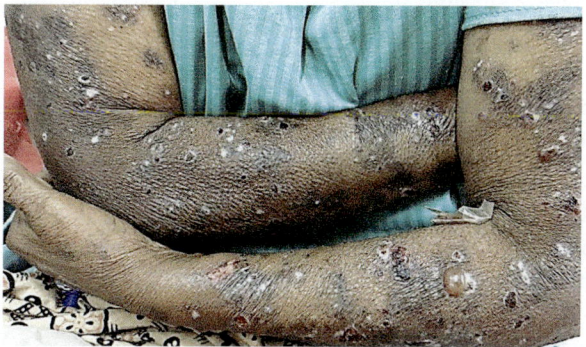

Fig. 12: Bullous pemphigoid: Tense bulla left forearm, erosions, hemorrhagic crusts and extensive prurigo like/excoriated lesions and lichenification seen over both upper limbs.
Courtesy: Dr Rishi Goyal, ESIPGIMSR, New Delhi.

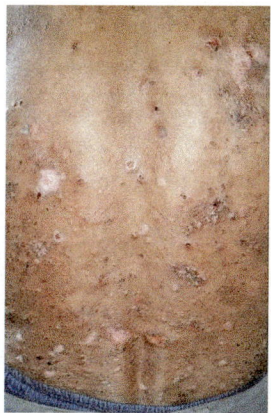

Fig. 13: Dermatitis herpetiformis having grouped excoriated papules present over back.

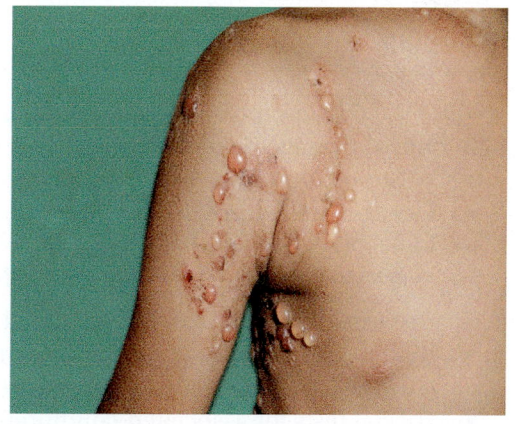

Fig. 14: Linear IgA disease adult having vesicles and bullae in annular configuration over arms and chest resembling string of pearls.
Courtesy: Dr Archana Lokhande, ESIPGIMSR, New Delhi.

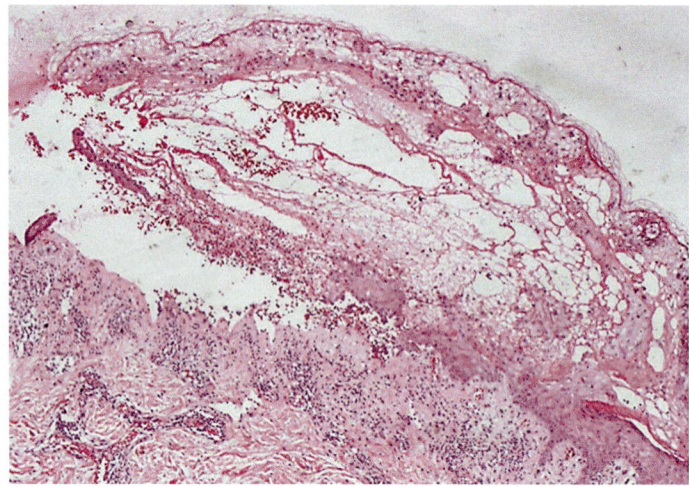

Fig. 15: Bullous pemphigoid: Subepidermal bullae filled with fibrin and inflammatory infiltrate consisting of RBC, lymphocytes and eosinophils.

Q.4 What investigations should be carried out to confirm the diagnosis and plan treatment?

Ans: Two major categories of investigations are called for:
1. To confirm the diagnosis
2. To plan and monitor treatment and to look for associated conditions.

To confirm diagnosis: If all facilities are available the following tests can be done:
- Bedside investigation
  - Tzanck smear.
- Skin biopsy
  - Hematoxylin and eosin examination
  - Direct immunofluorescence.
- Indirect immunofluorescence
- ELISA.

Tests listed below are only used for research purposes and have little relevance in routine management of patients:
- Western blotting, immunoprecipitation, immunoblotting
- Electron microscopy/immunoelectron microscopy
- Molecular diagnosis: Northern blot analysis, polymerase chain reaction, restriction fragment length polymorphism, epitope mapping analysis.

To plan treatment and look for associated conditions:
- Routine hematological, biochemical, radiological, electrocardiography and glucose-6-phosphate dehydrogenase (G6PD) levels
- Special tests for associated conditions: Potassium hydroxide (KOH) smear from skin and mucosal sites, bacterial cultures, antinuclear antibody, antithyroid microsomal antibodies; HLA-B8, DR3 and DQ2, serum IgA

autoantibodies to reticulin, gliadin and/or endomysium; iron and folate malabsorption studies and specific investigations for other systemic disorders and malignancies as per clinical clues.

Q.5 How can histopathological examination using light microscope help in diagnosis of vesiculobullous disease in middle age?

Ans: Histological findings provide a useful clue to differentiate between various types of vesiculobullous disorders by analyzing the following:
- Level of split-intraepidermal or subepidermal
  - Intraepidermal blisters: The clues can come on discerning various features of intraepidermal split
    - Site: Box 2 lists the site of split with common diseases
    - Mechanism of blister formation: The underlying mechanism of blister formation may be quite different in different diseases as can be seen in Box 3
    - Nature of inflammatory infiltrate: This may not be of great help in the diagnosis of intraepidermal blisters.
  - Subepidermal blisters
    - Mechanism of blister formation: It helps narrowing down the various disorders in which subepidermal blister is formed as can be seen in Box 4

BOX 2   Differentiating vesiculobullous disorders based on site of split.
- Intragranular zone: Pemphigus foliaceus, friction blister, impetigo
- Spinous zone: Allergic contact dermatitis, herpes infection
- Suprabasal: Pemphigus vulgaris, Hailey–Hailey disease

BOX 3   Differentiating vesiculobullous disorders based on mechanism of split.
- Spongiosis and intercellular edema: Allergic contact dermatitis, dyshidrotic dermatitis, some cases of erythema multiforme, Id reaction, insect bites
- Ballooning due to intracellular edema: Erythema multiforme, fixed drug eruption, herpes virus infections and irritant contact dermatitis
- Acantholysis due to dissolution of space between keratinocytes: Pemphigus group, Hailey–Hailey disease, Grover's disease

---

BOX 4   Differentiating vesiculobullous disorders based on mechanism of sub-epidermal split.
- Interface vacuolar dermatitis: Erythema multiforme, fixed drug eruption
- Secondary effects of immune complex deposits along dermoepidermal junction/dermal papilla: Bullous lupus erythematosus, dermatitis herpetiformis, linear IgA disease, bullous pemphigoid, pemphigoid gestationis
- Extensive papillary dermal edema: Polymorphous light eruption, sweet syndrome, allergic contact dermatitis

> **BOX 5   Differentiating vesiculobullous disorders based on inflammatory infiltrate.**
> - Lymphocytes: Erythema multiforme
> - Eosinophils: Bullous pemphigoid, pemphigoid gestationis, drug reactions, allergic contact dermatitis, insect bite (wedge shaped infiltrate), epidermolysis bullosa acquisita
> - Neutrophils: Dermatitis herpetiformis, adult linear IgA disease, bullous lupus erythematosus (also has nuclear dust with mucin in reticular dermis, presence of eosinophils essentially against the diagnosis of lupus erythematosus), epidermolysis bullosa acquisita
> - No/Scant inflammatory infiltrate: Porphyria cutanea tarda (also look for additional features like festooning of dermal papilla, presence of PAS-positive diastase-resistant fibrillar glycoprotein material in and around the upper dermal blood vessel walls and reduplication of the basement membrane)

– Nature of predominant inflammatory infiltrate: It may be very useful in differentiating between various causes of subepidermal blistering disorders which is described above in Box 5.
  o Both intraepidermal (spongiosis/ballooning) and subepidermal clefts: This can be found in important conditions like allergic contact dermatitis, herpes virus infections, bullous pemphigoid and erythema multiforme.

In situations like in the present patient who is likely a case of primary autoimmune bullous disorder, the histological findings which could be helpful in differentiating among the major autoimmune blistering diseases specially in the middle age is listed in Table 2.

Q.6   How does immunofluorescence help to differentiate further between primary autoimmune blistering diseases?

Ans: Nowadays immunofluorescence is considered to be the gold standard for the diagnosis of autoimmune diseases. Three types of immunofluorescence methods are used:
- Direct immunofluorescence (DIF) is the method to show the deposition of immunoreactants (in vivo bound autoantibodies) in skin or mucous membranes
- Indirect immunofluorescence (IIF) quantitates the respective circulating autoantibodies in the serum of the patient which are capable of binding to components of an epithelial specimen not from the patient
- Recent advances: Direct Immunofluorescence done on outer root sheath of telogen hair has been reported to be useful in the diagnosis of pemphigus vulgaris.

Immunofluorescence findings seen in autoimmune blistering disorders commonly presenting in middle age are listed in Table 3.

Q.7   Is there a role for electron microscopy and immune electron microscopy in blistering diseases?

Ans: Electron microscopy has been a great help in differentiating various forms of inherited epidermolysis bullosa where it was routinely used. This technique along with immune electron microscopy can be helpful in the various disorders (Tables 4 and 5) though at present, it is mainly used for research purposes only.

TABLE 2: Differentiating autoimmune blistering disorders on basis of histopathology.

Features	Pemphigus vulgaris	Pemphigus foliaceus	Paraneoplastic pemphigus	Bullous pemphigoid	Dermatitis herpetiformis	Linear IgA dermatosis	Epidermolysis bullosa acquisita
H and E findings	Suprabasal cleft with acantholysis (tombstone appearance); spongiosis; mixed perivascular chronic inflammatory infiltrate (Fig. 3b)	Intragranular/ subcorneal cleft with acantholysis and mixed perivascular inflammatory infiltrate	Suprabasal acantholysis, vacuolar interface dermatitis, dyskeratotic keratinocytes; superficial perivascular lymphocytic infiltrate	Eosinophilic spongiosis in early cases, subepidermal blistering with predominant eosinophilic dermal infiltrate. (Fig. 15)	Subepidermal vesicle with neutrophilic microabscesses in dermal papilla (Fig. 16)	Subepidermal blister with mixed papillary/ perivascular infiltrate with neutrophils and eosinophils	Subepidermal blister with minimal inflammatory infiltrate

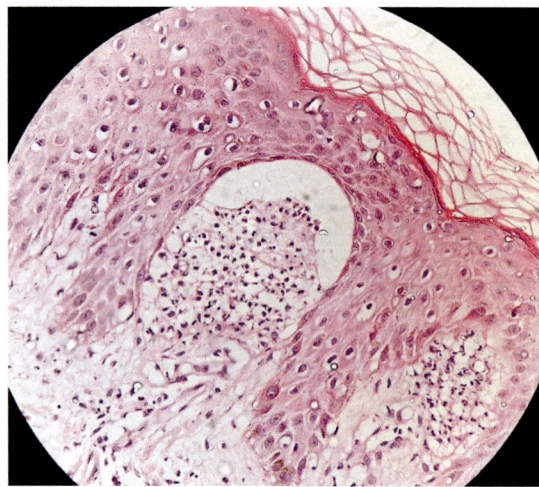

Fig. 16: Dermatitis herpetiformis: There is a characteristic focal collection of neutrophils forming a neutrophilic microabscess at the tip of the dermal papillae with a subepidermal cleft.

Q.8 How does ELISA test help in vesiculobullous disorders?

Ans: Specific ELISA assays may be used to detect antibodies in specific blistering diseases as mentioned in Table 6.
- Recent advances: Detection of desmoglein 3 IgG in saliva by ELISA shows good sensitivity and titers correlate with the oral disease activity in pemphigus vulgaris.

Q.9 What are the different types of pemphigus that one comes across in clinical practice?

Ans: Pemphigus is a group of chronic autoimmune disorders with different clinical forms, histopathology, immune reactant deposits and associations. They can be briefly described as follows:

Classical Types

Pemphigus Vulgaris Group
- Pemphigus vulgaris has already been described in details in the text above
- Pemphigus vegetans: Characterized by flaccid blisters and vegetative papillomatous proliferation mainly in the flexures. Cerebriform changes can be detected in the tongue of the affected patients. Two subtypes were initially described—the Neumann type (initial bullous lesions like pemphigus vulgaris) and the Hallopeau type (initial pustular lesions; benign course) which differ in clinical course and prognosis.

Pemphigus Foliaceus Group
- Pemphigus foliaceus: The salient features of this disease has been summarized in Tables 1, 2 and 3

TABLE 3: Differentiating autoimmune blistering disorders on basis of immunofluorescence.

Features	Pemphigus vulgaris*	Pemphigus foliaceus	Paraneoplastic pemphigus	Bullous pemphigoid	Dermatitis herpetiformis	Linear IgA disease	Epidermolysis bullosa acquisita
Direct Immuno-fluorescence	Intercellular IgG deposit throughout epidermis wiry/fishnet appearance (Fig. 3c)	Same as pemphigus vulgaris but fluorescence predominantly in superficial layers of epidermis	Intercellular IgG and C3 deposition. Linear C3 +/− IgG deposit can be seen at dermoepidermal junction in some patients	Linear continuous deposit of C3 and IgG along basement membrane zone. (Fig. 17)	IgA deposition in dermal papilla (granular pattern) (Fig. 18)	Linear IgA at basement membrane zone. Sometimes linear IgM, IgG and C3 deposits may also be seen (Fig. 19)	IgG and C3 at basement membrane zone (linear pattern)
Indirect immuno-fluorescence	Circulating IgG against keratinocyte surface in >80% patients; titers correlate with disease activity	Same as pemphigus vulgaris	Same as pemphigus vulgaris; antibodies also against columnar and transitional epithelium as IgG autoantibodies are directed against desmoplakin I and II which are present in stratified squamous epithelium and these other tissues	Antibasement zone IgG (upto 70% patients). Additional circulating autoantibodies of IgA, IgE and IgM can also be found	Routinely negative	Antibasement membrane IgA autoantibodies in serum in some cases	Antibasement zone IgG (30–50% patients). IIF most reliable methods of diagnosing EBA using 1M-NaCl split skin as a substrate. The immunoreactants can be seen in floor. of the split skin

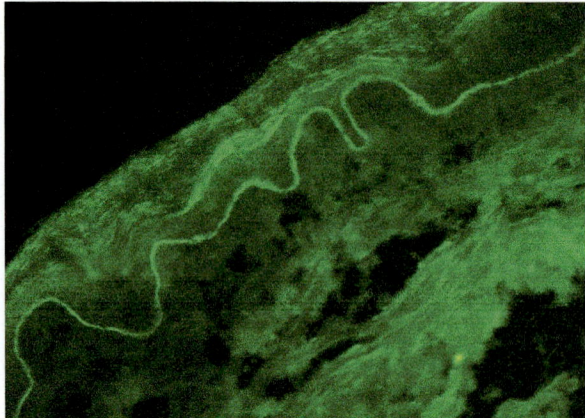

Fig. 17: Bullous pemphigoid: Direct immunofluorescence test reveals linear continuous deposits of C3 and IgG at basement membrane zone.

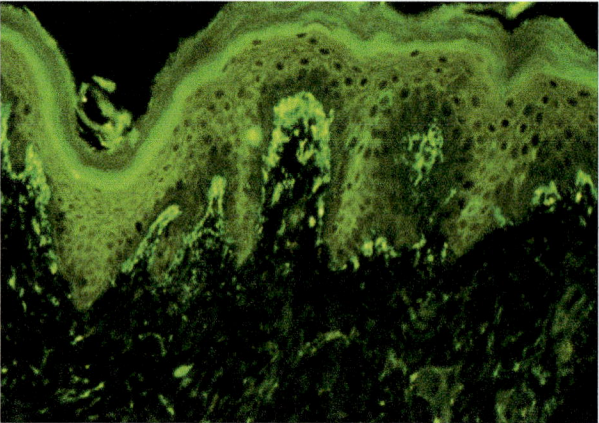

Fig. 18: Dermatitis herpetiformis: Direct immunofluorescence (DIF) test reveals presence of granular deposition of IgA at the tip of the dermal papillae.

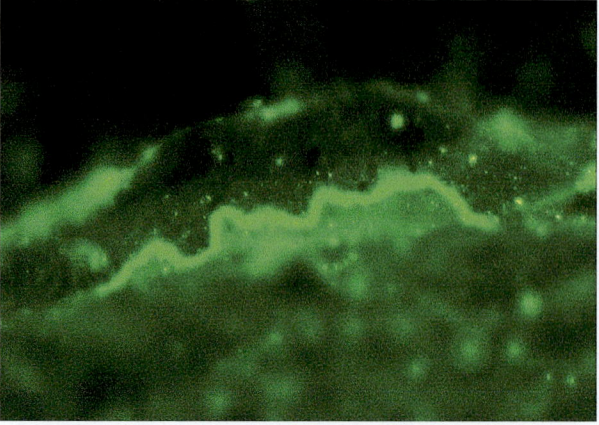

Fig. 19: Linear IgA disease : Direct immunofluorescence (DIF) test shows linear deposition of IgA along the basement membrane zone (BMZ).

TABLE 4: Electron microscopy for vesiculobullous disorders.

Disease	Electron microscopy features
Pemphigus vulgaris	Loss of the desmosomes preceded by a condensation of the tonofilaments and their separation from the desmosomes
Pemphigoid Gestationis	Basal cell degeneration, basement membrane zone split through lamina lucida
Bullous pemphigoid	Basement membrane zone dissolution through lamina lucida, mid basal cell degeneration, occasional lamina densa duplication/destruction
Epidermolysis bullosa acquisita	Dissolution of anchoring fibrils, basement membrane zone split below lamina densa, occasional through lamina lucida
Linear IgA disease	Split within lamina densa or beneath basal lamina as in dermatitis herpetiformis
Dermatitis herpetiformis	Neutrophilic abscess in dermal papilla; dissolution of tip of dermal papilla with split below basement membrane zone

TABLE 5: Immune electron microscopy for vesiculobullous disorders.

Disease	Immune electron microscopy features
Pemphigus vulgaris	IgG and C3 deposits over cell membrane of keratinocytes
Pemphigoid Gestationis	C3 and IgG in lamina lucida
Bullous pemphigoid	C3 and IgG in lamina lucida
Epidermolysis bullosa acquisita	IgG, C3, IgA, IgM in lower lamina densa and sub-lamina densa/anchoring fibrils
Linear IgA disease	IgA is detected at lamina lucida, lamina densa/sublamina densa, or both
Dermatitis herpetiformis	IgA and occasionally C3 on dermal microfibrils/elastic bundles in dermal papilla

TABLE 6: Enzyme-linked immunosorbent assay for vesiculobullous disorders.

Disease	EM features
Pemphigus vulgaris	IgG autoantibodies to desmoglein 1 (50%) and 3 (>90%). ELISA assays can monitor disease activity
Paraneoplastic pemphigus	IgG autoantibodies to envoplakin and periplakin besides other components
Bullous pemphigoid (BP)	ELISA using portions of BP180-specific and sensitive (70–98%); ELISA using BP 230 recombinant proteins-detect circulating autoantibodies in up to 5–10% of anti-BP 180-negative patients
Epidermolysis bullosa acquisita	Anti-type VII collagen autoantibodies. Serum levels correlate with the disease activity in patients
Dermatitis herpetiformis	Anti-tissue transglutaminase antibody, antiepidermal transglutaminase antibody

- Pemphigus erythematosus (localized): Considered as a localized form of pemphigus foliaceus characterized by scaly erythematous plaques with crust and erosions present predominantly over the malar region of face and other seborrheic sites. It has similar features as in Pemphigus foliaceus histologically and on immunofluorescence. In addition it may have circulating antinuclear antibodies similar to lupus erythematosus.

Nonclassical Types

Pemphigus Herpetiformis
It presents as erythematous annular plaques with grouped vesicles, blisters, erosions and crusts in a herpetiform pattern.

IgA Pemphigus
Flaccid vesicles and pustules overlying normal to erythematous skin coalesce to form an annular pattern with central crusting. Two subtypes—subcorneal pustular dermatosis (SPD) type and the intraepidermal neutrophilic (IEN) described.

Paraneoplastic Pemphigus
The features of paraneoplastic pemphigus have been already described. A new terminology "paraneoplastic autoimmune multiorgan syndrome (PAMS)" was coined for this type of pemphigus to highlight the involvement of multiple organs (kidney, lung etc.) in the disease.

Dyshidrosiform Pemphigus
It has pompholyx-like presentation with vesiculobullous lesions present on palms and soles.

Drug Induced Pemphigus
The main classes of drugs implicated are the thiol group (D-penicillamine, captopril), phenol group (rifampicin, cefadroxil) and non-thiol, non-phenol group (calcium channel blockers, angiotensin-converting enzyme inhibitors).

Q.10 What are the treatment options available in pemphigus vulgaris patients?

Ans. Broadly the aim of treatment in pemphigus vulgaris is to quickly control the disease activity (induction) followed by disease remission while attempting to minimize the side-effects of drugs. In the Indian scenario, goal of treatment has been to achieve permanent remission of the disease effectively leading to a cure by using pulse therapy combining different medications.

As per the consensus statement by the American Academy of Dermatology, the disease is under control when new lesions stop forming and the existing ones start to heal. This can be the beginning of consolidation phase. The end of consolidation phase is considered when no new lesions have developed for a minimum of 2 weeks, approximately 80% of lesions have healed and when most clinicians start to taper steroids. The patient then could be either in complete remission off therapy where absence of new or established lesions are present while the patient is off all systemic therapy for at least 2 months or could be in complete remission on therapy when absence of new or established lesions are there while the patient is receiving minimal therapy.

Therapeutic Management

General Principles
It includes adequate care of the hygiene, nutritional status and patient support.

Specific Therapy

First-line treatment
Systemic corticosteroids form the mainstay of treatment; however, the dosage and the duration varies from patient to patient. Following are some of the recent guidelines which could be helpful in guiding the treatment (Table 7).

Intravenous steroid pulse therapy
Pulse therapy refers to administration of large (suprapharmacologic) doses of drugs in an intermittent manner to enhance the therapeutic effects and reduce the side-effects. In pemphigus, use of following regimes of pulse therapy with their modifications have been documented:
- Dexamethasone-cyclophosphamide pulse (DCP): In this classic regimen, dexamethasone is given in a dose of 100 mg in 5% dextrose as a slow

TABLE 7: Treatment regimens for pemphigus vulgaris.

Oral steroid therapy	British guidelines, 2017	European Dermatology Forum guidelines, 2015
Starting dose of prednisolone	1 mg/kg/day in most cases	0.5–1.5 mg/kg/day
Increments	50–100% dose increments in 5–7 days if blistering continues	Dose could be increased up to 2 mg/kg/day if control not achieved in 2 weeks
Dose tapering once remission is induced and maintained	Taper daily dose by 5–10 mg every 2 weeks down to 20 mg daily followed by 2.5 mg every 2–4 weeks down to 10 mg daily (minimal therapy). Then the dose could be reduced slowly in increments of 1 mg	Taper daily dose by 25% bi-weekly till 20 mg daily, then proceed slowly
Dose modification in relapse	<ul><li>Going back to last dose at which control was there with 50% increments till control achieved</li><li>Consider adding adjuvant/changing existing adjuvant (if treatment failure criteria met of sufficient dose for 3 months)</li></ul>	Go two steps back in previous dose until control of the lesions is achieved within two weeks, then resume gradual decrease of systemic corticosteroids. If disease control is not reached go back to initial dose:<ul><li>Consider first line adjuvants if steroids given alone</li><li>Change in first line adjuvant/addition if second line adjuvant if already on steroid sparing drugs</li></ul>
Intravenous steroid pulse therapy	Consider in cases where >1 mg/kg/day oral prednisolone is required or as initial treatment in severe disease/in recalcitrant disease	No additional benefit of intravenous corticosteroid pulse

intravenous infusion over 2 hours for three consecutive days along with cyclophosphamide 500 mg infusion on one of the days. Cyclophosphamide 50 mg/day is given orally on the remaining days. It has four phases (induction, consolidation, remission, surveillance)
- Dexamethasone-azathioprine pulse (DAP): Here daily cyclophosphamide is replaced by 50 mg of azathioprine and there is no bolus adjuvant. It is recommended for unmarried patients as azathioprine does not cause gonadal toxicity
- Dexamethasone-methotrexate pulse (DMP): In this regimen cyclophosphamide is replaced by methotrexate in the dose of 7.5 mg/kg/week. It is recommended for patients not responding to DCP/DAP after 12 pulses in phase 1.

Immunosuppressive Adjuvants

They can be considered in refractory cases or as steroid-sparing agents at the start of therapy, particularly in cases of increased risk of corticosteroid therapy, complications due to expected prolonged use (>4 months) or dose dependency above minimal therapy (>10 mg/day).

First-line adjuvants:
- Azathioprine (1–3 mg/kg/day)
- Mycophenolate mofetil (2 g/day)
- Rituximab (2 × 1 g intravenous infusion 2 weeks apart; or 4 × 375 mg/m^2 infusions each 1 week apart) (British guidelines, 2017)

Second-line adjuvants:
- Intravenous immunoglobulins (IVIG, 2 g/kg/cycle)
- Immunoadsorption (2 cycles on 4 consecutive days, 4 weeks apart)
- Cyclophosphamide (500 mg as intravenous bolus or given orally at 2 mg/kg/day)
- Methotrexate (10–20 mg/week)
- Plasmapheresis (British guidelines only)
- Dapsone 100 mg/day or up to ≤1.5 mg/kg/day. (European Dermatology Forum guidelines only).

Management of Oral Lesions

Use of antiseptic mouthwash, local analgesic gel, topical potent steroids, intralesional steroids are few of the measures to accelerate healing. Maintenance of proper oral hygiene should be emphasized.

Q.11 When do you label a patient as a case of treatment failure?

Ans: There will be a subset of patients where there is a failure to control disease activity (relapse/flare) even with full therapeutic dose of various systemic drugs which include:
- 3 weeks of therapy on 1.5 mg/kg/day prednisone
- 12 weeks of 2 mg/kg/day cyclophosphamide
- 12 weeks of 2.5 mg/kg/day azathioprine
- 12 weeks of 20 mg/week methotrexate
- 12 weeks of 3 g/day of mycophenolate mofetil.

Q.12 What are the possible complications of this disorder?

Ans: The complications from pemphigus group of disorders are mainly related to high dosage of immunosuppressants used in the therapy.
- Secondary infection due to widespread erosions may lead to septicemia
- Adrenal suppression, cushingoid morphology, hypertension, fluid retention, bone mineral density (BMD) decline, diabetes, peptic ulcers, cataracts, glaucoma, increased susceptibility to infections and reactivation of tuberculosis due to long term corticosteroid use. There have been reports of deep vein thrombosis and pulmonary embolism arising due to the use of high-dose corticosteroids
- Bone marrow suppression due to the immunosuppressive agents may occur after a variable period of their use. It may be related to dosage of drugs used or in cases like azathioprine to the level of activity of thiopurine methyltransferase (TPMT) in an individual and can occur within weeks of institution of therapy
- Malignancies like leukemia, lymphomas, bladder carcinoma (in particular with cyclophosphamide), or of skin, liver, lungs and kidneys, etc. appear to increase with immunosuppressive medications used either alone or in combination. As these complications have been reported months to years after the use and even withdrawal of immunosuppressives, direct causal relationship is sometimes hard to establish
- Guidelines for individual immunosuppressive drugs should be followed for monitoring their use in pemphigus or for that matter in any immunosuppressive responsive dermatoses.

Q.13 How is the disease monitored?

Ans: Monitoring can be done by clinical examination and follow up of these patients. Cessation of appearance of new lesions and healing of existing erosions are useful clinical guide to assess the disease activity. Serological monitoring of disease activity can be done either by IIF or by sequential ELISA at 3 month interval.

CONCLUSION

A methodical step wise approach to a patient presenting with vesiculobullous disorders will usually lead to a correct diagnosis in majority of patients just on the basis of a good history and clinical examination along with some bed side procedures. In case of the autoimmune blistering group of disorders, an adequate biopsy subjected to both routine histopathology and direct immunofluorescence becomes mandatory. Serological investigations assist in determining disease activity in few of these disorders which will help in formulating proper treatment protocols. In disorders requiring long-term immunosuppressive therapy, timely monitoring of anticipated complications will prevent undesirable morbidity and mortality while ensuring disease control.

KEY POINTS

- Vesiculobullous disorders are an important group of dermatoses and require considerable clinical expertise for correct diagnose and appropriate management
- A diagnosis of pemphigus vulgaris should always be considered in a middle aged patient who presents with flaccid vesicles and bullae in skin, usually associated with painful oral erosions
- Simple bed side investigation, like demonstrating Tzanck cells in a Giemsa stain smear greatly help making provisional diagnosis
- Histopathology typically shows suprabasal cleft, row of tombstone appearance of basal layer and acantholytic cells
- Direct immunofluorescence shows deposition of immunoglobulins in "fishnet pattern" and is considered the gold standard tool for the diagnosis: Indirect immunofluorescence and demonstration of desmoglein 1 and 3 by ELISA are other useful diagnostic tools
- Systemic corticosteroids, in moderate to high doses (1–2 mg/kg/day, prednisolone equivalent), need to be used for a fairly long time depending on the severity to control the disease activity
- Use of suprapharmacological doses (pulse therapy, using dexamethasone or methyl prednisolone) have also been used very successfully in Indian studies
- A close monitoring to look for the adverse effects of corticosteroids, particularly the flare of infections like tuberculosis, metabolic complications and osteoporosis and bone necrosis should be done
- The use of steroid sparing agents, as an adjuvant, helps to reduce the cumulative dose and duration of corticosteroid administration and may help ensuring effective disease control and enhance safety
- Rituximab, a monoclonal antibody against CD20, that targets B-cells, is the latest advance in the therapy of refractory and recalcitrant pemphigus; however, the high cost of the therapy, is an important limitation for its routine use.

SUGGESTED READING

1. Abraham A, Roga G, Job AM. Pulse therapy in pemphigus: Ready reckoner. Indian J Dermatol. 2016;61:314-7.
2. Ackerman AB. An algorithmic method for diagnosis that employs pattern analysis. In: Ackerman AB, Böer A, Bennin B et al. Histologic diagnosis of inflammatory skin diseases, an algorithmic method based on pattern analysis. 3rd edn., New York: Ardor Scribendi; 2005.P.301-45.
3. Ahmed AR, Blose DA. Pemphigus vegetans. Neumann type and hallopeau type. Int J Dermatol. 1984;23:135-41.
4. Alonso-Llamazares J, Gibson LE, Rogers RS 3rd. Clinical, pathologic and immunopathologic features of dermatitis herpetiformis: Rreview of the Mayo Clinic experience. Int J Dermatol. 2007;46:910-19.
5. Amagai M, Komai A., Hashimoto T, et al. Usefulness of enzyme-linked immunosorbent assay using recombinant desmogleins 1 and 3 for serodiagnosis of pemphigus. Br J Dermatol. 1999;140(2):351-7.
6. Arya SR, Valand AG, Krishna K. A clinico-pathological study of 70 cases of pemphigus. Indian J Dermatol Venereol Leprol. 1999;65:168-71.
7. Atzmony L, Hodak E, Leshem YA, et al. The role of adjuvant therapy in pemphigus: Aa systematic review and meta-analysis. J Am Acad Dermatol. 2015;73(2):264-71.

8. Bernard P, Borradori L. Pemphigoid Group. In: Bolognia JL, Jorizzo JL, Schaffer JV (eds). Dermatology. 3rd ed. Elsevier Saunders, Philadelphia (USA). 2012; pp. 475-90.
9. Beutner EH, Chorzelski TP, Jablonska S. Immunofluorescence tests: Clinical significance of sera and skin in bullous diseases. Int J Dermatol. 1985;24:405-21.
10. Bickle KM, Roark TR, Hsu S. Autoimmune bullous dermatoses: A review. Am Fam Physician. 2002;65:1861-70.
11. Bonciolini V, Bonciani D, Verdelli A, et al. Newly described clinical and immunopathological feature of dermatitis herpetiformis. Clin Dev Immunol. 2012;2012:967974.2012; doi: 10.1155/2012/967974.
12. Brenner S, Srebrnik A, Goldberg I. Pemphigus can be induced by topical phenol as well as by foods and drugs that contain phenols or thiols. J Cosmet Dermatol. 2003;2:161-5.
13. Bressan AL, Silva RS, Fontenelle E, et al. Bressan Aline Lopes, Silva Roberto Souto da, Fontenelle Elisa, Gripp Alexandre Carlos. Immunosuppressive agents in Dermatology. An. Bras. Dermatol. 2010;85(1):9-22.
14. Chorzelski TP, Jablonska S, Maciejowska E. Linear IgA bullous dermatosis of adults. Clin Dermatol. 1991;9(3):383-92.
15. Cullen DR Genetic features of familial benign pemphigus. Br J Dermatol. 1965;77:20-3.
16. Cummins DL, Mimouni D, Anhalt GJ, et al. Oral cyclophosphamide for treatment of pemphigus vulgaris and foliaceus. J Am Acad Dermatol. 2003;49:276-80.
17. Daneshpazhooh M, Asgari M, Naraghi ZS, et al. A study on plucked hair as a substrate for direct immunofluorescence in pemphigus vulgaris. J Eur Acad Dermatol Venereol. 2009;23:129-31.
18. Düker I, Schaller J, Rose C, et al. Subcorneal pustular dermatosis-type IgA pemphigus with autoantibodies to desmocollins 1, 2, and 3. Arch Dermatol. 2009;145:1159-62.
19. Ertz-Archambault N, Kosiorek H, Taylor GE, et al. Association of therapy for autoimmune disease with myelodysplastic syndromes and acute myeloid leukemia. JAMA Oncol. 2017;3(7):936-43.
20. Fernandes JC, Dharan JB. Study of 100 cases of pemphigus. Indian J Dermatol Venerol Leprol. 1970;36:1-11.
21. Fleischli ME, Valek RH, Pandya AG. Pulse intravenous cyclophosphamide therapy in pemphigus. Arch Dermatol. 1999;135(1):57-61.
22. Georgi M, Jainta S, Bröcker EB, et al. Autoantigens of subepidermal bullous autoimmune dermatoses. Hautarzt. 2001;52:1079-89.
23. Gharami RC, Kumar P, Mondal A, et al. Dyshidrosiform pemphigus vulgaris: Report of an unusual case. Dermatol Online J. 2010;16:10.
24. Giurdanella F, Diercks GF, Jonkman MF, et al. Laboratory diagnosis of pemphigus: Direct immunofluorescence remains the gold standard. Br J Dermatol. 2016;175:185-6.
25. Hallaji Z, Mortazavi H, Lajevardi V, et al. Serum and salivary desmoglein 1 and 3 enzyme-linked immunosorbent assay in pemphigus vulgaris: correlation with phenotype and severity. J Eur Acad Dermatol Venereol 2010;24(3):275-80.
26. Hallel-Halevy D, Nadelman C, Chen M, et al. Epidermolysis bullosa acquisita: Update and review. Clin Dermatol. 2001;19:712-8.
27. Harman KE, Brown D, Exton LS, et al. British Association of Dermatologists. Guidelines for the management of pemphigus vulgaris 2017. Br J Dermatol. 2017;177(5):1170-1201.
28. Hertl M, Jedlickova H, Karpati S, et al. Pemphigus. S2 Guideline for diagnosis and treatment – guided by the European Dermatology Forum (EDF) in cooperation with the European Academy of Dermatology and Venereology (EADV). J Eur Acad Dermatol Venereol. 2015;29:405-14.
29. Hull C, Stratman E, Ofori AO. Approach to the patient with cutaneous blisters. UpToDate [Internet]. 2017. Available from: at https://www.uptodate.com/contents/approach-to-the-patient-with-cutaneous-blisters accessed on 20.1.2018.
30. Korman N. Pemphigus. J Am Acad Dermatol. 1988;18:1219-38.
31. Li-Kai Lo LK, Hung CM, Chen YF, et al. Azathioprine-induced severe bone marrow toxicity - A report of 3 cases. Dermatol Sinica. 2009;27:44-51.
32. Lionel FRY. Dermatitis herpetiformis: problems, progress and prospects. Eur J Dermatol. 2002;12: 523-31.

33. Murrell DF, Dick S, Ahmed AR, et al. Consensus statement on definitions of disease end points and therapeutic response for pemphigus. J Am Acad Dermatol. 2008;58:1043-6.
34. Ohata C, Koga H, Teye K, et al. Concurrence of bullous pemphigoid and herpetiform pemphigus with IgG antibodies to desmogleins 1/3 and desmocollins 1-3. Br J Dermatol. 2013;168(4):879-81.
35. Pasricha JS. Current regimen of pulse therapy for pemphigus: Minor modifications, improved results. Indian J Dermatol Venereol Leprol 2008;74:217-21.
36. Porro AM, Caetano L de VN, Maehara L de SN, et al. Non-classical forms of pemphigus: Pemphigus herpetiformis, IgA pemphigus, paraneoplastic pemphigus and IgG/IgA pemphigus. Anais Brasileiros de Dermatologia. 2014;89(1):96-106.
37. Radis CD, Kahl LE, Baker GL, et al. " Effects of cyclophosphamide on the development of malignancy and on long-term survival of patients with rheumatoid arthritis. A 20-year follow up study." Arthritis Rheum. 1995;38:1120-7.
38. Schmidt E, Zillikens D. Research in practice: diagnosis of subepidermal autoimmune bullous disorders. J Dtsch Dermatol Ges. 2009;7:296-300.
39. Valia RA, Ramesh V, Jerajani HR. Blistering Disorders. In: Valia RG, editor, Valia AR (eds). IADVL Textbook of Dermatology. 3rd ed. India: Bhalani Publishing House;. 2010;1087-152.
40. Venning VA. Linear IgA disease: Clinical presentation, diagnosis, and pathogenesis. Immunol Allergy Clin North Am. 2012;32(2):245-53.
41. Weaver JL. Establishing the carcinogenic risk of immunomodulatory drugs. toxicologic pathology. 2011;40(2):267-71.
42. Wieczorek M, Czernik A. Paraneoplastic pemphigus: Aa short review. Clinical, Cosmetic and Investigational Dermatology. 2016;9:291-5.
43. Wojnarowska F, Marsden RA, Bhogal B, et al. Chronic bullous disease of childhood, childhood cicatricial pemphigoid, and linear IgA disease of adults. A comparative study demonstrating clinical and immunopathologic overlap. J Am Acad Dermatol. 1988;19:792-805.
44. Zakka LB, Shetty SS, Ahmed AR. Rituximab in the treatment of pemphigus vulgaris. Dermatol Ther. 2012;2(1):17. doi: 10.1007/s13555-012-0017-3. Epub 2012 Nov 15.

CHAPTER 10

Erythroderma

Vijay P Zawar, Shrikant Kumavat

■ INTRODUCTION

Erythroderma is an inflammatory disorder characterized by generalized redness and scaling of skin affecting >90% of the body surface area.

In India incidence of erythroderma is 35 per 100,000 dermatologic patients. Male predominance is seen with mean age between 40 and 60 years.

It is a disorder with significant morbidity which, may develop serious complications such as cardiac failure, thermodysregulation and hypoproteinemia. This condition may become fatal in the absence of timely intervention. There are several etiologies; thus, a proper history and good clinical examination is important to establish the causative factor in order to provide specific treatment.

CASE REPORT

A 65-year-old male patient presented to us with scaling and redness involving skin of whole body. The rash started 3 weeks back over right leg which then gradually became generalized. Itching was moderate. On further enquiry patient revealed that he had scaly plaques over both the limbs for which he was applying some topical herbal medicine intermittently. Physical examination showed large scales and erythema over trunk (Fig. 1), arms and legs. Palms and soles showed (Fig. 2) severe sloughing of epidermis. Inguinal lymph nodes were grossly enlarged. Mild hepatomegaly was noted. Baseline investigations showed hemoglobin to be 10 g/dL (microcytosis, hypochromia), decreased serum albumin and raised erythrocyte sedimentation rate (ESR). Liver function test, renal function test, X-ray chest and ultrasonography were normal. Biopsy confirmed psoriatic pathology.

Patient was admitted and intravenous fluids were started. He was prescribed oral methotrexate 7.5 mg every week along with antihistaminics. White petroleum jelly was applied over the body twice a day. Patient responded well and was discharged in 2 weeks.

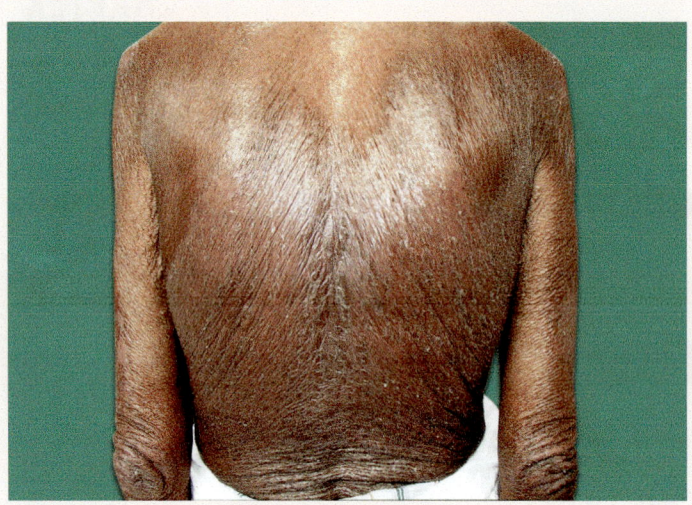

Fig. 1: Large scales and erythema over trunk.

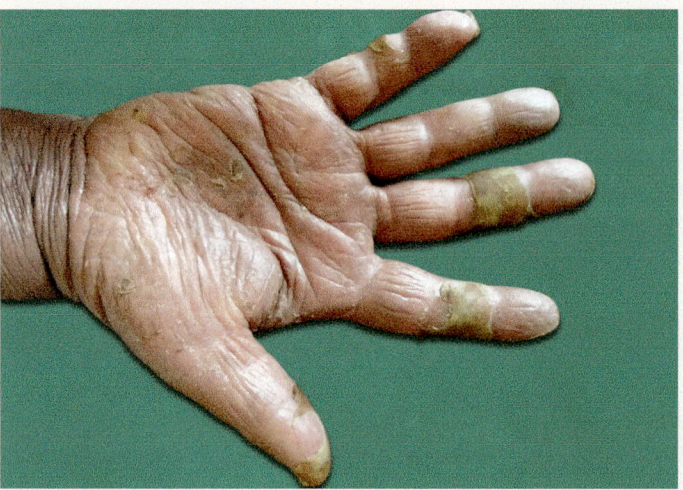

Fig. 2: Palm showing severe sloughing of epidermis.

INTERACTIVE TOPIC REVIEW

Q.1 **What are the different causes of erythroderma?**

Ans: When erythroderma occurs because of underlying systemic diseases or drugs, it is called as primary erythroderma; however, if it occurs because of pre-existing skin diseases it is called as secondary erythroderma.

Some of the important causes of erythroderma are given below:
- Infections:
  - Dermatophytosis
  - Candidiasis
  - Human immunodeficiency virus infection
  - Norwegian scabies.
- Keratinization disorders:
  - Eczema
  - Psoriasis
  - Pityriasis rubra pilaris
  - Ichthyosiform erythroderma.
- Bullous dermatoses:
  - Pemphigus foliaceus
  - Paraneoplastic pemphigus
  - Bullous pemphigoid.
- Drug induced
- Dermatitis:
  - Atopic dermatitis
  - Stasis dermatitis
  - Contact dermatitis
- Malignancies:
  - Cutaneous T-cell lymphoma
  - Hodgkin's disease
  - Leukemias.
- Idiopathic.

Q.2 What are most common causes of erythroderma?

Ans: According to incidence most common causes of erythroderma are:
- Idiopathic – 30%
- Drug allergy – 28%
- Lymphoma and leukemia – 14%
- Atopic dermatitis – 10%
- Psoriasis – 8%
- Contact dermatitis – 3%
- Seborrheic dermatitis – 2%.

Q.3 Can erythroderma occur in neonates? What are the common causes?

Ans: Yes, erythroderma can occur in neonates also. Some of the common causes of erythroderma in neonates are given below:
- Atopic dermatitis
- Congenital bullous and nonbullous ichthyosiform erythroderma
- Congenital syphilis
- Leiner's disease
- Infantile seborrheic dermatitis
- Widespread candidiasis.

Q.4 What are the triggering factors of erythroderma in psoriasis?

Ans: Triggering factors of erythroderma in psoriasis are application of irritants such as tar, salicylic acid and dithranol over plaques of psoriasis. Sudden withdrawal of topical as well as systemic steroids in patients of psoriasis may lead to erythroderma. Overdose of phototherapy and emotional stress also precipitate erythroderma.

Q.5 What are the clinical clues to diagnose psoriatic erythroderma?

Ans: History of psoriatic plaques somewhere on body before the onset of redness and scaling is many a times a clue to psoriatic etiology. Common nail changes associated with psoriasis patients like oil drop sign, pitting of nails, subungual hyperkeratosis and history of joint pain are important clues for the diagnosis of erythrodermic psoriasis.

Q.6 Which are the common drugs causing erythroderma?

Ans: Drug induced erythroderma is a relatively common variety. Commonly implicated drugs are:
- Phenylbutazone
- Hydantoin derivatives
- Carbamazepine
- Cimetidine
- Gold salts
- Lithium.

Q.7 What are the clinical features of drug-induced erythroderma?

Ans: Drug-induced erythroderma begins as morbilliform or scarlatiniform exanthem. Edema over the ankles and feet is common. It generally resolves within 2–6 weeks after stopping responsible drug.

Q.8 What is idiopathic erythroderma?

Ans: When no primary cause of erythroderma is found after clinical examination and laboratory investigations it is called as idiopathic erythroderma. It is also called as Red man syndrome which is a triad of palmoplantar keratoderma, dermopathic lymphadenopathy and raised serum immunoglobulin E (IgE). Idiopathic erythroderma has a chronic course as compared to other types of erythroderma.

Q.9 What are the nail changes seen in erythroderma?

Ans: Nail changes are seen in 40% of patients with erythroderma. Nails become shiny due to continuous rubbing of nails over the skin by patients because of pruritus. Also, there is a discoloration, brittleness, dullness, subungual hyperkeratosis, Beau's lines, paronychia and splinter hemorrhages can be seen in erythroderma. Nails can be totally shed in erythroderma.

Q.10 What is nose sign?

Ans: Sparing of nose and paranasal areas in erythroderma is called as nose sign or Pavithran sign.

Q.11 What are systemic manifestations of erythroderma?

Ans: Systems which may be involved in patients of erythroderma are shown in Table 1.

TABLE 1: Systems involved in erythroderma.	
System involved	Clinical features
Integumentary system	• Redness over skin • Itching and scaling over skin
Thermoregulatory system	• Chills and shivering
Cardiovascular system	• Tachycardia • Shortness of breath and easy fatigability
Urinary system	• Oliguria • Edema over feet
Digestive system	• Hepatomegaly • Splenomegaly
Lymphatic system	• Lymphadenopathy

Q.12 What laboratory findings are seen in patients of erythroderma?

Ans: Mild anemia, leukocytosis, eosinophilia, raised ESR, decreased serum albumin, increased uric acid, hypergammaglobulinemia and elevated IgE levels are seen commonly.

Q.13 What is acute skin failure?

Ans: Erythroderma is one of the causes of acute skin failure. Skin failure includes temperature dysregulation, increased loss of water and electrolytes through skin and failure of mechanical barrier function of skin.

Q.14 What are the complications of erythroderma?

Ans: The complications of erythroderma are elaborated in Table 2.

TABLE 2: Complications of erythroderma.	
Type of complication	Cause of complication
Hypoproteinemia	Loss of proteins in the form of scales
Renal failure	Increased transepidermal water loss and electrolyte imbalance
High output cardiac failure	Peripheral vasodilation
Hypothermia	Increased basal metabolic rate and compensatory hypermetabolism
Secondary skin infections	Decreased barrier function of skin

Q.15 How can we manage a case of erythroderma?

Ans: Hospitalization of patient is the first step. Correction of fluid and electrolyte imbalance is done according to Parkland's formula. Based on area of involvement the fluids to be administered are calculated.

Input = 4 mL/kg × body surface area involved with erythroderma

One half of this fluid is given in first 8 hours and remaining half is given over next 16 hours. Protein rich diet [2–3 g/kg (body weight)/ day] is given to patients to take care of hypoalbuminemia. If drug is suspected as a cause of erythroderma it should be removed immediately and also all nonessential drugs are stopped. Patient should be kept in temperature controlled room. Sedation and oral antihistaminics preferably hydroxyzine hydrochloride is given to control pruritus. Antibiotics should be administered if secondary infection is seen. To repair barrier function of skin good emollient and mild topical steroids should be applied repeatedly.

Systemic corticosteroids are given in drug induced erythroderma. Psoriatic erythroderma can be managed by methotrexate or cyclosporine. Biologics such as infliximab, etanercept are also tried in psoriatic erythroderma with good results. Treatment of underlying malignancy improves erythroderma.

CONCLUSION

Erythroderma is one of the emergencies in dermatology. If untreated, it may result in mortality in almost 15.6% of cases. Adequate monitoring of fluid and electrolyte balance in hospital is important in elderly and neonates. Determining the exact cause of erythroderma is challenging many times. Accurate history, clinical examination and laboratory investigations help to reduce complications and mortality in patients of erythroderma.

KEY POINTS

- Erythroderma is an important cause of skin failure and represents a significant morbidity and may lead to fatality if managed inappropriately
- Redness and scaling over more than 90% of skin surface is called as erythroderma
- Erythroderma arising from underlying systemic disorder or drug reaction is called as primary erythroderma
- Pre existing dermatosis leads to secondary erythroderma commonest cause being psoriasis vulgaris
- Large scales suggest acute stage of disease while smaller scales suggest chronicity.
- Systemic involvement is seen in the form of cardiac failure, renal failure, hypothermia and secondary skin infections
- Management involves hospitalization, thermoregulation and good monitoring of vital parameters
- Prognosis depends on underlying causative factors.

SUGGESTED READING

1. Chowdhury S, Podder I, Saha A, et al. Inpatient mortality resulting from dermatological disorders at a tertiary care center in Eastern India: A record-based observational study. Indian J Dermatol. 2017;62:626-9.
2. Inamdar AC, Palit A. Acute skin failure: Concept, causes, consequences and care. Indian J Dermatol Venerol Leprol. 2005;71:379-85.

3. Okoduwa C, Lambert WC, Schwartz RA, et al. Erythroderma: Review of a potentially life-threatening dermatosis. Indian J Dermatol. 2009;54:1-6.
4. Rothe MJ, Bernstein ML, Grant-Kels JM. Life-threatening erythroderma: Diagnosing and treating the "red man". Clinics in Dermatol. 2005;23:206-17.
5. Rym BM, Mourad M, Bechir Z, et al. Erythroderma in adults: A report of 80 cases. Int J Dermatol. 2005;44:731-5.
6. Sarkar R, Sharma RC, Koranne RV, et al. Erythroderma in children: A clinico-etiological study. J Dermatolol. 1999;26:507-11.
7. Umar SH. Medscape [Internet]. Erythroderma (Generalized exfoliative dermatitis); [cited 2018 March 20]. Available from: www.emedicine.medscape.com/article/1106906-overview#a3.

CHAPTER 11

Vaginal Discharge

Poonam Puri, Sushruta Kathuria

■ INTRODUCTION

Vaginal discharge is a common complaint of women in sexually transmitted disease clinic. The patient complains of whitish discharge per vagina which they often term as leukorrhea. It is essential to differentiate physiological vaginal discharge from pathological vaginal discharge. The origin of the vaginal discharge can be from vagina or cervix. Common sexually transmitted diseases (STDs) causing vaginal discharge are candidal vulvovaginitis, trichomoniasis, bacterial vaginosis, gonorrhea, and nongonococcal cervicitis. Besides STDs, vaginal discharge can be caused by various noninfective conditions.

CASE 1

History: A 40-year-old married, nonpregnant, heterosexual, diabetic female presented with complains of thick white discharge per vaginum for last 2 months. It was associated with significant itching, which was persistent throughout the day. The discharge was moderate in quantity requiring change of undergarments twice a day. There was no history of premarital or extramarital exposure nor was there any history of intake of oral contraceptives.

Examination: Moderate curdy-white discharge was seen at the vaginal introitus on inspection. Per speculum examination revealed thick curdy, white vaginal discharge coating the vaginal walls. The cervical opening was normal and no discharge was seen. On per vaginum examination, there was no free fluid in pouch of douglas or tenderness in the fornices.

Investigations: Gram stain of discharge showed pseudohyphae and budding yeast cells (Figs. 1 and 2). Culture on Sabouraud's dextrose medium from vaginal smear grew *Candida albicans*. Her fasting blood sugar was 135 mg/dL, postprandial blood sugar was 187 mg/dL, and HbA1c was 6.9% whereas pH of vagina was 4.7.

Treatment: Patient was treated with single dose of fluconazole 150 mg along with clotrimazole vaginal pessaries for night application. She was advised to practice local hygiene. Partner treatment was done in a similar way and abstinence was advised. Patient was instructed to report after a week for follow-up. A referral to endocrinologist was advised for control of diabetes.

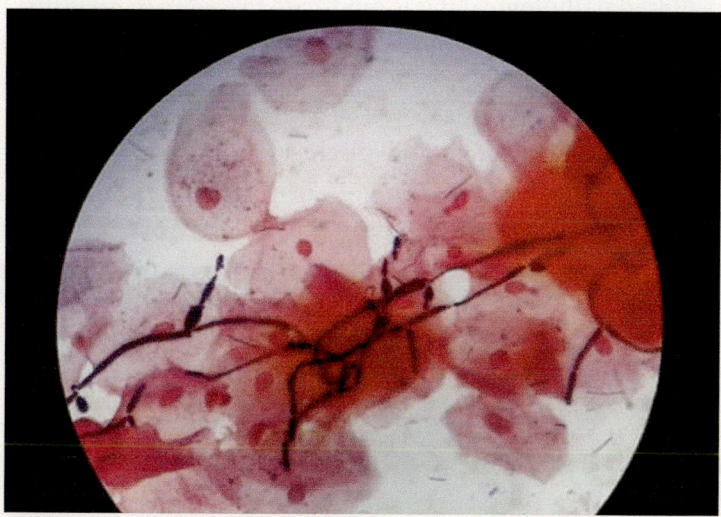

Fig. 1: *Candida albicans* (Gram stain) pseudohyphae.

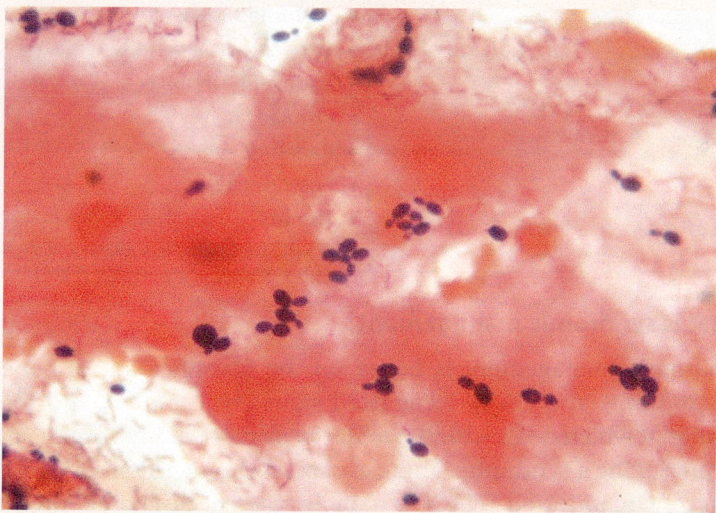

Fig. 2: *Candida albicans* (Gram stain) budding yeast cells.

INTERACTIVE TOPIC REVIEW

Q.1 What is abnormal vaginal discharge?

Ans. Vaginal discharge is of two types—physiological and pathological. Physiological discharge is small in amount, whitish in color, asymptomatic, and usually increase premenstrually or during midcycle. Vaginal discharge is considered pathological if it is moderate to severe in quantity, foul smelling, green or yellowish in color, mucopurulent or purulent or associated with itching. In this chapter, vaginal discharge will be referred as pathological vaginal discharge only.

Q.2 What is the etiology of vaginal discharge?

Ans: There are many infective and noninfective causes of vaginal discharge (Table 1).

TABLE 1: Etiology of abnormal vaginal discharge.

Infective	Noninfective
• Cervicitis • Genital herpes • *Gonococcus* • *Chlamydia trachomatis* • *Mycoplasma* • *Ureaplasma* • Vaginitis • Candidal vulvovaginitis • *Trichomonas vaginalis* • Bacterial vaginosis	• Gynecological conditions: Endocervical polyp, fistulae, tumors • Retained tampon • Intrauterine contraceptive device • Douches • Chemical irritants • Antiseptics • Deodorants • Bath additives • Detergent spermicide • Perfumed soaps • Gynecological conditions • Endocervical polyp • Fistulae • Radiation effects • Postoperative • Tumors • Medication and nutrition

Q.3 What is syndromic management?

Ans: Syndromic management is based on the identification of consistent groups of symptoms and easily recognized signs (syndromes), and the provision of treatment which deals with the majority or most serious organisms responsible for producing a syndrome. There are six syndromes identified by National AIDS Control Organisation (NACO), namely, vaginal discharge, urethral discharge, genital ulcer, lower abdominal pain, painful scrotal swelling and inguinal bubo.

The syndromic management of vaginal discharges mainly includes management of vulvovaginal candidiasis (VVC), bacterial vaginosis, trichomoniasis, gonorrhea and *Chlamydia*.

Advantages
- Prompt institution of treatment in a resource poor setting, based on clinical presentation
- No dependence on detailed investigations which may be time consuming
- Treatment can be provided at the first visit; most cases do not come for a second visit due to social stigma. No need for return visit
- Treatment can be dispensed by health care worker instead of a dermatologist and mixed infections are treated simultaneously.

Disadvantages
- Over diagnosis and over treatment
- Asymptomatic patients are missed
- Treatment is based on subjective assessment of the health care provider.

Q.4 How is vulvovaginal candidiasis classified?

Ans: Vulvovaginal candidiasis can be uncomplicated or complicated. Uncomplicated VVC is sporadic or infrequent, mild-to-moderate, likely to be due to *Candida albicans* and occurs in nonimmunocompromised women. Complicated VVC is recurrent, severe, and is due to non-*Candida albicans* species or seen in women with diabetes, immunocompromised conditions, debilitation or immunosuppressive therapy.

Q.5 What organisms cause vulvovaginal candidiasis?

Ans: Vulvovaginal candidiasis is caused by *Canidida albicans* in 85% cases, *Candida glabrata* in 15% and rarely *Candida krusei* and *Candida tropicalis*. The probability of a woman having VVC is 10% by the age of 25 years and 25% by 50 years. *Candida* spp. can also be found from asymptomatic women, these are endogenous in origin and should not be treated. VVC is not a pure sexually transmitted disease and can occur even without high risk behavior. A change in the normal vaginal flora leads to adherence of the organism to the vaginal epithelium and then its proliferation. Predisposing factors for development of VVC and recurrent VVC include pregnancy, oral contraceptive pill use, antibiotics, diabetes mellitus and immunosuppression.

Q.6 What are the symptoms of vaginal discharge?

Ans: The presenting complaint is usually increased vaginal discharge associated with itching. The different etiologies have certain characteristic features of discharge (Table 2).

Q.7 What investigations are done in a case of vaginal discharge?

Ans: After a detailed history and clinical examination, patient is made to lie in lithotomy position in a well-lighted room. All patients are subjected to human immunodeficiency virus (HIV) test and venereal disease research laboratory test for screening. Sample of the discharge is taken for the following tests (Table 3).

Q.8 What is point-of-care testing in management of vaginal discharge?

Ans: A big problem with patients with sexually transmitted disease is inhibition in coming to the doctor for treatment and accepting or declaring their personal and sexual issues. It has been observed that a second visit to the clinic by women

TABLE 2: Characteristics of vaginal discharge.

Organism	Symptoms	Characteristics of the discharge
Candida	Pruritus, vaginal soreness, dyspareunia, dysuria, excoriations, and fissures on vulva	Thick curdy white vaginal discharge
Trichomonas	Vulvar irritation may or may not be present, dysuria, vulvar soreness	Diffuse, malodorous, or yellow-green discharge
Bacterial vaginosis (caused by *Prevotella* species and *Mobiluncus* species *Gardnerella vaginalis*, *Ureaplasma*, *Mycoplasma*, and other anaerobes	Homogeneous, thin, white to grey discharge coating the vaginal walls. May or may not be associated with itching (Fig. 3)	pH >4.5, positive whiff test (fishy odor of vaginal discharge after addition of 10% KOH), clue cells (vaginal epithelial cells studded with adherent coccobacilli) on microscopic examination
Neisseria gonorrhoeae	Yellow purulent discharge. Maybe asymptomatic	Profuse, yellow purulent discharge coming out of the cervix, often obscuring the cervical os
Nongonococcal cervicitis (*Chlamydia, Mycoplasma, Ureaplasma*)	Dysuria, urethral pruritus, and mucoid, mucopurulent, or purulent discharge, occasionally intermenstrual bleeding	Mucoid, mucopurulent, or purulent discharge covering the os, sustained bleeding from the endocervix on gently passing a swab into the endocervical canal

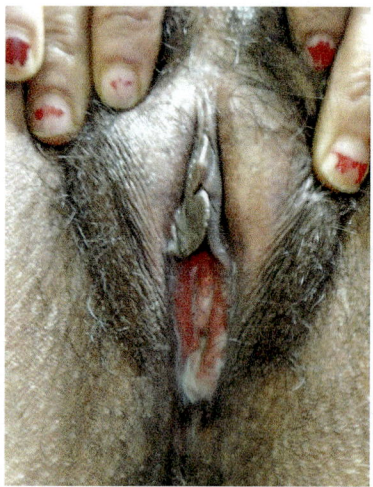

Fig. 3: Bacterial vaginosis

is much less. If treatment is not given at the first instance, there are chances that the patient will remain untreated. To avoid this, treatment based on syndromic management can be given, this again has the disadvantage of over treatment. To avoid this, there is requirement of point-of-care (POC) tests where the etiology can be confirmed within few minutes and treatment given accordingly.

TABLE 3: Investigations done in vaginal discharge.

Organism	Sample	Test	pH test	Culture
Candida	Vaginal smear collected from fornix and lateral vaginal walls	Wet mount with 10% KOH for budding yeasts and pseudohyphae. Sensitivity 70%	Normal <4.5	Sabouraud's dextrose agar for all symptomatic patients with inconclusive KOH report or for identification of species and antifungal drug sensitivity pattern
Trichomonas	Vaginal smear	Wet mount using normal saline for motile trichomonads, sensitivity of 51–65%, acridine orange stain, nucleic acid amplification test (NAAT) which is five times more sensitive [APTIMA test (trade name) is FDA approved]	Normal <4.5	Diamond's culture medium. Sensitivity 75–96%
Bacterial vaginosis	Vaginal smear	Whiff test, Gram stain for clue cells	>4.5	Not recommended
N. gonorrhoeae	Cervical smear	Gram stain for intracellular gram negative diplococci in polymorphs. Not very sensitive	–	Thayer-Martin, chocolate agar, GC agar at 35–36°C in a humid atmosphere (70% humidity) containing 5% carbon dioxide (CO_2)
	Endocervical swab, urine	NAAT	–	–
	Rectal, oropharyngeal swab	Gram stain not useful. NAAT is done	–	–
Non-gonococcal cervicitis (Chlamydia, Mycoplasma, Ureaplasma)	Vaginal discharge smear	Gram stain, methylene blue, or gentian violet stain showing >10 polymorphonuclear leukocytes without any gram-negative diplococci. Endocervical smear is not used as it does not have good positive predictive value		McCoy cell lines for Chlamydia (facilities not usually available)
	Vaginal cervical smear	NAAT, ELISA and direct fluorescent antibody technique for Chlamydia trachomatis	–	–

(NAAT: nucleic acid amplification testing; ELISA: enzyme-linked immunosorbent assay)

Commonly used POC tests are KOH preparation for *Candida*, Gram stain for bacterial vaginosis and gonococci, whiff test for bacterial vaginosis and wet mount for *Trichomonas*. Newer POC tests have been developed. Rapid vaginal yeast assay (SavvyCheck) can be used as POC test for *Candida* with 79% sensitivity as compared to culture. In bacterial vaginosis, rapid assays detecting the presence of proline amino peptidase and BV Blue, a chromogenic POC, based on elevated levels of sialidase, an enzyme produced by anaerobic flora including *Bacteroides*, *Prevotella* and *Gardnerella* species have been used. The sensitivity of Amsel's criteria remains highest for diagnosis of bacterial vaginosis. For trichomoniasis, POC antigen test (a lateral flow test strip that detects *T. vaginalis* membrane proteins) and transcription-mediated amplification (TMA), a nucleic acid amplification test (NAAT) that uses analyte-specific reagents (ASR) for *T. vaginalis* RNA, are available with 90% and 98% sensitivity respectively. These tests can be performed on clinician obtained or patient obtained vaginal samples with similar sensitivity, both being better than wet mount.[14] There are rapid tests commercially available using synthetic oligonucleotide probes to detect the presence of *Candida* species, *Gardnerella vaginalis* and *Trichomonas vaginalis* from a single vaginal swab with a sensitivity and specificity of 92% and 98% respectively.

Q.9 How will you approach a patient with vaginal discharge?

Ans: A patient with complaint of vaginal discharge should be made comfortable and should be completely evaluated. A thorough history regarding the duration and nature of symptoms, associated complaints, detailed sexual history, HIV-related complaints and symptoms of other sexually transmitted diseases must be recorded. General physical examination and local examination of genitals, inguinal lymph nodes and perianal area must be performed. Per speculum examination is done wherever possible. In a tertiary care centre, swabs are also taken from urethra, vagina and endocervix.

For urethral smear, labia majora is separated and a thin, water-moistened, swab (preferably calcium alginate or Dacron) is inserted into the urethral meatus and rotated 360° and removed. Urethral smear is collected for culture of *N. gonorrhoeae* and *Chlamydia*. Then a speculum is inserted to observe cervix, swabs are taken in and rotated all around the vaginal walls and fornices to collect vaginal smears for *Trichomonas*, bacterial vaginosis, pyogenic organisms and *Candida*. After this, cervical smears are taken for *Gonococcus*, *Chlamydia* (cytobrush preferred), *Mycoplasma* and *Ureaplasma*. An endocervical smear is taken by inserting swab 1–3 cm into the endocervical canal and slowly rotated 360° and withdrawn.

At a tertiary care center, where laboratory investigations are done, patient is called after 3 days with partner and treatment is given to both patient and partner. At the primary health care setup, syndromic management to both patient and partner is done.

Q.10 What is the treatment of vaginal discharge?

Ans: Any patient with abnormal vaginal discharge must be treated. It is advisable to give syndromic management because mixed infections are common and identification of the organism is not always possible due to scarcity of equipment and setup. NACO recommends syndromic management, whereas the Centers for Disease Control guidelines give treatment for individual organisms. Table 4 gives the recommended treatment options for vaginal discharge and Table 5 gives the alternative treatment options. Table 6 presents the syndromic management of vaginal discharge.

TABLE 4: CDC recommended treatment guidelines for vaginal discharge.

	CDC 2015
Vulvovaginal candidiasis	Clotrimazole 1% cream 5 g intravaginally daily for 7–14 days Or Clotrimazole 2% cream 5 g intravaginally daily for 3 days Or Miconazole 2% cream 5 g intravaginally daily for 7 days Or Miconazole 4% cream 5 g intravaginally daily for 3 days Or Miconazole 100 mg vaginal suppository, one suppository daily for 7 days Or Miconazole 200 mg vaginal suppository, one suppository for 3 days Or Miconazole 1,200 mg vaginal suppository, one suppository for 1 day Or Tioconazole 6.5% ointment 5 g intravaginally in a single application
Trichomoniasis	Metronidazole 2 g orally in a single dose Or Tinidazole 2 g orally in a single dose
Bacterial vaginosis	Metronidazole 500 mg orally twice a day for 7 days Or Metronidazole gel 0.75%, one full applicator (5 g) intravaginally, once a day for 5 days Or Clindamycin cream 2%, one full applicator (5 g) intravaginally at bedtime for 7 days
Gonorrhea	Ceftriaxone 250 mg intramuscularly in a single dose + Azithromycin 1 g orally in a single dose
Nongonococcal cervicitis	Azithromycin 1 g orally in a single dose Or Doxycycline 100 mg orally twice a day for 7 days

(CDC: Centers for Disease Control)

TABLE 5: Alternative treatment regimens.

	CDC 2015
Vulvovaginal candidiasis (VVC)	In recurrent VVC, oral weekly fluconazole 150 mg for 6 months For severe VVC, topical azole for 7–14 days Or Fluconazole 150 mg in two sequential oral doses (second dose 72 h after initial dose) is recommended. For non-*albicans* VVC, itraconazole or non-fluconazole azole regimen (oral or topical) for 7–14 days Or Boric acid 600 mg in a gelatin capsule administered vaginally once daily for 2 weeks
Trichomoniasis	Metronidazole 500 mg twice daily orally for 7 days
Bacterial vaginosis	Tinidazole 2 g orally once daily for 2 days Or Tinidazole 1 g orally once daily for 5 days Or Clindamycin 300 mg orally twice daily for 7 days Or Clindamycin ovules 100 mg intravaginally once at bedtime for 3 days
Gonorrhea	If ceftriaxone is not available: Cefixime 400 mg orally in a single dose + Azithromycin 1 g orally in a single dose
Nongonococcal cervicitis	Erythromycin base 500 mg orally four times a day for 7 days Or Erythromycin ethylsuccinate 800 mg orally four times a day for 7 days Or Levofloxacin 500 mg orally once daily for 7 days Or Ofloxacin 300 mg orally twice a day for 7 days

(CDC: Centers for Disease Control)

TABLE 6: Syndromic management of vaginal discharge (NACO, 2007).

Vaginitis	Tablet secnidazole 2 gm orally, single dose Or Tablet tinidazole 500 mg orally, twice daily for 5 days Tablet metoclopramide taken 30 minutes before tablet secnidazole, to prevent gastric intolerance + Tablet fluconazole 150 mg orally single dose Or Local clotrimazole 500 mg vaginal pessaries once at bedtime for seven nights
Cervical infection	Tablet cefixime 400 mg orally, single dose* + Tablet azithromycin 1 g, 1 h before lunch

*NACO 2007 treatment guidelines recommend cefixime 400 mg single oral dose along with azithromycin 1 g single oral dose. The Centers for Disease Control guidelines are more recent 2015 and are based on resistance and sensitivity patterns.

Q.11 What advice and precautions should be explained to patients while giving treatment?

Ans: In all patients, a baseline screening of HIV after pretest counseling and Venereal Disease Research Laboratory test (VDRL) is recommended. Patient should be advised regarding healthy sexual practices like single partner, use of condoms throughout the act, avoiding alcohol consumption, intravenous and oral drug abuse, and commercial sexual practices. Patient should also be advised to abstain from sex till all symptoms are resolved. Treatment of partner is also necessary to prevent reinfection in all cases of vaginal discharge except bacterial vaginosis. When patient is given metronidazole or tinidazole or secnidazole, she should be advised to stop alcohol consumption for at least 72 hours to avoid disulfiram-like reaction. If clindamycin cream or ovules are used, then one must advise the patient to abstain from sexual intercourse or use additional contraception other than condom because the oily base of topical clindamycin weakens the latex of condoms. Vaginal douching should be avoided. Reinfection is commonly seen in gonorrhea, so a repeat culture or NAAT should be repeated after 3 months of treatment for gonorrhea.

Q.12 What are the complications of vaginal discharge?

Ans: Vaginal discharge not only affects quality of life and sexual health, but also has other adverse effects also. Bacterial vaginosis and *Trichomonas vaginalis* increase risk of acquisition of HIV infection and are associated with adverse pregnancy outcomes like preterm delivery, low birth weight, premature rupture of membranes, and intrauterine death. Untreated gonococcal infection leads to pelvic inflammatory disease, infertility and ectopic pregnancy. *Chlaymdia, Mycoplasma* cervicitis lead to pelvic inflammatory disease and tubal blockage.

CASE 2

A 30-year-old pregnant woman presented with complaints of vaginal discharge with severe itching at 20 weeks. The discharge was thin and profuse. She also had dysuria. There was no history of premarital or extramarital exposure. HIV and VDRL tests was negative.

Examination: There was thin white discharge present at the introitus. Per speculum examination revealed discharge on all vaginal walls. Whiff test was negative.

Investigation: Vaginal smears from the discharge were made for Gram stain, wet mount, and KOH examination. Gram stain and KOH examination did not reveal any abnormality. Wet mount showed few motile trichomonads (Fig. 4).

Treatment: Patient was given metronidazole 500 mg tablet twice daily for 5 days. After a week there was significant improvement in discharge and pruritus subsided.

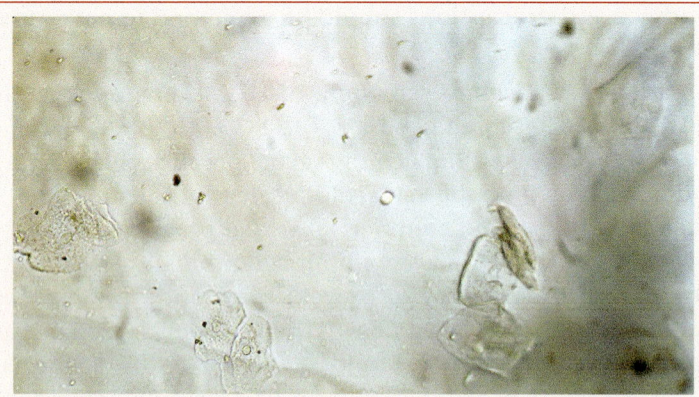

Fig. 4: *Trichomonas vaginalis* (wet smear).

▌ INTERATIVE TOPIC REVIEW

Q.1 What precautions have to be taken while examining a pregnant woman?

Ans: A pregnant woman must be made to feel comfortable during examination. Local examination must be done swiftly to avoid discomfort to the patient while lying down. Per vaginum examination is not done as it will not add much to the management. Per speculum examination may be done in any trimester, but endocervical smears are not taken for risk of abortion or infection.

Q.2 How does pregnancy affect vaginal discharge?

Ans: In pregnancy, due to increase in estrogen and progesterone, there is increased deposition of glycogen in vaginal epithelium. This favors increase in four *Lactobacillus* species (*L. crispatus, L. jensenii, L. gasseri* and *L. vaginalis*) and a decrease in the amount of anaerobic species. Risk of candidal colonization, bacterial vaginosis and trichomoniasis is increased.

Q.3 How does vaginal discharge affect pregnancy?

Ans: Vaginal discharge can have adverse outcomes in pregnancy. Vaginal candidiasis has been less frequently associated with preterm birth. However, a systematic meta-analysis shows that the risk of spontaneous abortions and preterm birth are significantly decreased when asymptomatic vulvovaginal candidiasis is treated. This meta-analysis is based on two randomized controlled trials with post hoc subgroup analysis, so the results must be interpreted with caution till a prospective randomized controlled trial is conducted. A systematic review and meta-analysis has shown that *T. vaginalis* was associated with an increased risk of preterm birth, preterm premature rupture of membranes, and small for gestational age infants. Premature rupture of membranes, preterm labor, preterm birth, intra-amniotic infection and postpartum endometritis have been associated with symptomatic bacterial vaginosis. There is conflicting data regarding treatment of asymptomatic trichomoniasis and bacterial vaginosis in pregnancy. So, it is not routine practice to screen all pregnant women for trichomonas or bacterial vaginosis.

Q.4 What is the treatment of vaginal discharge in pregnancy?

Ans: Intravaginal clotrimazole is category A drug for treatment of VVC in pregnancy and should be used as first line therapy for 7 days. Topical nystatin 100,000 units intravaginally once daily for 2 weeks is a safe alternative as it does not get absorbed or cause congenital malformations. Use of fluconazole in first trimester does not appear to increase risk of congenital malformations.

Bacterial vaginosis in pregnancy is treated with metronidazole. Metronidazole 250 mg or 500 mg can be given twice daily for 7 days. Metronidazole is safe in pregnancy and has not been found to cause adverse pregnancy outcomes. Metronidazole vaginal gel 0.75% for 5 days or metronidazole 1.3% single dose intravaginally, clindamycin gel and oral clindamycin are other safe options. Mothers treated with oral medicines have lesser neonatal admission rates. Trichomoniasis is treated with metronidazole 2 g single dose.

Gonococcal and nongonococcal cervicitis should be treated together with ceftriaxone 250 mg in a single intramuscular dose and azithromycin 1 g orally as a single dose.

CASE 3

A 32-year-old woman presented with yellowish discharge per vaginum for 3 days. It was associated with dysuria and itching. She is working as a commercial sex worker for the last 3 years and was also an occasional alcohol drinker. There was no history of fever, weight loss, joint pains, oral ulcers, diarrhea, genital ulcers, or other systemic complaints.

Examination: Patient was of thin built. No significant lymphadenopathy was found. Oral cavity examination and palms and soles were normal. There was profuse purulent discharge coming out of cervical os (Fig. 5). Per rectal examination was normal.

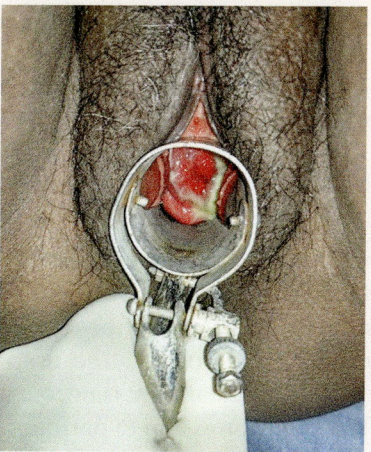

Fig. 5: Gonorrhoea. Purulent discharge coming out of cervical os.

Investigations: Gram stain from the discharge revealed multiple polymorphonuclear leukocytes with gram-negative intracellular diplococcic (Fig. 6). KOH and wet mount did not reveal any organism. Culture on chocolate agar grew colonies consistent with *N. gonorrhoeae*.

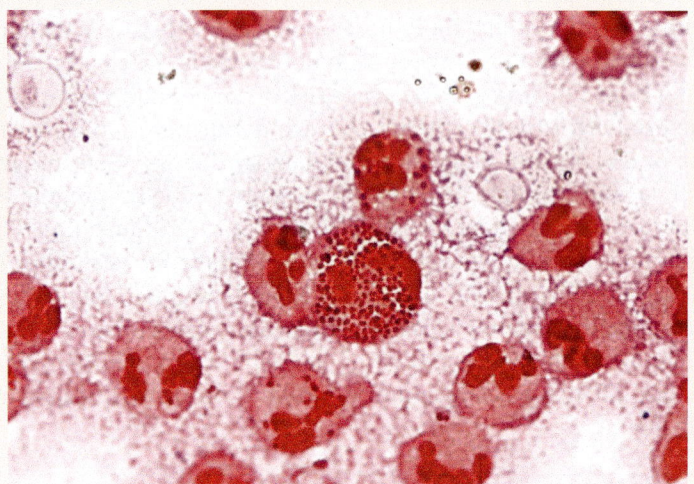

Fig. 6: N. *gonorrhoeae* (Gram stain). Gram-negative intracellular diplococci.

The HIV test was positive for HIV-1, VDRL was negative, CD4+ T-cell count was 578 cells/mm^3.

Treatment: She was treated with dual therapy of injection ceftriaxone 250 mg intramuscular with tablet azithromycin 1 g single oral dose. Patient was reviewed after one week for resolution of symptoms. She was advised to give same treatment to her recent partners and was also counseled about safe sexual practices.

▌INTERACTIVE TOPIC REVIEW

Q.1 What is the management of vaginal discharge in seropositive (HIV positive) patient?

Ans: In a retroviral-positive patient with vaginal discharge, it is necessary to record the stage of HIV and CD4+ T-cell counts. If possible, viral counts should be performed. Universal precautions must be followed while taking vaginal discharge sample for smear and culture. The used speculum has to be put separately for disinfection. Early treatment is necessary in HIV-positive patients because of increased risk of transmission to partner.

Treatment options for HIV-positive patient is given in Table 7.

TABLE 7: Treatment of vaginal discharge in HIV-positive patient (CDC guidelines 2015).

Etiology	Treatment
Candidal vulvovaginitis	Same as non-HIV treatment Clotrimazole 1% cream 5 g intravaginally daily for 7–14 days Or Clotrimazole 2% cream 5 g intravaginally daily for 3 days Or Miconazole 2% cream 5 g intravaginally daily for 7 days Or Miconazole 4% cream 5 g intravaginally daily for 3 days Or Miconazole 100 mg vaginal suppository, one suppository daily for 7 days Or Miconazole 200 mg vaginal suppository, one suppository for 3 days Or Miconazole 1,200 mg vaginal suppository, one suppository for 1 day Or Tioconazole 6.5% ointment 5 g intravaginally in a single application
Bacterial vaginosis	Same as non-HIV patient Metronidazole 500 mg orally twice a day for 7 days Or Metronidazole gel 0.75%, one full applicator (5 g) intravaginally, once a day for 5 days Or Clindamycin cream 2%, one full applicator (5 g) intravaginally at bedtime for 7 days
Trichomoniasis	Metronidazole 500 mg orally twice daily for 7 days (rather than 2 g single dose of metronidazole)
Gonococcal cervicitis	Same as non-HIV patient Ceftriaxone 250 mg intramuscularly in a single dose* + Azithromycin 1 g orally in a single dose
Nongonococcal cervicitis	Same as non-HIV patients Azithromycin 1 g orally in a single dose Or Doxycycline 100 mg orally twice a day for 7 days

*NACO 2007 treatment guidelines recommend cefixime 400 mg single oral dose along with azithromycin 1 g single oral dose. CDC guidelines are more recent 2015 and are based on resistance and sensitivity patterns.
(CDC: Centers for Disease Control)

CONCLUSION

Vaginal discharge is one of the most common presenting complaints of women of sexually reproductive age group. It is associated with decreased quality of life as well as obstetric and gynecological complications. The treatment of vaginal discharge can be syndromic in a resource poor setting or based on laboratory tests and culture in a tertiary care centre. Various POC rapid tests are being developed to avoid the risk of overtreatment and delay in providing treatment.

KEY POINTS

- Vaginal discharge can be pathological or physiological
- In the various cause of vaginal discharge sexually transmitted diseases form an important subgroup
- It is mandatory to screen every patient for HIV and VDRL and do partner management
- In a resource poor setting, syndromic management offers good cure, but in tertiary care setup, laboratory based treatment should be encouraged.

SUGGESTED READING

1. Alsaad AM, Kaplan YC, Koren G. Exposure to fluconazole and risk of congenital malformations in the offspring: A systematic review and meta-analysis. Reprod Toxicol. 2015;52:78-82.
2. Aptima Trichomonas vaginalis Assay (Panther™ System) http://www.hologic.com/sites/default/files/package%20inserts/503797-IFU-PI_001_01.pdf
3. Brocklehurst P, Gordon A, Heatley E, et al. Antibiotics for treating bacterial vaginosis in pregnancy. Cochrane Database Syst Rev. 2013;1:CD000262.
4. Dan M, Leshem Y, Yeshaya A. Performance of a rapid yeast test in detecting Candida spp. in the vagina. Diagn Microbiol Infect Dis. 2010;67:52-5.
5. Foxman B, Muraglia R, Dietz JP, et al. Prevalence of recurrent vulvovaginal candidiasis in 5 European countries and the United States: Results from an internet panel survey. J Low Genit Tract Dis. 2013;17:340-5.
6. Huppert JS, Hesse E, Kim G, et al. Adolescent women can perform a point-of-care test for trichomoniasis as accurately as clinicians. Sex Transm Infect. 2010;86:514-9.
7. Huppert JS, Mortensen JE, Reed JL, et al. Rapid antigen testing compares favorably with transcription-mediated amplification assay for the detection of Trichomonas vaginalis in young women. Clin Infect Dis. 2007;45:194-8.
8. Joesoef MR, Hillier SL, Wiknjosastro G, et al. Intravaginal clindamycin treatment for bacterial vaginosis: Effects on preterm delivery and low birth weight. Am J Obstet Gynecol. 1995;173:1527-31.
9. Laboratory diagnosis of sexually transmitted infections, including human immunodeficiency virus by WHO 2013.
10. Laboratory manual for diagnosis of sexually transmitted and reproductive tract infections by NACO, Ministry of Health and Family Welfare. NACO. Available from: naco.gov.in/sites/default/files/STI_Lab%20manual_09-01-2014.pdf
11. Lamont RF, Duncan SL, Mandal D, et al. Intravaginal clindamycin to reduce preterm birth in women with abnormal genital tract flora. Obstet Gynecol. 2003;101:516-22.
12. Madhivanan P, Krupp K, Li T, et al. Performance of BV Blue rapid test in detecting bacterial vaginosis among women in Mysore, India. Infect Dis Obstet Gynecol. 2014;2014:908313.
13. McGregor JA, French JI, Jones W, et al. Bacterial vaginosis is associated with prematurity and vaginal fluid mucinase and sialidase-results of a controlled trial of topical clindamycin cream. Am J Obstet Gynecol. 1994;170:1048-60.
14. National guidelines on prevention, management and control of reproductive tract infections including sexually transmitted infections by NACO 2007. Available from: http://naco.gov.in/sites/default/files/National_Guidelines_on_PMC_of_RTI_Including_STI%201.pdf
15. Nye MB, Schwebke JR, Body BA. Comparison of APTIMA Trichomonas vaginalis transcription-mediated amplification to wet mount microscopy, culture, and polymerase chain reaction for diagnosis of trichomoniasis in men and women. Am J Obstet Gynecol. 2009;200:e181-7.

16. Roberts CL, Algert CS, Rickard KL, et al. Treatment of vaginal candidiasis for the prevention of preterm birth: A systematic review and meta-analysis. Syst Rev. 2015;4:31.
17. Schwebke JR, Hobbs MM, Taylor SN, et al. Molecular testing for Trichomonas vaginalis in women: Results from a prospective U.S. clinical trial. J Clin Microbiol. 2011;49:4106-11.
18. Sexually transmitted diseases treatment guidelines 2015 by CDC. MMWR. 2015;64:51-81. Available from: https://www.cdc.gov/std/tg2015/tg-2015-print.pdf
19. Sheehy O, Santos F, Ferreira E, et al. The use of metronidazole during pregnancy: A review of evidence. Curr Drug Saf. 2015;10:170-9.
20. Silver BJ, Guy RJ, Kaldor JM, et al. Trichomonas vaginalis as a cause of perinatal morbidity: A systematic review and meta-analysis. Sex Transm Dis. 2014;41:369-76.
21. Sobel JD. Vaginitis. N Engl J Med 1997;337(26):1896-1903.
22. Sobel JD. Vulvovaginal candidosis. Lancet. 2007;369:1961-71.
23. Soong D, Einarson A. Vaginal yeast infections during pregnancy. Can Fam Physician. 2009;55:255-6.
24. Yudin MH, Money DM. No. 211-Screening and Management of Bacterial Vaginosis in Pregnancy. J Obstet Gynaecol Can. 2017;39:e184-e191.

CHAPTER 12

Urethral Discharge

Taru Garg, Mahima Agrawal

■ INTRODUCTION

Urethral discharge is characterized by mucoid, mucopurulent or purulent discharge from the urethra. This is a manifestation of male urethritis and is commonly encountered in a Dermatology-Venereology setup. Sexually transmitted urethritis can be broadly categorized into two types—gonococcal urethritis (GU) caused by *Neisseria gonorrhoeae* and nongonococcal urethritis (NGU). The NGU is further attributed to multiple organisms, most common being *Chlamydia trachomatis* and *Mycoplasma* species; however, it can be caused by other bacteria and rarely by viruses and protozoa.

A thorough knowledge about managing urethral discharge is important because of the constantly evolving drug resistant organisms and in turn shifting treatment paradigms. Successful treatment of urethral discharge not only reduces substantial morbidity in the patient, but also breaks the chain of transmission of this sexually transmitted infection (STI) and thereby preventing long-term sequelae in female partners.

CASE 1

A 24-year-old unmarried male, tea stall owner by occupation, presented with sudden onset moderate yellowish discharge from the urethra for 2 days. This was associated with severe pain and burning particularly while passing urine and increased frequency of urination. There was no history of prior urethral instrumentation or any systemic complaints. Sexual history revealed unprotected peno-vaginal intercourse with an unknown female sexual worker 4 days prior to the onset of symptoms and multiple sexual contacts with both known and unknown partners in the past. He denied any history of homosexuality or past history of similar complaints. There was no history suggestive of any other STI or immunosuppression.

Local examination revealed profuse yellowish purulent discharge from the urethra accompanied by perimeatal erythema. There was no inguinal lymphadenopathy, testicular or epididymal swelling or tenderness. Systemic examination was within normal limits.

Investigations: The discharge was smeared on a glass slide and smears were prepared for Gram staining. It was examined under oil immersion microscope (1000x) with several of them showing field full of polymorphonuclear lymphocytes (PMNLs) and several of them showed intracellular gram-negative diplococci suggestive of GU. He was also advised serological testing for syphilis and enzyme-linked immunosorbent assay (ELISA) for human immunodeficiency virus (HIV) 1 and 2.

Treatment: Patient was treated as per National AIDS control organization (NACO) guidelines and prescribed Kit 1 (grey colored kit) for the syndromic management of urethral discharge comprising of tablet cefixime 400 mg and tablet azithromycin 1 g stat and asked to review again after 1 week. He was also advised sexual abstinence during the period of treatment and counseled for safe sex practices. He was asked to inform the partner for evaluation and treatment. On the follow-up visit after 1 week, patient was free of symptoms and serological tests for syphilis and HIV were nonreactive. The safe sex practices were reinforced and repeat testing for HIV was scheduled after 3 months.

Case Review in a Nutshell

A case of discharge from the urethra presenting in an STI clinic is not an uncommon presenting complaint amongst men. It is important to be aware of the common causes and their treatment of choice in order to relieve the patient of this distressing condition and its complications and to prevent further infection to the sexual partners.

The patient in the aforementioned case was suspected to have urethritis, either gonococcal or nongonococcal or mixed in etiology. He was confirmed to be having GU due to the presence of intracellularly located gram-negative diplococci. However, on reviewing the clinical history and examination there were several pointers that had bent the index of suspicion towards GU, which were:
- Abrupt onset
- Onset of symptoms within 2–6 days of the high risk sexual contact (corroborative with the incubation period of gonorrhea)
- Severe symptoms
- Profuse amount of discharge
- Purulent discharge.

These clinical features are the hallmarks of gonococcal infection. An extensive search to look for anorectal discharge and pharyngitis was not carried out as this patient denied history of homosexuality. This patient was further advised serological testing for syphilis and HIV in keeping with the NACO guidelines.

He was offered treatment for both GU and NGU as per NACO guidelines. *Chlamydia* has been isolated very commonly in patients of gonorrhea and they are known to co-exist. Treating solely for gonorrhea can often result in incomplete resolution of symptoms due to persistence of chlamydial component of the infection. Another advantage of using two antibiotics to treat the infection is prevention of antibiotic resistant gonorrhea species as two antibiotics active against gonorrhea are used concurrently.

Patient was advised sexual abstinence during the course of treatment, provided condoms, educated about correct and consistent use of condoms. Counseling also included information about limiting the number of partners and alternatives to penetrative sex. Contact tracing is an important constituent of any STI management and in a case of urethral discharge it is essential to evaluate the partner(s) and treat them appropriately. It may be advisable to treat the partners at the first visit if detailed examination and testing is not possible as they may be lost to follow-up therefore missing out on an opportunity to intervene.

CASE 2

A 30-year-old married male presented with history of urethral discharge for 7–10 days associated with mild burning sensation. There was no past history of similar complaints. He gave history of extramarital unprotected penovaginal contact with a known married female partner 2 weeks prior to the onset of symptoms. There was no history of receiving any prior treatment. There was no history suggestive of any other STI, immunosuppression or similar complaints in any of the sexual partners.

On local examination there was no urethral discharge. The urethra was milked from the root to the tip of the penis but no discharge was obtained. The patient was then asked to review again the next day after 4 hours of holding the urine. The following morning slight mucoid discharge was noticed per urethra. Rest of the genital and systemic examination was normal.

Investigations: The discharge was smeared on a glass slide and stained with Gram stain. It showed 15–20 PMNLs per oil immersion field. There was absence of any intracellular gram-negative diplococci. A diagnosis of NGU was made.

Treatment: Patient was treated as per NACO guidelines and prescribed kit 1 (gray colored kit) for the syndromic management of urethral discharge comprising of tablet cefixime 400 mg and tablet azithromycin 1 g stat and asked to review again after 1 week. He was also advised sexual abstinence during the period of treatment and counseled for safe sex practices. He was asked to inform the partner for evaluation and treatment. On the follow-up visit after 1 week, patient was free of symptoms and serological tests for syphilis and HIV were nonreactive. The safe sex practices were reinforced and repeat testing for HIV was scheduled after 3 months.

Case Review in a Nutshell

The salient points of this case are as follows:
- Mild burning sensation
- Minimal amount of discharge
- Mucoid discharge
- 15–20 PMNLs per oil immersion field
- Absence of gram-negative intracellular diplococci.

In contrast to case 1, this patient presented with milder symptoms and the nature of the discharge also differed significantly. Clinically, this presentation would prompt a diagnosis of NGU. The number of PMNLs per oil immersion field fulfilled the criteria required to make a diagnosis of urethritis. Furthermore absence of gram-negative intracelullar diplococci tilted the diagnosis finally to NGU.

Urethral Discharge | 175

This patient like case 1, received the treatment according to the NACO guidelines and showed complete resolution after 1 week. It is important to note here that in this case diagnosed as NGU, treatment for gonorrhea is also recommended because absence of intracellular gram-negative diplococci on Gram stain does not rule out gonococcal infection.

CASE 3

A 28-year-old unmarried male presented with urethral discharge of 10 days duration associated with minor symptoms. He was diagnosed as a case of NGU at the first visit, which was 7 days back and treated as per NACO guidelines with kit 1. At the second visit 7 days after the administration of the kit there was not much improvement in the discharge. Last sexual contact was 2 weeks prior to the onset of discharge, which was unprotected peno-vaginal contact with a known female partner. He denied any history of sexual re-exposure or urethral instrumentation in the last 1 week. There was also no additional systemic symptom at this visit.

Local examination revealed minimal thin homogeneous discharge from the urethra without any other local or systemic finding.

Investigations: A wet mount preparation was prepared in view of persistence of the symptoms despite receiving kit 1 and the preparation was immediately examined under the microscope. Few motile flagellate organisms were seen under the oil immersion microscope. A diagnosis of *Trichomonas* urethritis was made.

Treatment: Patient was prescribed tablet secnidazole 2 g stat as per NACO syndromic management guidelines for urethral discharge and asked to review after 1 week, while re-emphasizing on abstinence from sexual intercourse. The partner was also treated with the same. The serologies for syphilis and HIV were negative so the patient was made to review after 1 more week.

After another 1 week patient reported complete resolution of symptoms.

Case Review in a Nutshell

This patient complained of persistence of symptoms despite receiving treatment against gonorrhea and chlamydial infection in kit 1. This would occur in the following settings:
- Possibility 1: In case of reinfection
- Possibility 2: In case of another pathogen responsible for symptoms (Trichomonas vaginalis)
- Possibility 3: In case of antimicrobial resistance.

Patient denied history of repeat sexual contact, thereby eliminating possibility 1. NACO guidelines recommend treatment for *Trichomonas* infection in this situation and demonstration of motile organisms in the wet mount confirmed the *Trichomonas* infection. No further evaluation for antifungal resistance was done because of demonstration of the organism and complete resolution with secnidazole treatment.

■ INTERACTIVE TOPIC REVIEW

Q.1 Can urethritis manifest without urethral discharge?

Ans: Yes, both GU and NGU can be asymptomatic or minimally symptomatic. Community studies have shown that up to two-thirds of men who had no symptoms were found to have urethral gonorrhea by routine screening, some had minor symptoms, which were ignored.

Q.2 What are the causes of urethral discharge?

Ans: The causes of urethral discharge maybe sexually transmitted infections or may comprise of nonsexually transmitted causes as enlisted in Table 1.

TABLE 1: Causes of urethral discharge.

Sexually transmitted infectious causes	Nonsexually transmitted causes
• Bacteria: 　○ *N. gonorrhoeae* 　○ *Chlamydia trachomatis* 　○ *Mycoplasma genitalium* 　○ *Ureaplasma urealyticum* 　○ *Hemophilus* species 　○ Coliform species	• Urinary tract infection • Bacterial prostatitis • Urethral stricture • Phimosis • Urethral instrumentation • Congenital defects • Chemical irritation
• Virus: 　○ Herpes simplex virus 　○ Adenovirus 　○ Epstein–Barr virus	• Tumors • Stevens–Johnson syndrome • Pemphigus
• Protozoa: 　○ *Trichomonas vaginalis*	

Q.3 Enumerate the causative organisms of urethral discharge. Which are the commonest causes?

Ans: The organisms are mostly bacterial, including *N. gonorrhoeae, C. trachomatis, M. genitalium, Ureaplasma urealyticum, Hemophilus* species and some coliform species (important in homosexual men). Other occasional causes include viruses like herpes simplex virus, Epstein–Barr virus and adenovirus and protozoa like *Trichomonas vaginalis*. The two most common causes are *N. gonorrhoeae* and *C. trachomatis*.

Q.4 What are the point-of-care tests for urethritis?

Ans: Point-of-care tests for urethritis include examining urethral discharge smears for Gram, methylene blue or gentian violet stains under the microscope, microscopy of the first void urine and leukocyte esterase testing.

Q.5 In what percentage of cases of GU, we may not be able to detect intracellular gram-negative diplococci?

Ans: It is possible that in about 5% of GU cases intracellular gram-negative diploccoci may not be visible.

Q.6 What is the pathomechanism of GU?

Ans: Gonococci express pili, by which the organism adheres to the host epithelial cell. This is followed by either entry of the organism into the submucosal space through the intercellular spaces or through the epidermal cell. This is in turn followed by inflammatory reaction which manifests as epidermal shedding and pus discharge.

Q.7 How are the *C. trachomatis* serovars classified?

Ans: *C. trachomatis* serovars are divided into three groups A–C, D–K, and L1–L3. Out of these serovars A–C cause trachoma and L1–L3 are responsible for lymphogranuloma venereum. The serovars D–K are responsible for genital infections like urethritis.

Q.8 Describe briefly the developmental cycle of *C. trachomatis*.

Ans: *C. trachomatis* has two stages in the development cycle after entry into the host, which includes an infectious elementary body (EB) and a reproductive reticulate body (RB). Initially the organism enters into the host cells as EBs which are located inside a vacuole, termed as inclusion. These EBs convert into active form known as RBs, which are the replicative forms and multiply to form multiple RBs. These RBs are again cycled into EBs which release from cells and are capable of infecting other cells.

Q.9 When is culture required in cases of GU? How do you send the sample for culture?

Ans: Culture remains the gold standard for gonococcal infections, although it may not be required routinely in cases of GU as the diagnosis is established on the basis of Gram stained smears showing gram-negative intracellular diplococci. We should opt for culture of the organism in cases of treatment failure to standard antibiotics when we suspect antimicrobial resistance and sensitivity testing is required. For symptomatic heterosexual men, culture of the urethral exudate suffices, but in cases of men having sex with men, with history of peno-oral intercourse, pharyngeal cultures are required. Urethral exudate is obtained by inserting a thin, water-moistened swab (calcium alginate or dacron) or a platinum loop inserted 3–4 cm into the urethra, rotated slowly and withdrawn gently. Ideally, the specimens should be inoculated onto culture medium (modified Thayer-Martin medium) immediately after collection to preserve the viability of gonococci for isolation. In cases of nonavailability of the specific media, a transport medium maybe used (e.g. Amie's transport medium or Stuart transport medium).

Q.10 What is the 3-glass test used for urethritis?

Ans: In the 3-glass test the patient is asked to void the urine into three different clear glasses. The first glass comprises of the initial 10 mL of urine, the second glass would contain the midstream portion of a noninterrupted stream and the final portion has the very last end of the stream. Leukocyturia in the first glass indicates an inflammation in the urethra, in the second glass a general inflammation in the urinary bladder and/or upper urinary tract and in the third glass an inflammation in the prostate.

Q.11 What is postgonococcal urethritis?

Ans: It is the persistence of symptoms in case of optimum treatment of GU. It occurs due to the fact that *Chlamydia* and *gonorrhoeae* coinfection commonly exists and treatment targeted only against gonorrhea leads to persistence of urethral discharge or other symptoms of urethritis due to persistent chlamydial component. Gonorrhea has a shorter incubation period than chlamydia so men with both the infections can present with gonococcal symptoms meanwhile the chlamydial infection is still incubating.

Q.12 When do we suspect *Trichomonas* as a cause of urethral discharge?

Ans: We suspect *Trichomonas* as a cause of urethral discharge when even after optimum treatment of discharge for gonorrhea and *Chlamydia* in the patient as well as the partner, there is no resolution of symptoms after 7 days especially in high prevalence areas. This should prompt a search for other less common causes of urethritis and warrants a wet mount preparation from the discharge to look for motile organisms and preferably a culture in Diamond's medium.

Q.13 Can urethral discharge occur due to nonsexually transmitted causes? If yes, then which causes?

Ans: Urethritis can occur in association with urinary tract infection, bacterial prostatitis, urethral stricture, phimosis, or urethral instrumentation. Rare causes include congenital defects, chemical irritation, or tumors. It may also occur as a part of Stevens-Johnson syndrome mucosal involvement.

Q.14 How do you examine a patient of urethral discharge?

Ans: Refer to Flowchart 1 for the clinical diagnosis of urethral discharge. The discharge is evaluated in terms of quantity and quality. It can be profuse (dribbling from the urethra spontaneously), scanty (not visible without milking the urethra) or intermediate (between profuse and scanty). The color and consistency is determined, it can be yellow, gray-white or greenish and the consistency can range from frank purulent in consistency to mucoid or mixed or rarely clear. Associated penile edema and inguinal lymphadenopathy must be looked for. In case a patient presents without active discharge, the urethra should be "milked" from root to tip and observed for discharge. Even if this manoeuver does not reveal discharge, the patient must be called the next day after not voiding urine overnight (or a minimum of 4 h at least) to enhance the likelihood of reaching a firm diagnosis.

Q.15 How do you investigate a patient for urethral discharge?

Ans: Investigation for urethral discharge includes point of care tests like Gram stain preparation from the discharge. Additional investigations include urine sediment evaluation of first void urine, leukocyte esterase testing on first void urine specimen and cultures. Nucleic acid amplification testing (NAAT) for detection of gonococcal, chlamydial, *Mycoplasma* and *Trichomonas* urethritis can also be carried out and offers higher specificity and sensitivity. Specimen of

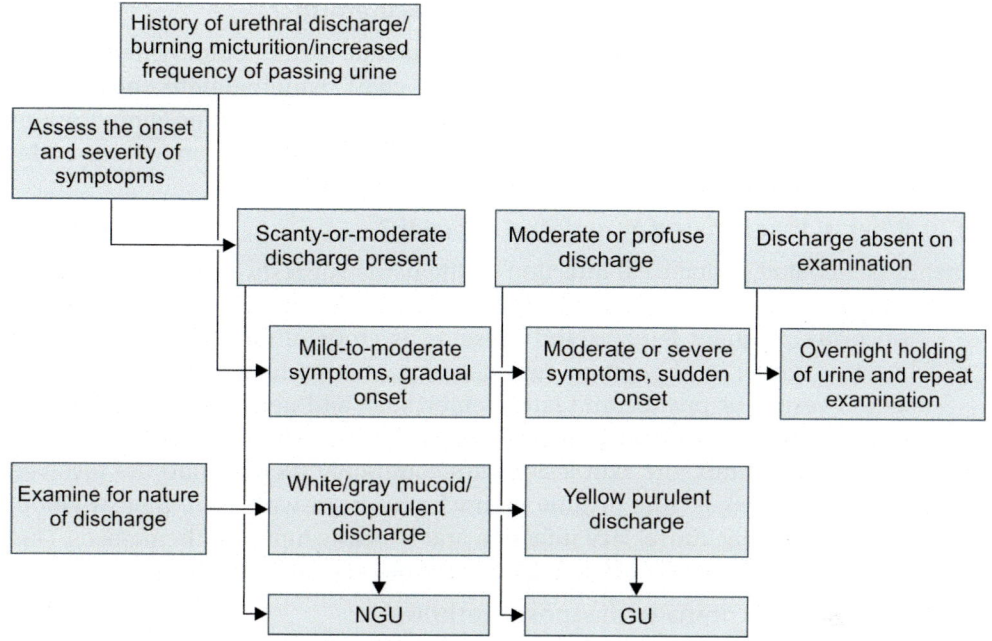

(GU: gonococcal urethritis; NGU: nongonococcal urethritis)
Flowchart 1: Clinical diagnosis of urethral discharge.

choice for NAAT in men is urine. NACO recommendations include testing every patient for serology of syphilis (VDRL test) and HIV.

Q.16 Are there clinical differences between GU and NGU?

Ans: Although it is difficult to distinguish between the two on clinical grounds, yet some differences exist. Both may cause urethral discharge, dysuria, or urethral itching; however, the presentation is more severe and discharge is purulent and profuse and abrupt in onset in case of GU, whereas it is scant, mucoid and less abrupt in onset in cases of NGU. Another important difference is the chronological association with sexual intercourse, while gonorrhea develops within 2–6 days after exposure, NGU usually takes between 1 and 5 weeks.

Q.17 What are the other manifestations of urethritis?

Ans: They include conjunctivitis (probably as a result of autoinoculation in cases of gonorrhea and *Chlamydia*), epididymitis, and reactive arthritis. Other local manifestations include penile shaft edema, rarely periurethral abscess and prostatitis.

Q.18 Are there any other sites which should be examined?

Ans: In cases of peno-oral contact the pharynx of the recipient partner should be examined for gonococcal pharyngitis and in cases of peno-anal contact the recipient partner should undergo a proctoscopic examination to look for rectal involvement.

Q.19 What are the complications of gonococcal urethritis?

Ans: The complications maybe local which include acute epididymitis, penile lymphangitis, penile edema (bull-headed clap), lymphadenitis, postinflammatory urethral strictures, periurethral abscess, etc. The systemic complications are rare and include disseminated gonococcal infection, gonococcal endocarditis and meningitis.

Q.20 What is disseminated gonococcal infection?

Ans: Disseminated gonococcal infection as the name suggests occurs due to blood borne dissemination of gonococcal infection. It is seen primarily in females, especially pregnant females and presents as crops of necrotic lesions which begin as tender erythematous macules or papules, which eventually develop central vesicle or pustule and later hemorrhage and necrosis ensues. Patients also present with migratory polyarthralgia, thereby the synonym dermatitis-arthritis syndrome. The skin lesions are commonly seen around the involved joints. Other risk factors include men who have sex with men, menstruation, intravenous drug abuse, HIV infection and systemic lupus erythematosus. Due to hematogenous mode of spread, often the blood culture yields positive result.

Q.21 What are the criteria to diagnose urethritis?

Ans: Presence of intracellular gram-negative diplococci is consistent with GU. Gram stained smears must show >5 PMNLs per oil immersion field in urethral smear or >10 PMNLs per high power field in the sediment of first void urine in case of NGU. The Centers for Disease Control and Prevention (CDC) (2015) guidelines differ in this regard and recommends that urethritis can be documented in men whose Gram stain of urethral secretion demonstrates ≥2 white blood cells per oil immersion field. Other tests include positive leukocyte esterase test in first void urine.

Q.22 How do you treat GU and NGU?

Ans: Treatment options for GU include—tablet cefixime 400 mg orally in a single dose (NACO recommendation) or intramuscular injection of ceftriaxone 250 mg in a single dose.

Treatment options for NGU include—tablet azithromycin 1 g orally in a single dose (NACO recommendation) or tablet doxycycline 100 mg orally twice a day for 7 days or alternative regimens include—tablet erythromycin base 500 mg orally four times a day for 7 days or tablet erythromycin ethylsuccinate 800 mg orally four times a day for 7 days or tablet levofloxacin 500 mg orally once a day for 7 days or tablet ofloxacin 300 mg twice a day for 7 days.

Treatment options for *Trichomonas* urethritis—tablet secnidazole 2 g orally in a single dose or tablet metronidazole 2 g orally in a single dose or tablet tinidazole 2 g orally in a single dose.

Q.23 What is GISP? Discuss antimicrobial resistant *N. gonorrhoeae*.

Ans: It is Gonococcal Isolate Surveillance Project (GISP) established in 1986 in the United States of America to monitor trends of antimicrobial susceptibilities of urethral *N. gonorrhoeae* strains. In 2007 fluoroquinolone resistance was an emerging concern and subsequent to this CDC guidelines recommended the use of cephalosporins for the treatment of gonococcal infection. Another step to combat the rising resistance was introduction of dual therapy, even in chlamydial NAAT negative patients of GU with azithromycin and cefixime so as to use two drugs active against gonorrhea. In the latter half of 2000–2010 rising minimum inhibitory concentratons were noted for cefixime thus, also rendering it less effective. Consequently intramuscular ceftriaxone along with oral azithromycin is the recommended regimen for GU according to CDC. It is predicted that cephalosporin resistance will have a rising trend in future too. The GISP isolates have also documented tetracycline resistance, although in case of azithromycin allergy, doxycyline remains the preferred second drug in place of azithromycin.

Q.24 Is treatment of sex partners warranted?

Ans: Yes, all sexual partners of patients with urethral discharge within 60 days before the onset of symptoms or diagnosis of infection should be evaluated and treated for urethral discharge syndrome.

Q.25 What is the most common cause of persistent or recurrent urethritis?

Ans: Men who have persistent symptoms after treatment of urethritis have been shown to have infection most commonly due to *Mycoplasma genitalium* especially following doxycycline therapy. In case of primary treatment by doxycyline, azithromycin should be offered to such patients. In case of failure to azithromycin, retreatment with moxifloxacin should be done. Other causes of persistent or recurrent urethritis include *Trichomonas vaginalis* especially in heterosexual men in high prevalence areas for *Trichomonas*. Such setting warrants a wet mount examination and treatment with agents like metronidazole or tinidazole or secnidazole.

CONCLUSION

Urethral discharge is a common presentation of sexually transmitted infection in males. It may vary in symptomatology and the type and amount of discharge. Sound clinical knowledge and a step-wise methodical approach towards these cases can help us delineate different etiologies and help in appropriate line of management. Treatment of these cases is not only important to alleviate the symptoms of the patients but also to prevent various complications and transmission to female partners and protect the latter from long-term consequences like infertility.

KEY POINTS

- Urethral discharge can be caused by bacterial (*N. gonorrhoeae, C. trachomatis, M. genitalium, Ureaplasma urealyticum, Haemophilus* species), viral (herpes simplex virus, Epstein–Barr virus, adenovirus) and protozoan (Trichomonas) causes
- Commonly urethral discharge is divided into gonococcal and non-gonococcal causes

- Gonococcal urethritis is more severe and discharge is purulent and profuse and abrupt in onset, whereas it is scant, mucoid and less abrupt in onset in cases of nongonococcal urethritis
- Gram stained smears must show >5 PMNLs per oil immersion field in urethral smear or >10 PMNLs per high power field in the sediment of first void urine in case of urethritis
- The complications include acute epididymitis, penile lymphangitis, penile-edema (bull-headed clap), lymphadenitis, postinflammatory urethral strictures, periurethral abscess, disseminated gonococcal infection, gonococcal endocarditis and meningitis.

SUGGESTED READING

1. Centers for Disease Control and Prevention. Sexually transmitted diseases treatment guidelines, 2015. MMWR. 2015;64(RR3):1-137.
2. Holmes KK, Sparling PF, Stamm WE. Sexually Transmitted Diseases, 4th edition. New York: McGraw-Hill Professional; 2007.
3. National AIDS Control Organization. National Guidelines on Prevention, Management and Control of Reproductive Tract Infection and Sexually Transmitted Infection. New Delhi: NACO, Ministry of Health and Family Welfare, Government of India; 2014.

CHAPTER 13

Granulomatous Disorders

Geeti Khullar, V Ramesh

■ INTRODUCTION

Granulomatous disorders are characterized by unique inflammatory reaction pattern comprising of granulomas on histology. A granuloma is a focal, compact collection of epithelioid cells, admixed with different types of multinucleate giant cells and other inflammatory cells, formed in response to a persistent inciting antigen. Granulomatous disorders often pose a diagnostic challenge due to overlapping clinical and histological features. Clinicopathological correlation in conjunction with ancillary investigations often aid in reaching the final diagnosis. Broadly, granulomatous disorders are classified as infectious and noninfectious.

CASE 1

A 32-year-old woman presented with an asymptomatic erythematous, indurated plaque of size 4 × 1 cm with overlying brownish crusting on the right upper arm for last 3 years (Fig. 1). There was no regional lymphadenopathy. The patient denied any history of preceding trauma or systemic symptoms.

Investigations: Histopathologic examination revealed irregular acanthosis of the epidermis. The upper dermis showed confluent epithelioid cell granulomas with dense cuffing of lymphocytes and few Langhans type of giant cells abutting the epidermis (Figs. 2a and 2b). Some discrete granulomas were present in the mid-dermis (Fig. 2c). Ziehl–Neelsen (ZN), Fite, Giemsa and periodic acid–Schiff stains were all negative. Tissue cultures for *M. tuberculosis* and fungus were negative. Slit skin smears for lepra bacilli and Leishman-Donovan bodies were negative. Potassium hydroxide (KOH) 10% smear was also negative. Mantoux test was strongly positive with a reading of 35 × 25 mm at 48 hours. Chest radiograph was normal. Based on the clinical presentation, histopathology and strongly positive Mantoux test, a final diagnosis of lupus vulgaris (plaque type) was made.

Treatment: She was started on 4-drug antitubercular treatment (ATT), had shown good response after a month of therapy and is currently on follow-up.

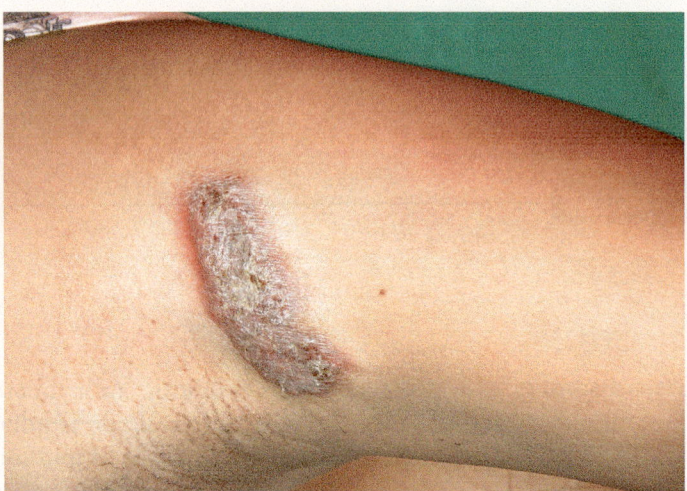

Fig. 1: A well-defined erythematous indurated plaque of size 4 × 1 cm with overlying greyish-brown crusting on the lateral aspect of the right upper arm.

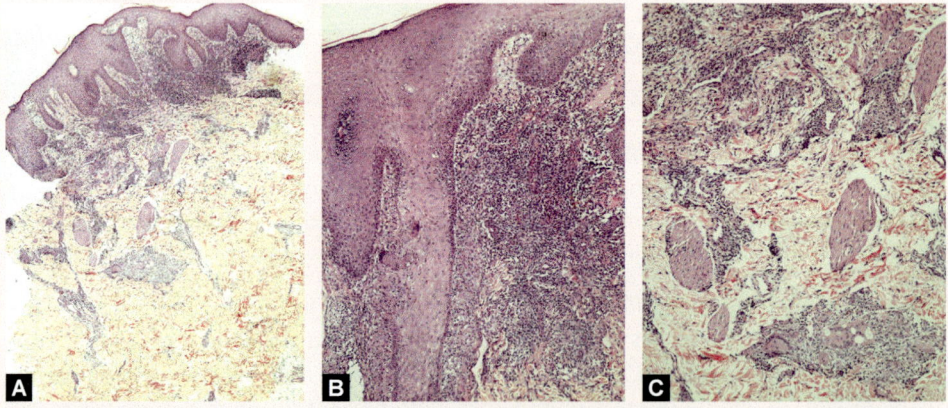

Fig. 2: (A) The epidermis shows irregular acanthosis. Moderate degree of inflammatory infiltrate is present in the papillary dermis extending into the mid-dermis (H&E, 4x); (B) Confluent granulomas composed of epithelioid cells, dense infiltrate of lymphocytes and Langhans giant cells are present abutting the acanthotic epidermis (H&E, 10x); (C) Discrete epithelioid cell granulomas with multinucleate giant cells present in the mid-dermis (H&E, 10x).

INTERACTIVE TOPIC REVIEW

Q.1 What are the differential diagnoses that can be considered clinically in this case?

Ans: Deep fungal infections such as fixed cutaneous sporotrichosis and chromoblastomycosis, borderline tuberculoid leprosy and cutaneous leishmaniasis.

Q.2 How can one differentiate them histopathologically?

Ans: The salient histological features of various infectious granulomatous conditions are described in Table 1.

TABLE 1: Histopathological findings in infectious granulomatous dermatoses.

Diagnosis	Light microscopic features
Lupus vulgaris	• Epidermis: Hyperplastic, atrophic or ulcerated • Dermis: Confluent granulomas in upper and mid-dermis and discrete granulomas in lower dermis • Granulomas comprise of epithelioid cells, Langhans giant cells and peripheral cuff of lymphocytes. Caseation necrosis may be present. Varying degree of fibrosis may be seen. Ziehl–Neelsen stain is usually negative
Deep fungal infection	• Epidermis: Pseudoepitheliomatous hyperplasia, intraepidermal microabscesses • Dermis: Tuberculoid or suppurative granulomas. Yeast like cells or cigar bodies are rarely seen in sporotrichosis. Sporothrix asteroid is a yeast cell in the center surrounded by eosinophilic hyaline material with ray like processes extending from center. Round, thick walled, septate, golden brown sclerotic bodies within giant cells or lying free are seen in chromoblastomycosis
Borderline tuberculoid leprosy	• Epidermis: Thinned out or normal • Dermis: Noncaseating, oblong/curvilinear epithelioid cell granulomas in perineural, periappendageal and peri-erector pilorum muscle distribution • The granulomas contain multinucleate giant cells and lymphocytes. Cutaneous nerve bundles are infiltrated and even destroyed by the granulomas. Fite Faraco stain for acid-fast bacilli is usually negative
Cutaneous leishmaniasis	• Epidermis: Acanthotic, atrophic or ulcerated • Dermal infiltrate of lymphocytes, plasma cells, macrophages and occasional giant cells • Parasites are usually present within the macrophages as small (2–4 microns), round to oval basophilic structures with an eccentric kinetoplast. As the lesions become chronic, the number of parasitized macrophages decrease and tuberculoid granulomas appear. Giemsa stain may be used to demonstrate the Leishman-Donovan bodies

Q.3 How are granulomas classified histologically?

Ans: The histological subtypes of granulomas are enlisted in Table 2.

TABLE 2: Histopathological classification of granulomas.

Type of granuloma	Salient features
Tuberculoid	Composed of epithelioid cells, giant cells (Langhans and foreign body type) and cuffing by dense infiltrate of lymphocytes. Tend to become confluent. Caseation may sometimes be present
Suppurative	Composed of epithelioid cells, giant cells, centrally distributed neutrophils and peripheral rim of lymphocytes and plasma cells
Sarcoidal	Discrete granulomas composed of epithelioid cells, giant cells (Langhans or foreign body type) with a sparse rim of lymphocytes and plasma cells (naked granulomas). Giant cells may contain asteroid and Schaumann bodies
Necrobiotic/ collagenolytic	Necrobiosis refers to areas of altered dermal collagen characterized by loss of definition of collagen fibers which appear more basophilic or eosinophilic on light microscopy. Poorly formed granulomas with necrobiotic areas surrounded by a rim of histiocytes and giant cells forming a palisade
Foreign body	Composed of epithelioid cells, foreign body giant cells and other inflammatory cells. Foreign material is usually identifiable
Xanthogranuloma	Composed of foamy/pale histiocytes, Touton giant cells and some inflammatory cells

Q.4 How to classify cutaneous tuberculosis?

Ans: Cutaneous tuberculosis has been classified in many ways taking various facets of its presentation and mode of spread. A simple one has been described in Table 3.

TABLE 3: Classification of cutaneous tuberculosis.

Host immunity	Route of entry	Morphologic type
Paucibacillary		
High	Exogenous/hematogenous/contiguous	Lupus vulgaris
High	Exogenous	Tuberculosis *Verrucosa* cutis
High	Hematogenous	Tuberculids
Naïve	Exogenous	Tuberculosis secondary to BCG vaccine (primary complex-like reaction, perforating lymphadenitis, lupus vulgaris, scrofuloderma, lichen scrofulosorum)
Multibacillary		
Naïve	Exogenous	Tuberculous chancre
Low	Contiguous	Scrofuloderma
Low	Autoinoculation	Orificial tuberculosis
Low	Hematogenous	Acute cutaneous miliary
Low	Hematogenous	Tuberculous gumma

Q.5 What are the clinical variants of lupus vulgaris?

Ans: The clinical forms of lupus vulgaris include:
- Plaque type
- Ulcerative and mutilating
- Vegetative
- Tumor-like
- Papular and nodular
- Giant.

Q.6 Enumerate the complications of lupus vulgaris.

Ans: Complications of lupus vulgaris include scarring which may be atrophic or keloidal, contractures, destruction of auricular or nasal cartilage, ectropion, microstomia, laryngeal stenosis, malignant transformation into squamous cell carcinoma (SCC) in situ or invasive, basal cell carcinoma, melanoma, lymphoma and sarcoma. The incidence of SCC arising in lupus vulgaris varies from 0.5% to 10.5%, with a mean of around 4%. Malignant transformation may result from free radicals produced due to chronic inflammation, immunosuppression due to ultraviolet radiation (in sun-exposed lesions) and mutations in *p53* gene.

Q.7 What investigations are done in a suspected case of cutaneous tuberculosis?

Ans: Routine investigations like complete hemogram, liver and renal function tests, urine routine and microscopy and erythrocyte sedimentation rate. Specific investigations like skin biopsy for histopathology and culture, direct microscopy for acid fast bacilli, chest radiograph and tuberculin skin test. The HIV serology should be done particularly in adults with multifocal cutaneous lesions or multibacillary systemic disease. Sputum for acid fast bacilli and radiological imaging for other organ involvement (abdomen, central nervous system, lymph nodes, bones and joints) should be done where indicated. KOH and slit skin smear (Giemsa and modified ZN staining), fungal and Leishmania cultures are done to exclude other differential diagnoses. As the smears and cultures are often negative in cutaneous tuberculosis owing to its paucibacillary nature, a therapeutic trial of 4-6 weeks of The ATT is often used to confirm or refute the diagnosis in difficult cases. Based on the histopathology and strongly positive Mantoux reaction in the present patient, we considered the diagnosis of lupus vulgaris (plaque type) and started her on ATT. She showed good response after 1 month of therapy.

Q.8 Discuss the role of tuberculin skin test and interferon-γ release assays (IGRAs) in the diagnosis of cutaneous tuberculosis.

Ans: Tuberculin skin test (Mantoux method) is done by injecting 0.1 mL of purified protein derivative (PPD) [or 5 tuberculin units] intradermally into the volar aspect of the forearm with a 27 gauge needle. The diameter of the induration is measured at 48–72 hours. It detects delayed type of hypersensitivity reaction to mycobacterial antigens. As PPD shares antigens with *M. bovis* (BCG vaccine) and nontuberculous mycobacteria, Mantoux test suffers from low specificity.

It can be false negative in tuberculous chancre, gumma, miliary tuberculosis, malnutrition, HIV infection, in patients treated with immunosuppressants, advanced age and pregnancy. In a study by Ramam et al. the sensitivity and specificity of the test have been reported to be 58.97% and 62.5%, respectively, when 10 mm was used as the cut off value, thereby making it less accurate in confirming the diagnosis in equivocal cases. According to Index TB guidelines on extrapulmonary tuberculosis from India, Mantoux test may be done as an ancillary investigation in doubtful cases and the result must be correlated with clinical findings and other investigations. A reading of 22 mm or more is said to support the diagnosis of cutaneous tuberculosis.

The IGRAs (Quantiferon-TB Gold In-Tube Test and T-SPOT TB test) are more specific than tuberculin test as they are based on measurement of T-cell responses to antigens namely, early secretory protein 6 and culture filtrate protein 10, which are absent in BCG strains and most nontuberculous mycobacteria. They are useful for diagnosing latent tuberculosis infection in BCG vaccinated individuals.

Q.9 **What is the role of mycobacterial polymerase chain reaction (PCR) in the diagnosis of cutaneous tuberculosis?**

Ans: The current evidence suggests that PCR cannot be recommended for routine diagnosis of cutaneous tuberculosis. In a recent Indian study of 49 cases of cutaneous tuberculosis, DNA-PCR for *M. tuberculosis* showed a sensitivity of 24.5%. The sensitivity has been shown to vary from 4.5 to 88% in different studies, attributable to laboratory variation. It is suggested that PCR should be preferred over culture in cases with inconclusive histopathology. It also has the advantage of yielding rapid results within 24 hours. Most commonly, insertion sequence IS6110 has been used because of its repetitive nature in the *M. tuberculosis* genome. Other gene targets include *16s rRNA* gene or genes encoding MPB-64, 38 kDa and 65 kDa proteins. Multiplex PCR using combination of two or more gene targets has also been studied. The disadvantages of PCR include false positive and false negative results, risk of contamination, high cost and availability issues.

Q.10 **Discuss about drug resistance in cutaneous tuberculosis.**

Ans: Multidrug resistant (MDR) tuberculosis is defined as resistance to isoniazid and rifampicin with or without resistance to other anti-tubercular drugs. Multi-drug resistant cutaneous tuberculosis should be suspected when there is no response and/or clinical deterioration on first line ATT and when alternative diagnoses are unlikely. Culture and drug susceptibility testing should be performed where facilities are available. However, owing to paucibacillary nature of cutaneous tuberculosis, organisms are often not isolated on culture and therefore demonstration of drug resistance is difficult. In such cases where no other diagnosis is forthcoming, the patient's condition shows signs of deterioration and attempts to culture are unsuccessful, a trial of second line ATT may be justified for a period of 2 months and subsequently continued for 24 months in those showing response.

Q.11 What is the treatment regimen for cutaneous tuberculosis?

Ans: The standard ATT regimen for a newly diagnosed case of cutaneous tuberculosis is of 6 months duration, with an initial intensive phase of 2 months and a continuation phase of 4 months. The drugs administered in intensive phase are isoniazid (300 mg), rifampicin (450 mg if weight is <60 kg and 600 mg if ≥60 kg), pyrazinamide (1500 mg) and ethambutol (1200 mg) and in continuation phase are isoniazid, rifampicin and ethambutol. It is currently recommended that daily dosing should be used in both intensive and continuation phases of treatment rather than thrice weekly dosing because of higher rates of treatment failure, relapse and acquired drug resistance associated with the intermittent dosing schedule. Appropriate laboratory tests should be done to monitor the side-effects of the drugs.

Q.12 What are tuberculids?

Ans: Tuberculids are defined as cutaneous hypersensitivity reactions to hematogenous dissemination of *M. tuberculosis* or its antigens from a primary focus in individuals with strong cell mediated immunity. The criteria to diagnose them include strongly positive Mantoux test, negative smear and culture for *M. tuberculosis*, tuberculoid granulomas on histology and response to ATT. However, mycobacterial DNA has been demonstrated by PCR in tuberculids. Tuberculids are categorized as:
- Micropapular—lichen scrofulosorum
- Papular—papulonecrotic tuberculid
- Nodular—erythema induratum of Bazin.

CASE 2

A 40-year-old woman presented with asymptomatic erythematous annular plaques on the face for 2 years (Fig. 3). She had no systemic complaints. There was no lesional sensory loss on examination.

Investigations: Routine investigations including hemogram, liver and renal function tests and urine microscopy were within normal limits. Her skin biopsy showed thinned out epidermis and presence of compact granulomas in the dermis (Fig. 3). The granulomas were composed of epithelioid cells, multinucleated giant cells and sparse infiltrate of lymphocytes in the periphery (Fig. 4). Chest radiograph showed no abnormality. Mantoux test and slit skin smear for lepra bacilli were negative.

Treatment: She was treated with mid-potency topical corticosteroids and showed good improvement after 2 months.

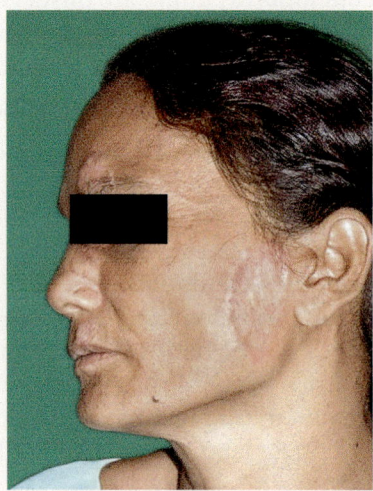

Fig. 3: Erythematous annular plaques with raised indurated borders and mild central atrophy on the left eyebrow, left preauricular area and above upper lip.

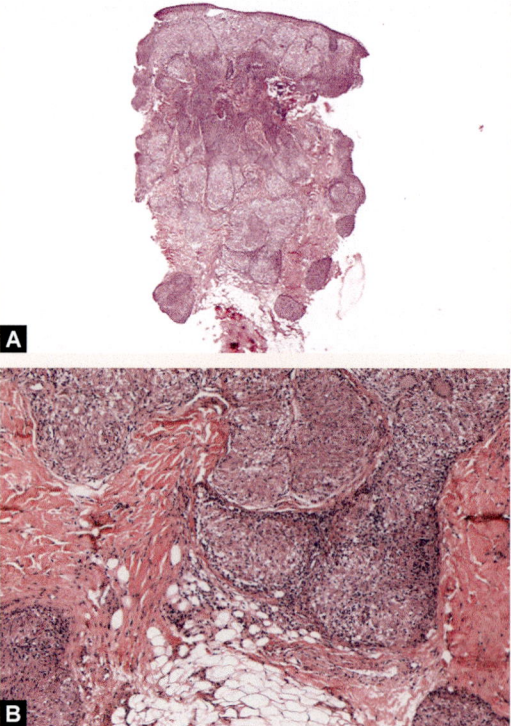

Fig. 4: (A) Scanner view showing thinned out epidermis and presence of discrete, compact granulomas distributed throughout the dermis (H&E, 2x); (B) Dermis showing naked granulomas composed of epithelioid cells, Langhans giant cells and sparse lymphocyte cuffing (H&E, 10x).

INTERACTIVE CASE REVIEW

Q.1 What are the clinical differential diagnoses for this case?

Ans: Borderline tuberculoid leprosy, granuloma annulare.

Q.2 Enumerate the clinical variants of cutaneous sarcoidosis.

Ans: The more frequent specific lesions include maculopapular, nodular, plaque, lupus pernio, scar sarcoidosis and subcutaneous sarcoidosis. The less common forms include angiolupoid, lichenoid, ulcerative, hypopigmented, psoriasiform, ichthyosiform, verrucous and erythrodermic.

Q.3 What is lupus pernio?

Ans: It is a distinct form of cutaneous sarcoidosis that is frequently seen in older black women. Clinically it presents as infiltrated erythematous to violaceous plaques distributed on the nose, cheeks, forehead, ears, lips and fingers. It can be disfiguring but does not ulcerate. Lupus pernio is associated with sarcoidosis of the upper respiratory tract in about half the cases. Other associations include chronic uveitis, pulmonary fibrosis and bony cysts of the terminal phalanges. It usually runs a chronic course.

Q.4 What are the nonspecific cutaneous lesions seen in sarcoidosis?

Ans: Erythema nodosum (EN) is the most common nonspecific cutaneous lesion associated with sarcoidosis, in almost 20% of the cases. It is often the initial presentation of the disease and heralds a good prognosis and a benign disease course. When associated with bilateral hilar and right paratracheal lymphadenopathy, fever, arthralgia and uveitis it is known as Lofgren syndrome. Other nonspecific cutaneous manifestations include Sweet's syndrome, pyoderma gangrenosum, prurigo nodularis-like lesions, drug reaction or viral exanthema-like rash, erythema multiforme, erythroderma and lower limb swelling.

Q.5 What are important systemic manifestations of sarcoidosis?

Ans: Systemic manifestations of sarcoidosis are enlisted in Table 4.

TABLE 4: Systemic involvement in sarcoidosis.

System	Manifestations
Pulmonary	Dry cough, dyspnea, bilateral hilar lymphadenopathy, pulmonary fibrosis and hypertension
Eye	Anterior/posterior uveitis, chorioretinitis, papilloedema, retinal hemorrhage, secondary glaucoma and cataract
Reticuloendothelial system	Peripheral lymphadenopathy, rarely splenomegaly and bone marrow involvement
Liver	Hepatomegaly, noncaseating granulomas and cholestasis
Heart	Supraventricular and ventricular arrhythmias, complete heart block and congestive heart failure
Nervous system	Cranial nerve involvement (facial paralysis, optic nerve), aseptic meningitis, seizures, pyramidal tract signs and diabetes insipidus
Others	Nephrocalcinosis, nephrolithiasis, hypercalcemia and parotid involvement

Q.6 Which other conditions can show sarcoidal granulomas on histopathology?

Ans: Blau's syndrome, reaction to foreign materials (silica, silicon, tattoo pigment, zirconium, interferon injections), granuloma annulare, metastatic Crohn's disease, orofacial granulomatosis and sezary syndrome. Certain infections notably tuberculosis, leprosy and secondary syphilis may also demonstrate sarcoidal granulomas.

Q.7 What are asteroid and Schaumann bodies and in which other diseases they are seen?

Ans: Asteroid bodies contain an eosinophilic central core surrounded by radiating spicules. They are formed from trapped collagen bundles or components of cytoskeleton. Schaumann (conchoidal) bodies are basophilic, concentric, round to oval lamellar structures containing lipomucoglycoproteins impregnated with calcium and iron. Both the bodies are seen within multinucleated giant cells. Besides sarcoidosis, they are seen in other granulomatous conditions like tuberculosis, leprosy, Crohn's disease and berylliosis.

Q.8 What investigations would you advise in a patient of sarcoidosis?

Ans: Complete hemogram, liver and renal function tests, chest radiograph, pulmonary function tests including diffusion capacity for carbon monoxide, urine analysis, electrocardiogram, ophthalmologic examination, serum angiotensin converting enzyme level, serum and urine calcium and tuberculin skin test. High resolution contrast tomography may be required in cases with atypical chest radiograph findings.

Q.9 Discuss the management of cutaneous sarcoidosis.

Ans: In patients with systemic disease, cutaneous lesions usually respond to oral corticosteroids with/without antimalarials or other immunosuppressants. First line treatment for mild cutaneous lesions is topical corticosteroids. Intralesional injections of triamcinolone acetonide (5–20 mg/mL) can also be administered in localized disease. In lupus pernio or disfiguring skin lesions, oral corticosteroids (0.5–1 mg/kg/day for 1–3 months) are recommended, which are gradually tapered to the lowest effective dose. Second line therapies like antimalarials, methotrexate and tetracyclines are indicated when oral corticosteroids are contraindicated and as corticosteroid sparing agents in lupus pernio. Anti-tumor necrosis factor-α agents like infliximab and adalimumab are third line agents for refractory cutaneous sarcoidosis.

Q.10 What are idiopathic facial granulomatous eruptions that may mimic sarcoidosis clinically?

Ans: Idiopathic facial granulomatous eruptions include granulomatous rosacea (GR), lupus miliaris disseminatus faciei (LMDF) and granulomatous periorificial dermatitis (GPD). These entities have been grouped together as they exhibit similar clinico-histopathological features. The salient clinical features of these three disorders in relation to sarcoidosis are enlisted in Table 5. Histologically, they are characterized by perivascular and perifollicular epithelioid cell granulomas or sometimes a diffuse lymphohistiocytic infiltrate. Caseation is a distinguishing finding in LMDF and rarely GR. All

TABLE 5: Idiopathic facial granulomatous disorders.[4]

Clinical features	Granulomatous rosacea	Lupus miliaris disseminatus faciei	Granulomatous periorificial dermatitis	Sarcoidosis
Age	20–50 years	Young adults	Prepubertal children	Young to middle aged
Race and gender	Usually in white females, can be seen in anyone	Often in males	Usually in blacks, both genders	More in blacks, females
Cutaneous lesions	Dull red-brown papules on a background of erythema and thickened skin	Dull red-brown papules, central necrosis may be seen. Typically resolve with scarring	Multiple discrete tiny yellow-brown papules	Micropapules, papules, nodules, plaques
Facial sites	Central and lateral areas	Central area	Periocular, perinasal and perioral	Anywhere, may be localized
Vascular findings	Less than rosacea	Absent	Mild	Absent
Extrafacial sites	Uncommon	Rare	May occur	Common
Ocular involvement	Blepharitis and conjunctivitis	Absent	Rarely blepharitis	Uveitis, scleritis episcleritis
Systemic disease	Absent	Absent	Absent	Present
Spontaneous regression	Not seen	Usual	Usual	Seen in acute forms

three disorders are treated similarly, on the lines of rosacea. It is essential to follow-up these facial idiopathic granulomatous disorders as long standing lesions, involvement of extrafacial sites, annular, deep-seated plaques and systemic manifestations raise the possibility of sarcoidosis, which can be confirmed on further investigations.

Q.11 What is the classification of necrobiotic granulomas?

Ans: Necrobiotic granulomas are classified in Table 6.

TABLE 6: Lynch and Barrett classification of necrobiotic granulomas.

Blue	Red
Granuloma annulare	Necrobiosis lipoidica
Wegener's granulomatosis	Necrobiotic xanthogranuloma
Rheumatoid vasculitis	Rheumatoid nodule
	Pseudorheumatoid nodule
	Churg–Strauss syndrome
	Eosinophilic cellulitis

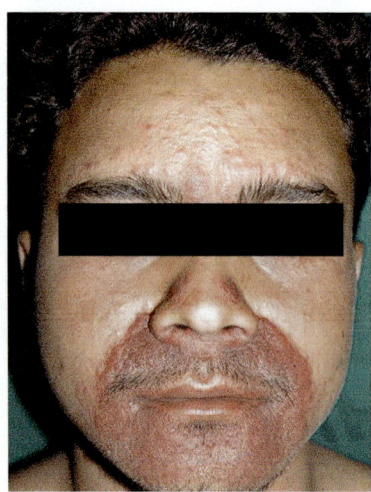

Fig. 5: Multiple discrete erythematous papules on the forehead and periocular areas, coalescing to form plaques on the glabella, along with erythematous infiltrated plaques on the lateral aspect of the nose and extending below to involve the nasal vestibules, perinasal, perioral areas and the chin.

Q.12 What are the clinical variants of granuloma annulare?

Ans: These include localized form which is the most common, generalized, perforating and subcutaneous types. Less frequent variants include patch type, papular umbilicated, linear, follicular and generalized pustular perforating types.

Q.13 What are the histological patterns described in granuloma annulare?

Ans: Three histological patterns are seen in granuloma annulare—interstitial or incomplete type which is the most common, necrobiotic palisading and sarcoidal or tuberculoid type, which is the least common.

Orofacial granulomatosis (OFG) is a descriptive term that encompasses conditions which present clinically as recurrent or persistent orofacial swelling and histologically as noncaseating granulomas. It may be categorized as primary/idiopathic (Fig. 5) and secondary. The various etiologies for OFG are Crohn's disease, sarcoidosis, tuberculosis, rosacea and allergy to food additives and dental materials. However, the cause in majority of the cases remains unknown and these cases are grouped under primary OFG. The latter is used synonymously with granulomatous cheilitis and Melkersson–Rosenthal syndrome (triad of granulomatous cheilits, facial nerve palsy and fissured tongue).

▮ CONCLUSION

Granulomatous disorders are a broad group of conditions characterized histologically by discrete collections of histiocytes admixed with multinucleate giant cells and varied number of other inflammatory cells. They can be classified as infectious and noninfectious. It is often challenging to distinguish them clinically and hence histopathological features like arrangement and composition of granulomas, presence of caseation, necrobiosis, suppuration, foreign body and micro-organisms are important clues that aid in making a definite diagnosis in majority of the cases. In others, relevant laboratory investigations and response to treatment may also be considered to support the diagnosis.

KEY POINTS

- Granulomatous disorders frequently present a diagnostic challenge, both clinically and histologically and the diagnosis is best formulated based on clinico-pathological correlation in most of the cases
- In Indian scenario, infectious granulomatous dermatoses are more frequent than noninfectious conditions. In infectious conditions, the type and pattern of granuloma on histopathology is an important determinant in arriving at the diagnosis
- Demonstration of organisms on histopathology using special stains and/or isolation on culture, confirms the diagnosis, but are less often rewarding
- Ancillary tests and response to treatment often help in supporting the diagnosis in difficult cases where histopathology and microbiology results are inconclusive.

SUGGESTED READING

1. Agarwal P, Singh EN, Agarwal US, et al. The role of DNA polymerase chain reaction, culture and histopathology in the diagnosis of cutaneous tuberculosis. Int J Dermatol. 2017;56:1119-24.
2. Griffiths C, Barker J, Bleiker T, et al. Rook's Textbook of Dermatology. 9th ed. UK: John Wiley and Sons, Ltd; 2016.
3. Kumaran MS, Narang T, Jitendriya M, et al. Cutaneous squamous cell carcinoma in lupus vulgaris caused by drug resistant Mycobacterium tuberculosis. Indian Dermatol Online J. 2017;8:257-60.
4. Makkar R, Ramesh V. On the diagnosis of facial granulomatous disorders of obscure origin. Int J Dermatol. 2005;44:606-9.
5. Miest R, Bruce A, Rogers RS 3rd. Orofacial granulomatosis. Clin Dermatol. 2016;34:505-13.
6. Patterson J, editor. Weedon's Skin Pathology 4th ed. UK: Elsevier; 2015.
7. Ramam M, Malhotra A, Tejasvi T, et al. How useful is the Mantoux test in the diagnosis of doubtful cases of cutaneous tuberculosis? Int J Dermatol. 2011;50:1379-8.
8. Ramam M, Mittal R, Ramesh V. How soon does cutaneous tuberculosis respond to treatment? Implications for a therapeutic test of diagnosis. Int J Dermatol. 2005;44:121-4.
9. Ramam M, Tejasvi T, Manchanda Y, et al. What is the appropriate duration of a therapeutic trial in cutaneous tuberculosis? Further observations. Indian J Dermatol Venereol Leprol. 2007;73:243-6.
10. Ramesh V, Kumar J. Cutaneous tuberculosis. Expert Rev Dermatol. 2010;5:417-31.
11. Ramesh V, Sen MK, Sethuraman G, et al. Cutaneous tuberculosis due to multidrug-resistant tubercle bacilli and difficulties in clinical diagnosis. Indian J Dermatol Venereol Leprol. 2015;81:380-4.
12. Ramesh V. Orofacial granulomatosis due to tuberculosis. Pediatr Dermatol. 2009;26:108-9.
13. Sharma SK, Ryan H, Khaparde S, et al. Index-TB Guidelines: Guidelines on extra-pulmonary tuberculosis for India. Indian J Med Res. 2017;145:448-463.

CHAPTER 14

Diffuse Hair Loss

Bela J Shah, Deval B Mistry

■ INTRODUCTION

Diffuse hair shedding can be quite distressing, affecting any age or sex. Interruptions of the normal hair cycle results in diffuse hair loss. Triggers responsible for the same include various physiological or emotional stresses, hormonal imbalances, dietary deficiencies, etc. Elaborate history taking and physical examination are required to find the cause and thereby effectively manage this problem. Patient education is of utmost importance in the management of diffuse hair loss.

CASE 1

A 30-year-old female presented to the outpatient department (OPD) clinic with complaints of diffuse hair loss since 2 weeks. The hair fall was abrupt in onset, continuous, rapid and diffuse. The patient gave history of hospital admission for pyrexia which was diagnosed as typhoid fever and received treatment for the same about 2 months ago. The patient did not reveal any history of recent surgery, childbirth, psychological stress, thyroid, renal or liver disorder, or any other chronic disease. The menstrual history was normal. Dietary history was insignificant. The patient did not give any history of taking over the counter medications or any alternative medications. The patient did not have any family history of pattern hair loss, alopecia areata, or thyroid disorder.

Clinical examination revealed positive hair pull test over all the areas of scalp. There were no signs suggestive of anemia or thyroid dysfunction. Trichoscopy did not reveal any characteristic findings apart from reduction in hair density. A trichogram showed significant increase in telogen hairs. Scalp biopsy was not performed.

A clinical diagnosis of acute telogen effluvium was made and the patient was given reassurance and supportive treatment. She was explained that the condition is because of excessive hair shedding and that regrowth of hair would occur and there will not be any resultant baldness from this condition.

Significant regrowth was obtained in this patient within a period of 3 months, however, for the patient, cosmetically acceptable regrowth took about 5 months.

Diffuse Hair Loss | 197

Case Review in a Nutshell (Figs. 1 and 2)

Diffuse hair loss is very common amongst all age groups. For any diffuse hair loss case presenting to the OPD, it is imperative to know all the common clinical differentials to reach a correct diagnosis and enable appropriate treatment. In the author's case, the following entities were considered:
- Telogen effluvium (acute/chronic)
- Female pattern hair loss
- Diffuse type of alopecia areata/alopecia areata incognita
- Anagen hair loss.

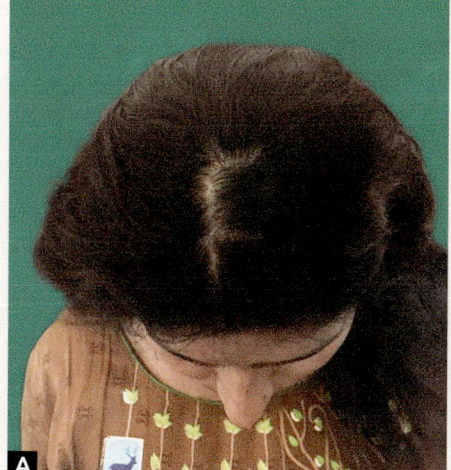
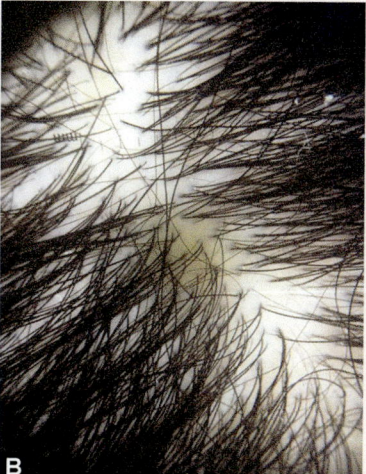

Fig. 1: (A) Diffuse hair loss for the past 2 weeks; (B) Trichoscopy normal.

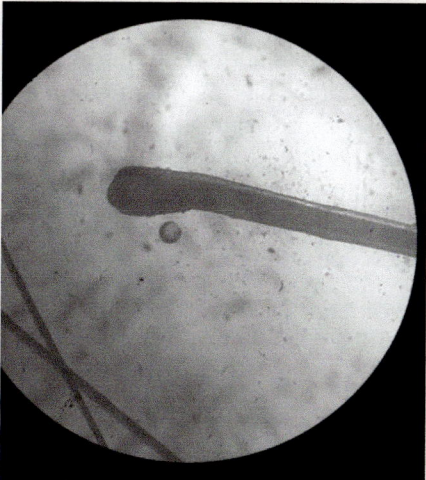

Fig. 2: Telogen hair follicle with club shaped bulb.

Keeping in mind the history and more importantly the chronology of events, the first differential considered was acute telogen effluvium. Abrupt onset of rapid and diffuse hair fall following 2 months after a stress factor (typhoid fever in our case) with a positive hair pull test, no specific trichoscopy findings and significant increase in telogen hairs on trichogram makes the diagnosis of acute telogen effluvium very likely. Chronic telogen effluvium is considered when the hair loss lasts for a duration of 6 or more months.

Episodes of telogen hair shedding may occur in early stages of androgenetic alopecia, before the typical clinical presentation sets in. However, in the absence of any trichoscopy or trichogram findings supporting this diagnosis, a positive hair pull test and a negative family history, pattern hair loss was not considered.

Diffuse type of alopecia areata was also not considered in view of the trichoscopy and trichogram findings. Anagen hair loss would present as severe diffuse scalp alopecia within a short period (1–2 weeks) of an acute, severe metabolic insult (like chemotherapeutic drugs/cytotoxic agents) and other body hair may also be affected. In absence of any history or clinical findings supporting this diagnosis, anagen hair loss was also ruled out.

The patient was given appropriate explanation, supportive treatment and reassurance and she showed significant hair growth within 3 months as the cause for telogen effluvium was already treated. Complete recovery was obtained within a period of 5 months.

■ INTERACTIVE TOPIC REVIEW

Q.1 What is the normal hair cycle?

Ans: Scalp hair grows in cycles, with each hair follicle undergoing 10–30 cycles in its lifetime. The basic etiology of diffuse hair shedding is disruption of any phase of the hair cycle, i.e. anagen (active hair growth), catagen (involution), or telogen (resting). The duration of anagen phase is 2–8 years, the catagen phase lasts 4–6 weeks, while telogen phase lasts 2–3 months. The exogen phase in which there is release of dead hair, coincides with the end of the telogen phase.

Normally, each hair follicle has an independent cycle. So, at any given time, there are some hair follicles in resting stage, some will be growing while some will be in the phase of shedding. This is how the number of hair and its density is maintained steadily. Most people have about 100,000 scalp hairs, out of which on a normal basis 10–15% will be in the telogen phase. Shedding of 100–150 telogen hairs per day is considered normal. However, anagen hair loss is never normal.

Q.2 What is the most common type of diffuse hair loss?

Ans: The most common type of diffuse hair fall is telogen effluvium. Here, there is premature transition of hair follicles from anagen to telogen phase. This results in increased hair shedding at the end of the telogen phase 2–3 months later. Telogen effluvium is a sign of some underlying pathology and hence it is not a complete diagnosis per se.

Q.3 What is the differential diagnosis of diffuse hair loss?

Ans: Differential diagnosis of diffuse hair loss:
- Telogen hair loss (acute and chronic): A variety of factors can cause telogen effluvium. It can be acute (lasting <6 months), chronic (6 months or more), or chronic-repetitive. The type of trigger determines the duration of hair loss, viz., acute short-lived triggers cause acute telogen effluvium, while repetitive, continuous, or sequential triggers can cause chronic hair loss
- Androgenetic alopecia: Early androgenetic alopecia (pattern hair loss) is an important differential diagnosis in telogen hair shedding. It may present as episodic telogen hair loss before any distinctive pattern is seen
- Anagen hair loss: Premature termination of anagen hair growth or anagen arrest can cause anagen hair loss. This occurs after an acute and severe metabolic insult. It is commonly iatrogenic due to treatment with radiation or cytotoxic drugs
- Alopecia areata incognita/diffuse type of alopecia areata: The clinical picture seen here closely resembles telogen effluvium, however, specific clinical findings as well as dermoscopic picture of alopecia areata will be present along the course of the disease
- Other rare causes: Apart from the above mentioned causes, other uncommon causes of diffuse hair loss include loose anagen hair syndrome, congenital hypotrichosis, congenital atrichia as well as hair shaft abnormalities (hair breakage, unruly hairs).

Q.4 What are the triggers of diffuse telogen hair fall?

Ans: Triggers of diffuse telogen hair fall:
- Physiological stress: Factors such as surgical trauma, high fever, chronic systemic illness and hemorrhage can cause telogen effluvium 2–3 months after the insult. Telogen hair loss can also be seen 2–4 months after childbirth (telogen gravidarum)
- Emotional stress: The relationship between emotional stress and hair loss is difficult to identify and hair loss itself is stressful to the patient. There is association between severe stress and hair fall, which is acute and reversible. However, the relationship between chronic diffuse hair loss and psychological stress is controversial. Evidence for this association appears to be weak, as daily stresses are not likely to trigger hair loss
- Medical disorders: Thyroid disorder (both hypothyroidism and hyperthyroidism) can cause diffuse telogen hair loss. Once the patient becomes euthyroid, hair fall usually is reversible. Chronic systemic disorders-like hepatic failure, chronic renal failure, systemic amyloidosis, inflammatory bowel disease and lymphoproliferative disorders can cause telogen hair shedding. Various infections like human immunodeficiency virus and secondary syphilis as well as connective tissue disorders like systemic lupus erythematosus and dermatomyositis can cause telogen hair loss. Psoriasis, seborrheic dermatitis, allergic contact dermatitis and various other inflammatory disorders can all cause diffuse telogen hair loss

- Dietary factors: Severe protein and caloric restriction with chronic starvation and crash dieting can lead to diffuse telogen hair loss. Nutritional deficiencies of zinc and iron can cause telogen hair loss. Malabsorption syndromes, pancreatic disease and essential fatty acid deficiency can also precipitate telogen hair shedding. Vitamin D deficiency may be associated with diffuse hair loss. Very rarely, biotin deficiency can result in alopecia
- Drugs: Drugs can cause telogen hair loss. It usually begins about 12 weeks after initiation and continues while on therapy. Dosing changes can also precipitate hair shedding. Any medication including over-the-counter products or alternative medicines the patient is taking should be suspected in hair loss
- Drugs known to cause telogen effluvium are oral contraceptive pills, angiotensin-converting enzyme inhibitors, β-blockers, retinoids, anticonvulsants, androgens, antithyroid drugs, antidepressants and anticoagulants like heparin and warfarin
- Hair care procedures/cosmetics: Various procedures that are done on the hair for cosmetic purpose like smoothening, straightening, perming, spa therapy, ironing, etc., can lead to diffuse hair loss of various degrees.

Q.5 How to identify the triggers of diffuse telogen hair loss?

Ans: Normal hair shedding usually goes unnoticed. However, with telogen effluvium, there is 25% increase in hair shedding. To determine the exact trigger of telogen hair loss, the relationship between the trigger and the hair loss must be reproducible. Hence, on addition or removal of trigger, hair loss should worsen or revert accordingly.

In acute onset of telogen hair loss 2–3 months after an acute, short-lived triggering event, a detailed history is crucial to determine accurate sequence of events by analyzing the timeline. Even then, no trigger is identified in many cases. Regrowth may not be visible for 4–6 months. Recovery is likely to be complete if the triggering factor is determined and removed.

In chronic diffuse telogen hair loss (lasts >6 months), a variety of factors are implicated in precipitating shedding. It is idiopathic or secondary to prolonged, sequential, or repeated triggers and hair loss may be less pronounced than in acute telogen effluvium.

Chronic telogen effluvium is an idiopathic condition where telogen hair loss lasts longer than 6 months. The disease course is fluctuating, over many years and without any identifiable cause. Patients may present with a full head of hair or with bitemporal recession without midline widening. Histology shows absence of miniaturization of hair follicles. Chronic telogen effluvium is a diagnosis of exclusion reached by ruling out all causes of diffuse telogen hair loss, including pattern hair loss.

Q.6 What is the clinical presentation of androgenetic alopecia in women?

Ans: Androgenetic alopecia or pattern hair loss usually presents as well-defined, patterned hair loss in patients who may have a similar family history. Diffuse hair loss over the vertex and widening of the central part in women, with or without frontal accentuation ("Christmas tree" pattern), is characteristic.

The mechanism is related to progressive miniaturization of the hair follicles and anagen phase shortening. Sometimes, androgenetic alopecia can also present as diffuse scalp hair loss with episodic telogen hair shedding, which may cause confusion in reaching a clinical diagnosis.

Q.7 When is a hormonal profile indicated in diffuse hair loss?

Ans: Androgen excess disorders can cause diffuse scalp hair loss or patterned hair loss although most women with hair loss will have normal androgen levels. Signs of hyperandrogenism include hirsutism, oligomenorrhea, severe or recalcitrant acne, infertility, acanthosis nigricans and galactorrhea. Women in whom androgenetic alopecia is severe, abrupt, rapidly progressive, or associated with severe bitemporal recession, or women with clinical signs and symptoms suggestive of hyperandrogenism, would require hormonal screening tests. These tests help us in ruling out underlying causes like polycystic ovarian disease and adrenal or ovarian tumors. Basic tests include total and free testosterone and dehydroepiandrosterone sulfate. A comprehensive screening panel includes FSH, LH, T3, T4, TSH, prolactin and ultrasound for ovaries and adrenal glands in addition to the above tests.

Q.8 What are the clinical features of anagen hair loss?

Ans: Anagen hair loss, a result of interruption of the anagen hair cycle, presents as abrupt anagen hair shedding with severe diffuse scalp alopecia. A severe insult may cause up to 80% loss of scalp hair. Following an insult to hair follicles, anagen effluvium is evident within days to weeks as opposed to telogen effluvium. The hair-pull test is positive for dystrophic anagen hairs with tapered ends. Hair regrowth starts within weeks if the insult ceases.

The common causes include chemotherapy and alopecia areata. Antimitotic chemotherapeutic drugs cause anagen phase arrest due to an insult to the rapidly dividing hair matrix. Hair loss is usually seen 1–2 weeks after chemotherapy and is most visible by 1–2 months. The scalp hair is commonly affected, but all body hair could also be involved. Chemotherapeutic agents commonly implicated in causing hair loss include cisplatin, carboplatin, cyclophosphamide, docetaxel, paclitaxel, fluorouracil, epirubicin, gemcitabine, vincristine, etc. Anagen hair loss can also result due to radiation, heavy-metal poisoning and boric acid poisoning.

Another cause of anagen hair loss is alopecia areata. Having an autoimmune etiology, it may lead to patchy hair loss, or may result in complete loss of scalp hair (alopecia subtotalis and totalis), or complete loss of scalp as well as body hair (alopecia universalis).

Q.9 What are the important points for history taking in a case of diffuse hair loss?

Ans: Important points for history taking in a case of diffuse hair loss:
- Hair loss duration
- Continuous or episodic hair loss
- Determining percentage hair lost

- Identifying triggers and their temporal relationship to hair loss
- Recent fever or other illness, surgery, psychological stress, childbirth
- Menstrual history
- Weight loss and diet history
- History of chronic disease, infection, malignancy, liver or renal disease, autoimmune disease
- Medication history including over-the-counter products and alternative medicines
- Family history of androgenetic alopecia, alopecia areata, thyroid disorder and autoimmune disease
- Hair care procedures/cosmetics
- Heavy metal exposure or history of radiotherapy.

Q.10 How is the hair-pull test performed?

Ans: It is advisable to perform the hair-pull test in all patients with hair loss. It involves gentle traction/pulling from the base to the tips of a group of hairs (approximately 50–60) by grasping between the thumb and the index and middle fingers. A negative test (≤6 hairs extracted) is indicative of normal hair loss and a positive test (>6 hairs extracted) indicates active hair shedding.

In acute telogen effluvium, usually >10% of the total hairs pulled are easily extracted from all regions of the scalp (provided the patient has not shampooed the hairs for >24 hours). This test is usually negative in pattern hair loss.

Q.11 What is the importance of laboratory investigations in diffuse hair loss?

Ans: A laboratory work-up with a minimum battery of investigations helps in identifying various causes of diffuse hair loss. This includes:
- A complete blood count, routine urine, serum ferritin
- A thyroid profile (TSH, T3 and T4)
- An extensive metabolic workup to rule out chronic renal or liver disease in suspected patients.

If the history and examination points to a specific disorder, appropriate tests can be performed. A hormonal profile is indicated if the patient shows signs of hyperandrogenism or if a hormonal cause is suspected. Zinc and biotin may be related to hair loss, however their quantification does not have a scientific basis and hence not measured.

Q.12 What are the indications of scalp biopsy in diffuse hair fall?

Ans: Lack of identifiable triggers, chronic hair loss, miniaturized hair shafts and failure to exclude alopecia areata are all indications for scalp biopsy.

Scalp biopsy should be done in a direction parallel to hair growth. This is done to avoid transecting the follicles which will prevent development of a patch of alopecia. Also the biopsy should reach the subcutis to include the bulbs of terminal follicles. At least a 4 mm punch is to be used for biopsy. Usually two biopsies are preferred, one each for vertical and horizontal sectioning.

Vellus and terminal hair count is done and the anagen-telogen hair ratio is calculated. In acute telogen effluvium, a reversal of the normal anagen-telogen ratio can be seen. The proportion of normal telogen follicles in excess of 15% is considered suggestive of telogen effluvium, while a level of 25% or more is considered definitive. Normal telogen counts are typically in the range of 6–13%. Androgenetic alopecia shows miniaturization of the hair shafts and decreased terminal to vellus hair counts. In alopecia areata, characteristic peribulbar lymphocytic infiltration can be seen.

Q.13 What are the general measures for managing diffuse hair loss?

Ans: General measures for managing diffuse hair loss:
- Determining and treating underlying cause
- Reassurance and explanation
- Evaluation and treatment of iron deficiency and thyroid disorder
- Monthly assessment of the case
- Optimum diet and avoidance of drugs related to hair loss.

Q.14 What is the treatment for telogen hair loss and pattern hair loss?

Ans: Acute telogen effluvium is self-limiting and usually resolves within 3–6 months if the causative factor is identified and removed. No specific drug treatment is required for the same. Complete recovery could take a longer time.

Topical minoxidil 2–5% has been used in expectation that it will prolong anagen phase of hair growth. Chronic telogen effluvium may be a self-limiting process and may resolve spontaneously in 3–10 years, however, the evidence for this remains poor. The natural history remains poorly characterized and the prognosis is uncertain.

In patients of pattern hair loss, the various treatment options available include:
- Minoxidil topical solution 2–10%
- Oral finasteride/dutasteride
- Hair transplantation (FUE, FUT)
- Hormonal therapy (anti-androgens like cyproterone acetate) for women
- Topical biomimetic peptides
- Saw palmetto extracts (topical and oral)
- Topical procapil
- Topical Capixyl
- Topical Caffeine
- Topical Aminexil
- Platelet-rich plasma therapy
- Microneedling
- Micropigmentation
- Hair dust/spray
- Hair bonding and weaving
- Hair prosthesis-like wigs

Q.15 What is HAIR-AN syndrome?

Ans: The HAIR-AN syndrome is the combination of hyperandrogenism, insulin resistance and acanthosis nigricans (AN). It is an uncommon disease and may be considered a subset of polycystic ovary syndrome. Hyperandrogenism in women usually presents as hirsutism, menstrual irregularities, acne and uncommonly, clitorimegaly, pattern hair loss, muscle mass changes and voice deepening. Insulin resistance results in high levels of insulin but normal glucose levels in some patients, while others have glucose levels in the diabetic range. Symptoms of diabetes including polydipsia, polyuria and weight loss are present sometimes. Other related symptoms are increased libido, increased blood pressure, infertility and obesity.

Q.16 What is SAHA syndrome?

Ans: The combination of seborrhea, acne, hirsutism and alopecia in women is termed SAHA syndrome. Polycystic ovary syndrome, cystic mastitis, obesity and infertility can be associated with SAHA syndrome. It usually presents in young to middle-aged women with the patient having elevated androgen levels or increased peripheral response to androgen with normal androgen levels in blood. It is crucial to find the cause of peripheral hyperandrogenism and exclude androgen-secreting tumors by a comprehensive history, examination and laboratory investigations. Treatment depends on the underlying cause, whereas the aim in idiopathic cases is to improve the clinical features.

Q.17 What is the clinical picture of alopecia in syphilis?

Ans: Although other associated clinical features of secondary syphilis may facilitate diagnosis, "moth-eaten" alopecia can be the only presenting feature of syphilis. The frequency of hair loss in secondary syphilis ranges from 2.9 to 7%. The exact pathogenesis still remains to be elucidated. Alopecia seen in syphilis is nonscarring and can be diffuse or moth-eaten or both. It may also affect hair-bearing areas apart from the scalp. On biopsy, a noninflammatory picture or changes indistinguishable from alopecia areata may be seen. The hair loss is expected to resolve after appropriate treatment within three months.

Q.18 What are the trichoscopic features in various diffuse alopecias?

Ans: Trichoscopy is the dermoscopic evaluation of the scalp and hair. This relatively new diagnostic modality is simple, noninvasive and quite useful as a bed side tool for the diagnosis of common disorders of hair and scalp.
- Anagen effluvium: Trichoscopy of anagen effluvium is characterized by the presence of black dots, monilethrix—like hairs or Pohl-Pinkus constrictions
- Telogen effluvium: There are no specific findings in telogen effluvium and it is a diagnosis of exclusion on trichoscopy. It can be suspected when there is decreased hair density with presence of empty hair follicles over the entire scalp area with no site predilection and absence of characteristic features of other scalp disorders
- Androgenetic alopecia: The characteristic trichoscopic features of androgenetic alopecia include hair shaft diameter variation of >20% (anisotrichosis), peripilar halo (early stages), increased vellus hairs, an increased proportion of follicular units with single hair shaft and sebaceous gland hypertrophy. These findings are most prominent in the frontal scalp.

A decreased ratio of terminal to vellus hairs in androgen dependent scalp areas is also characteristic. The most significant finding is the hair diameter variability, which reflects hair follicle miniaturization
- Alopecia areata: The various trichoscopic findings include yellow dots with short vellus, dystrophic and tapered hairs, black dots (cadaverized broken hairs), exclamation mark hairs, caudability hairs (hairs of normal length with a narrowed proximal shaft), hypopigmented vellus hairs. Exclamation mark hairs may be considered specific for active alopecia areata. Yellow dots show high sensitivity but low specificity for alopecia areata.

CONCLUSION

Diffuse hair loss is extremely common. Clinical diagnosis is established after an elaborate history, with special focus on the chronology of events, scalp examination and evaluation of the shed hair-bulbs, along with a few simple laboratory investigations. Appropriate treatment will arrest the hair loss in majority of cases except probably chronic telogen effluvium.

KEY POINTS

- Diffuse hair loss, a multifactorial condition, requires a comprehensive history, thorough clinical examination and appropriate investigations for identification of causative factors and appropriate management
- Early androgenetic alopecia may present as episodic telogen hair shedding, before any distinctive pattern is seen
- Telogen effluvium is a sign of some underlying pathology and hence not a complete diagnosis in itself
- Acute cases of telogen effluvium are usually self-limited, resolving within 3–6 months if the cause or trigger is identified and removed or treated, while the prognosis of chronic cases is uncertain and may take many years for resolution.

SUGGESTED READING

1. Bergfeld WF, Mulinari-Brenner F. Shedding: how to manage a common cause of hair loss. Cleve Clin J Med. 2001;68(3):256-61.
2. Bergfeld WF. Telogen effluvium. In: McMichael J, Hordin MK, editors. Hair and scalp diseases: Medical, surgical, and cosmetic treatments. London, UK: Informa Health Care; 2008. pp. 119-36.
3. Care H. Hair loss solution. South African Pharmaceutical and Cosmetic Review. 2012;39(6):21.
4. Dhurat R, Sukesh MS, Avhad G, et al. A randomized evaluator blinded study of effect of microneedling in androgenetic alopecia: A pilot study. Int J Trichology. 2013;5(1):6.
5. Fiedler VC, Gray AC. Diffuse alopecia: Telogen hair loss. Disorders of hair growth: Diagnosis and treatment. 2003;2:303-20.
6. Fischer TW, Hipler UC, Elsner P. Effect of caffeine and testosterone on the proliferation of human hair follicles in vitro. Int J Dermatol. 2007;46(1):27-35.
7. Goette DK, Odom RB. Alopecia in crash dieters. JAMA. 1976;235(24):2622-3.
8. Harrison S, Bergfeld W. Diffuse hair loss: its triggers and management. Cleve Clin J Med. 2009;76(6):361-7.
9. Harrison S, Sinclair R. Telogen effluvium. Clin Exp Dermatol. 2002;27(5):389-95.
10. Headington JT. Telogen effluvium: New concepts and review. Arch Dermatol. 1993;129(3):356-63.

11. Jain N, Doshi B, Khopkar U. Trichoscopy in alopecias: Diagnosis simplified. Int J Trichology. 2013;5(4):170.
12. Kadowaki H, Kadowaki T. HAIR-AN syndrome. Nihon Rinsho. 1994;52(10):2648-52.
13. Kaliyadan F, Nambiar A, Vijayaraghavan S. Androgenetic alopecia: An update. Indian J Dermatol Venereol Leprol. 2013;79(5):613.
14. Khatu SS, More YE, Gokhale NR, et al. Platelet-rich plasma in androgenic alopecia: Myth or an effective tool. J Cutan Aesthet Surg. 2014;7(2):107.
15. Kligman AM. Pathologic dynamics of human hair loss: I. Telogen effluvium. Arch Dermatol. 1961;83(2):175-98.
16. Kutlubay Z, Serdaroglu S. Trichoscopy and trichogram. In Hair and Scalp Disorders 2017. InTech.
17. Lacarrubba F, Dall'Oglio F, Nasca MR, et al. Videodermatoscopy enhances diagnostic capability in some forms of hair loss. Am J Clin Dermatol. 2004;5(3):205-8.
18. Madani S, Shapiro J. Alopecia areata update. J Am Acad Dermatol. 2000;42(4):549-66.
19. Mas-Chamberlin C, Mondon P, Lamy F, et al. Reduction of hair-loss: Matrikines and plant molecules to the rescue. In Proceedings of the 7th Scientific Conference of the Asian Society of Cosmetic Chemists (ASCS): Toward a New Horizon: Uniting Cosmetic Science with Oriental Wisdom 2005 Mar 7.
20. Olsen EA, Messenger AG, Shapiro J, et al. Evaluation and treatment of male and female pattern hair loss. J Am Acad Dermatol. 2005;52(2):301-11.
21. Orfanos CE, Adler YD, Zouboulis CC. The SAHA syndrome. Horm Res. 2000;54(5-6):251-8.
22. Paus R, Cotsarelis G. The biology of hair follicles. N Engl J Med. 1999;341(7):491-7.
23. Prager N, Bickett K, French N, et al. A randomized, double-blind, placebo-controlled trial to determine the effectiveness of botanically derived inhibitors of 5-alpha-reductase in the treatment of androgenetic alopecia. J Altern Complement Med. 2002;8(2):143-52.
24. Qiao J, Fang H. Moth-eaten alopecia: A sign of secondary syphilis. CMAJ. 2013;185(1):61.
25. Rook A, Dawber R. The comparative physiology, embryology and physiology of human hair. In: Rook A, Dawber R, editors. Diseases of the hair and scalp. Oxford, UK: Blackwell Science Publications; 1982. pp. 1-17.
26. Rook A, Dawber R. Diffuse alopecia: endocrine, metabolic and chemical influences on the follicular cycle. In: Rook A, Dawber R, editors. Diseases of the hair and scalp. Oxford, UK: Blackwell Science Publications; 1982:115-45.
27. Sellheyer K, Bergfeld WF. Histopathologic evaluation of alopecias. Am J Dermatopathol. 2006;28(3):236-59.
28. Shapiro J, Wiseman M, Lui H. Practical management of hair loss. Can Fam Physician. 2000;46(7):1469-77.
29. Shrivastava SB. Diffuse hair loss in an adult female: approach to diagnosis and management. Indian J Dermatol Venereol Leprol. 2009;75(1):20.
30. Sinclair R, Grossman KL, Kvedar JC. Anagen hair loss. In: Olsen EA, editor. Disorders of hair growth: Diagnosis and treatment. 2nd ed. New York, NY: McGraw-Hill Publishing; 2003. pp. 275-302.
31. Sinclair RD, Dawber RP. Androgenetic alopecia in men and women. Clin Dermatol. 2001;19(2):167-78.
32. Sperling LC. Hair and systematic disease. Dermatologic Clin. 2001;19(4):711-26.
33. Thai KE, Sinclair RD. Finasteride for female androgenetic alopecia. Br J Dermatol. 2002;147(4):812-3.
34. Tosti A, Misciali C, Piraccini BM, et al. Drug-induced hair loss and hair growth. Drug Safety. 1994;10(4):310-7.
35. Tosti A, Pazzaglia M. Drug reactions affecting hair: diagnosis. Dermatol Clin. 2007;25(2):223-31.
36. van Zuuren EJ, Fedorowicz Z, Carter B, et al. Interventions for female pattern hair loss. Cochrane Database Syst Rev. 2012;5.
37. Whiting DA. Chronic telogen effluvium. Dermatologic clinics. 1996;14(4):723-31.
38. Whiting DA. Chronic telogen effluvium: Increased scalp hair shedding in middle-aged women. J Am Acad Dermatol. 1996;35(6):899-906.

CHAPTER 15

Scalp Pruritus

Poonam Puri, Sushruta Kathuria

INTRODUCTION

Scalp pruritus is a broad term where patient complains of itchy scalp. Scalp dysesthesia, also known as burning scalp syndrome encompasses burning, stinging and pruritic sensation of the scalp without a primary skin condition. Scalp dysesthesia is classified as one of the chronic pain syndromes, which also include burning mouth syndrome, brachioradial pruritus, notalgia paresthetica, meralgia paresthetica and trigeminal trophic syndrome. There are many etiologies of scalp pruritus, in some an underlying dermatological disease may be found while in others no obvious disease is seen. Scalp pruritus is disabling and can affect concentration in work, social interaction, sleep and lifestyle. Hence, correct evaluation, diagnosis and management is necessary.

CASE 1

A 40-year-old lady presented with severe itching of the scalp for 3 months. The itch was persistent throughout the day and occasionally was associated with burning sensation in the scalp. There was no history of hair fall, patchy hair loss or any systemic complaints. There was no history of itching elsewhere on the body, fever, or muscle weakness. She was not able to sleep at night due to her itching and recently, her daughter had noticed lack of social interaction. Family history of itching on scalp was absent. Her husband died 6 months back. Patient was taking antihistamines with partial improvement.

Examination: There were no hair shaft abnormalities or hair loss. Scalp was normal without any evidence of underlying skin disease or ectoparasites. Hair pull test was negative and rest of the skin examination was also normal.

Investigations: Trichoscopy of five areas of the scalp did not reveal any abnormality. A psychiatric evaluation showed her to be suffering from generalized anxiety disorder.

Treatment: The patient was diagnosed as a case of psychosomatic pruritus of the scalp and was started on pregabalin 75 mg/day increased to 150 mg/day along with levocetirizine 5 mg twice daily. There was significant improvement in her symptoms after two weeks.

> **Case Review in a Nutshell**
>
> The patient was suffering for severe scalp pruritus which was hampering her daily lifestyle and sleep. Despite taking regular antihistamines, there was no improvement in her symptoms. In her case, an important history was that her husband had died few months ago following which she developed these symptoms. On clinical examination, no dermatological or systemic cause could be identified for scalp pruritus. In such cases, where no cause is found and there is a history of change in behavior, a psychiatric evaluation should be done. The patient was diagnosed as a case of generalized anxiety disorder and was treated accordingly. Her scalp pruritus was due to somatization of her anxiety disorder and therefore it responded to pregabalin.

■ INTERACTIVE TOPIC REVIEW

Q.1 What are the various etiologies of scalp pruritus?

Ans: Scalp pruritus has various etiologies including dermatological, systemic, neurogenic and psychogenic causes. The causes of scalp pruritus is given in Table 1.

TABLE 1: Causes of scalp pruritus.

Etiology	Diseases	
Dermatological	• Seborrheic dermatitis • Psoriasis • Urticaria • Atopic dermatitis • Allergic contact dermatitis	• Alopecia areata • Lichen planopilaris (Fig. 1) • Infection and infestation • Folliculitis • Cicatricial alopecia
Systemic	• Dermatomyositis • Chronic renal failure • Chronic liver disease	• Thyroid dysfunction • Hematological malignancy • Drug induced
Neurological	• Diabetic neuropathy • Postherpetic neuralgia • Migraine • Atypical facial neuralgia	• Brain and spinal cord injury • Wallenberg syndrome • Brain tumor
Psychogenic/psychosomatic	Somatoform pruritus with comorbidity of psychiatric disease	

Q.2 What is trichodynia and trichokinesis?

Ans: Trichodynia is painful burning sensation, whereas trichokinesis is itch triggered by touching the hair.

Q.3 What are the various mediators involved in the pathogenesis of scalp pruritus?

Ans: The mediators are released from mast cells [histamine, histamine 4 receptor (H4R), nerve growth factor (NGF), leukotriene B4, neurokinin 1 receptor,

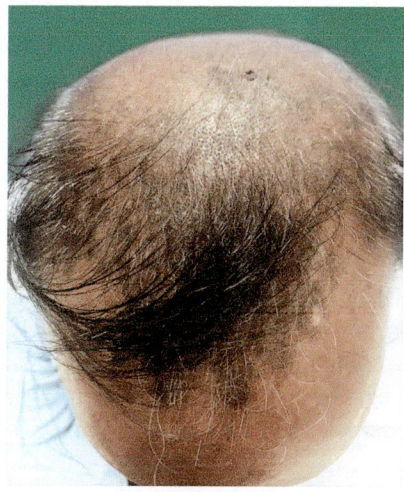

Fig. 1: Lichen planopilaris.

protease (tryptase), endothelin receptor A (ETAR), Prostaglandin D_2 (PGD_2), and interleukin-2 (IL-2), basophils (histamine, H4R, IL-4), eosinophils [(H4R, nerve growth factor (NGF), neurotrophins-3 (NT-3), Brain-derived neurotrophic factor (BDNF), eosinophil-derived neurotoxin (EDN), eosinophil cationic protein (ECP)], and T-cells (IL-31, H4R). Pruritus due to scalp folliculitis caused by *Staphylococcus aureus* is mediated by IL-31.

Q.4 What are the various etiologies proposed for scalp pruritus?

Ans: In majority of scalp pruritus due to alopecia, psoriasis and seborrheic dermatitis, there are aggregates of mast cells which release mediators causing pruritus. A study by Kim et al. shows that in scalp psoriasis the intraepidermal nerve fiber density is increased.

A case report of dermatomyositis causing severe scalp pruritus revealed decreased density of epidermal nerve fibers and abnormal nerve morphology (small fiber neuropathy).

Q.5 What is the etiology of psychogenic/psychosomatic scalp pruritus or scalp dysesthesias?

Ans: There is very little data on epidemiology and pathogenesis of psychogenic scalp pruritus and scalp dysesthesias. Psychogenic/psychosomatic scalp pruritus refers to only pruritus caused due to an underlying psychiatric condition. However, scalp dysesthesias includes burning, stinging, sensations on scalp with or without pruritus. In both the conditions, underlying dermatological disease is not seen. Causes of psychogenic scalp pruritus and scalp dysesthesias may be similar. Scalp dysesthesias are seen in three subcategories of patients mainly those with psychiatric condition, cervical spine disease and/or a history of a facial or brow lift. However, there is no clear cut association between the level of stress/psychiatric disease and the scalp dysesthesia and whether the psychiatric comorbidity is the causative agent or a confounding factor.

The psychiatric disorders known to be associated with scalp pruritus are dysthymic disorder, generalized anxiety and somatization. The hypothesis behind cervical spinal disease causing scalp dysesthesia is that a cervical spondylosis or pathology causing impingement of the C5 and C6 nerves leads to tension in the occipitofrontalis muscle and scalp aponeurosis which in turn leads to abnormal sensations of the scalp. Similarly, a facial or brow lift causes injury to the nerves of the scalp leading to dysesthesias.

Q.6 What is a sensitive scalp?

Ans: The occurrence of pricking, burning, or tingling sensation on scalp due to physical (heat, cold, ultraviolet radiation), chemical (cosmetics, soap, water), hormonal (premenstrual) or psychological factors (stress) is known as "sensitive scalp". Pruritus and erythema may or may not be associated. Usually a causative agent is found in sensitive scalp unlike scalp pruritus. It is a part of sensitive skin syndrome.

Q.7 What are the complications of scalp pruritus?

Ans: Various complications secondary to scratching such as lichenification, secondary folliculitis, chronic excoriated papules and nodules can occur.

Q.8 What are the investigations to be done in scalp pruritus?

Ans: Any case of scalp pruritus maybe classified into one of the three categories: Pruritus on diseased skin, pruritus on nondiseased skin and pruritus with chronic scratch lesions.

Category 1 (patient with pruritus on diseased skin): In such a patient, a thorough history and clinical examination must be done to ascertain the primary dermatological disease. Table 2 tabulates the various investigations.

TABLE 2: Investigations in scalp pruritus with diseased skin.	
Disease	Suggested investigations
Pediculosis	Saline mount of nits and lice
Tinea capitis (Fig. 2)	KOH microscopy
Folliculitis	Gram stain and pus culture sensitivity
Allergic contact dermatitis	Patch test
Scarring and nonscarring alopecia	Scalp biopsy
Dermatomysositis	Scalp biopsy, CPK, ANA

(KOH: potassium hydroxide; CPK: creatine phosphokinase; ANA: antinuclear antibody)

Category 2 (patients with pruritus without diseased skin): In such patients, the investigation is usually according to the suspected systemic disease. A complete blood count, liver and kidney function tests, thyroid function test, malignancy screen, cervical spine computed tomography scan and psychological evaluation are some of the tests which may be done according to the patient's symptoms.

Category 3 (patients with pruritus having chronic scratch lesions): Same investigations as discussed in category 1 and 2 should be performed.

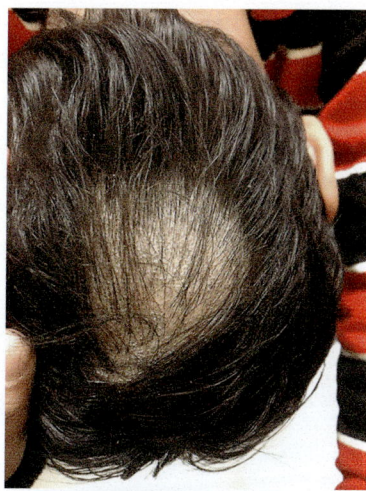

Fig. 2: Tinea capitis.

Q.9 What is the role of trichoscopy in scalp pruritus?

Ans: Trichoscopy is dermoscopy of hair and scalp. It can help in diagnosing specific dermatological conditions like tinea capitis (Fig. 2), psoriasis, alopecia areata and cicatricial alopecia. In scalp dysesthesia, areas with short hair, brownish discoloration, trichoptilosis, bloom hair, block hair and trichorrhexis nodosa is seen.

Q.10 What is the treatment of scalp pruritus?

Ans: Treatment of scalp pruritus is directed at the treatment of underlying dermatological or systemic disease. Symptomatic management which includes antihistamines must be advocated. Patient must be advised to wash hair regularly and properly. In scalp dysesthesias or psychogenic scalp pruritus, low dose antidepressants should be added.

Q.11 What is the treatment of pediculosis?

Ans: Pediculosis is a common cause of scalp pruritus especially in school going children and teenagers. A thorough examination to check for nits and lice must be done in all patients complaining of scalp pruritus. The treatment is using permethrin 1% lotion on scalp for 15–30 minutes followed by washing it. Permethrin is a good pediculicide which kills the adult lice as well as the nits. All family members especially those with medium to long length of hair must be treated simultaneously. Most of the commercially available permethrin scalp lotions are shampoo based, so additionally shampoo must not be used. A repeat application after 1 week is recommended to clear any remaining nits.

CASE 2

A 35-year-old man presented with itching and white flakes on the scalp (Fig. 3). The itching was mild to moderate, persisting throughout the day. It did not affect his sleep or daily activities. However, he felt embarrassed on meeting people because of the white scales which used to shed on his clothes. On examination, there were thin, ill-defined erythematous plaques on entire scalp with adherent yellowish white scales.

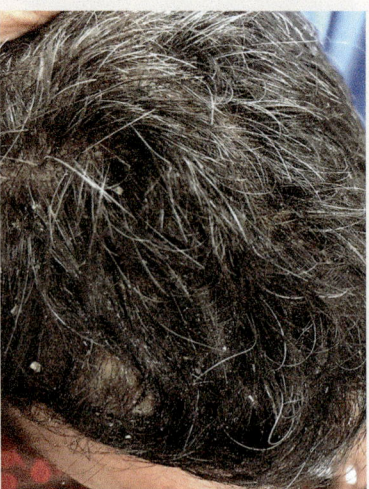

Fig. 3: Seborrheic dermatitis.

Treatment: Patient was treated with ketoconazole and zinc pyrithione shampoo and advised to stop application of hair oil. Levocetirizine 5 mg was added. Patient had significant improvement after 4 weeks of treatment.

Case Review in a Nutshell

The patient was diagnosed as a case of mild seborrheic dermatitis. The diagnosis of seborrheic dermatitis is made on clinical signs and symptoms. The presence of ill-defined plaques with greasy scales is suggestive of seborrheic dermatitis. Treatment includes use of antifungal shampoos in mild cases.

▌INTERACTIVE TOPIC REVIEW

Q.1 What is dandruff?

Ans: Dandruff is a common term used by patients to indicate flaky scaling of the scalp with or without erythema and is usually associated with pruritus. It represents mild to moderate form of seborrheic dermatitis.

Q.2 What is the pathogenesis of seborrheic dermatitis?

Ans: The exact etiology of seborrheic dermatitis is not clear. It is caused by interaction of various factors such as sebaceous secretions, skin surface fungal colonization and individual susceptibility. All the three factors are equally important in causing seborrheic dermatitis. In majority of cases, it is linked to *Malassezia* species which is a commensal. *M. furfur, M. globosa* and M. restricta subtypes have been implicated most commonly in pathogenesis of seborrheic dermatitis. Under normal conditions, *Malassezia* species are in high concentrations in the infundibulum of scalp hair. When the balance of scalp commensals is disturbed, *Malassezia* species also tend to grow on scalp. The lipases and phospholipases produced by *Malassezia* leads to formation of oleic acid which is responsible for desquamation of scalp skin and manifests as dandruff. It has been observed that oleic acid can cause dandruff only in genetically susceptible individuals. The composition of skin surface lipids is the most important factor for development of seborrheic dermatitis. Keratinocytes also produce pro-inflammatory cytokines such as IL-1α, IL-6, IL-8 and IL-12 after stimulation from *Malassezia*. Scalp pruritus is caused by increased levels of Cathepsin S and histamine.

Q.3 Is the sebum excretion rate increased in seborrheic dermatitis?

Ans: Studies have shown that increased sebum excretion rate does not occur in seborrheic dermatitis.

Q.4 What are the common seborrheic sites?

Ans: The seborrheic sites are scalp, medial end of eyebrows, nasolabial folds, external ear canal, retroauricular area, under the nose area, chin, presternal region, midline of back, umbilicus, axillae, groin and pubic area (Fig. 4).

Q.5 What underlying conditions can lead to new onset seborrheic dermatitis or aggravate pre-existing seborrheic dermatitis?

Ans: Immunocompromised conditions such as HIV/AIDS, organ transplant, lymphomas, neurological disorders and psychiatric diseases (Parkinson's disease, neuroleptic-induced parkinsonism, tardive dyskinesia, traumatic brain injury, epilepsy, facial nerve palsy, spinal cord injury and mood depression), chronic alcoholic pancreatitis, hepatitis C virus and Down syndrome are some aggravating or precipitating conditions.

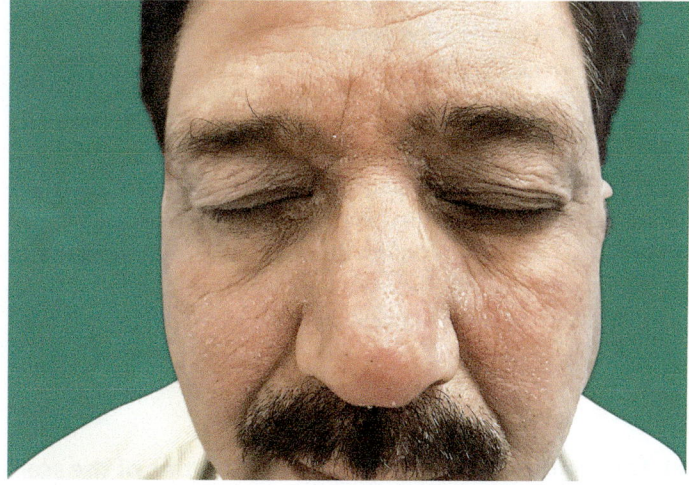

Fig. 4: Seborrheic dermatitis of eyebrows and nasolabial folds.

Q.6 What is the treatment of seborrheic dermatitis of scalp?

Ans: The mainstay of treatment of seborrheic dermatitis is use of antifungal-based shampoos. In mild cases, only antifungal shampoos are sufficient. The various antifungal shampoos used are ketoconazole 2%, bifonazole 1%, ciclopiroxamine oleate 1.5% and selenium sulphide 2.5%. Relapse is common on stopping treatment, so antifungal shampoos should continue for a longer time. Second-line treatment includes zinc pyrithione and tar-based shampoos. Regular and proper shampooing of the hair with normal shampoo also reduces colonization of *Malassezia* and symptoms of scalp pruritus.

If the scaling or eczema is severe, then moderate to potent topical corticosteroid preparations or nonsteroidal immunosuppressants (tacrolimus or pimecrolimus) can be added at bedtime. In resistant or extensive cases, short course of oral ketoconazole, oral itraconazole, or oral terbinafine is given. Low-dose isotretinoin 10 mg/day also reduces seborrhea and seborrheic dermatitis.

CASE 3

A 55-year-old female presented with complaints of severe itching of scalp along with excoriated papules and plaques on nape of neck and sides of neck for 8 months. On detailed history, she mentioned that pruritus increased 2 days after application of hair dye. She had been using black colored hair dye for last 3 years once every 15 days. On examination, patient had staining of scalp with black hair dye, excoriated erythematous papules and plaques of varying size over nape of neck and sides of neck. Few papules could be seen on vertex of scalp. There were no other deformities of hair shaft or hair loss. Lesions on the body were not seen.

Patient was patch tested with Indian standard series and was found to be 2+ to para-phenylene diamine (PPD) after 96 hours. She was diagnosed as a case of allergic contact dermatitis to hair dye and was advised to stop hair dye application. Topical potent corticosteroid was given at bedtime application along with levocetirizine 5 mg twice daily. For coloring of hair, she was advised to use PPD-free vegetable hair dyes. After one month of follow-up, considerable improvement was seen.

Case Review in a Nutshell

This lady presented with papules and plaques around the neck along with scalp pruritus. The location of the plaques and staining of scalp with hair dye are quite suggestive of contact dermatitis to hair dye. Also, she gave a history of aggravation of pruritus following application of hair dye. To confirm the diagnosis, patch test was done which was confirmatory of hair dye dermatitis. The main treatment is resolution of the symptoms by topical corticosteroid and stopping application of PPD-based dyes.

■ INTERACTIVE TOPIC REVIEW

Q.1 What are the common causes of contact dermatitis of the scalp?

Ans: The common causes of contact dermatitis of scalp are tabulated in Table 3.

TABLE 3: Common causes of scalp dermatitis.

Allergen	Source
Metals: • Nickel, cobalt • Potassium dichromate	• Hair clips and clasps • Textile dye fixing agents, leather clips
Fragrances: • Balsam of Peru • Fragrance mix • Rubber accelerator • Carba mix	• Hair cosmetics and shampoo • Hair cosmetics and shampoo • Hair brush handles, bathing caps, rubber hair nets, hat bands
Vehicles: • Propylene glycol	• Hair products
Hair coloring: • Para-phenylene diamine (PPD) • Disperse blue dye	• Hair dye • Cross-sensitivity to PPD
Preservatives: • Kathon CG • Methyldibromoglutaronitrile • Thiomersal • Quaternium-15	• Hair products • Hair products • Hair products • Hair products

Q.2 What are the common sites of affliction in hair dye dermatitis?

Ans: The common sites of involvement are margins of the scalp, nape of neck, ears, periorbital area, around eyebrows, forehead, sides of cheek, upper back. The whole of the scalp especially vertex of the scalp is less commonly involved probably because scalp skin is thick and rich in pilosebaceous units. Hair dressers and people who apply hair dye themselves can also have dermatitis of the fingertips.

Q.3 What is the etiology of hair dye dermatitis?

Ans: Allergic contact dermatitis is caused by PPD and toluene 2,5-diamine (PTD) which are aniline derivatives. Normally, these are packaged in unoxidized form and are colorless. On mixing with hydrogen peroxide, PPD and PTD become oxidized and give color. However, the oxidized and polymerized forms are nonallergenic. Therefore, hair dye dermatitis is caused when less-experienced people do not perform proper mixing to form completely oxidized PPD and PTD. The allergen causes type IV delayed hypersensitivity response leading to erythematous plaques and papules.

Q.4 What is the best investigation to confirm hair dye dermatitis?

Ans: Patch testing with common allergen series is the best test for diagnosis of hair dye dermatitis. If the patient also complains of photosensitivity or there is suspicion of photoaggravated or photocontact dermatitis, then photopatch test should be done.

Q.5 How is patch test done?

Ans: A patch test is done in suspected patients with hair dye dermatitis. The common series of allergens (Indian standard series) is applied on the upper back. The allergens (liquid and semi-soild paste) come in tubes. Around 2–3 mm length of allergen is applied lengthwise on aluminium chambers (Finn chambers) stuck on hypoallergenic adhesive tapes. If the allergen is aqueous or alcohol based, few drops are put on a filter paper disc and placed on the aluminium chamber. These tapes are then applied on clean uninflamed back of the patient. Over these tapes, gauze packs are applied and are stuck on firmly using adhesive tapes or dynaplast.

The patient is advised not to sleep on the back, not to scratch, bathe and remove dressing. After 48 hours, the patch is removed and reading is taken after 30 minutes (Table 4). The second reading is taken at 96 hours following the same instructions as above.

TABLE 4: Reading patch test results according to International Contact Dermatitis Research Group.

Negative	Normal appearing skin
Doubtful reaction?	Faint erythema only
1+ reaction (weak positive)	Mild erythema, infiltrated, questionable papules
2+ reaction (strong positive)	Erythema infiltration, papules, vesicles
3+ reaction (extreme positive)	Intense erythema and infiltration, coalescing vesicles
–	Negative reaction
IR	Irritant reaction
NT	Not tested

Q.6 What allergen is used in Indian standard series to test for hair dye dermatitis?

Ans: Para-phenylene diamine 1% in petrolatum base is used in Indian standard series. It is the preferred test allergen.

Q.7 What are disadvantages of patch test?

Ans: The disadvantages of patch test include risk of active sensitization, severe or fiery reaction at the patch test site, flare of existing dermatitis, depigmentation, hyperpigmentation and granuloma at test site.

Q.8 What is the treatment of contact dermatitis to hair dye?

Ans: The first and foremost treatment is to stop use of hair dye. Any hair dye or coloring agent which will contain PPD or gives black color to hair will cause hair dye dermatitis. Instead alternative vegetable dyes or PPD-free dyes must be advised to the patient. Dyes containing 2-Methoxymethyl-P-Phenylenediamine (Me-PPD) are also better tolerated in patients with allergic contact dermatitis to hair dye.

In mild to moderate cases, treatment includes moderate to highly potent topical corticosteroid and antihistamines. Topical nonsteroidal immuno-suppressants like tacrolimus 0.1% cream or pimecrolimus can be used instead of corticosteroids. In severe eczematous cases, addition of short course of oral corticosteroid started at 0.75–1 mg/kg/day tapered over 4 weeks will help in resolution of the symptoms.

Q.9 How can a patient prevent hair dye dermatitis?

Ans: It is recommended that before application of any hair dye, self-test with the product must be done. The self-test method is described on the instructions leaflet of all commercially available hair dyes. However, the methodology, the amount of hair dye applied, location and size of the application area, number of applications, whether or not rinsing was performed after application, the reading times, varies in different products.

CONCLUSION

Scalp pruritus is a broad term which refers to itching on scalp associated with or without burning sensation. It has various etiologies both dermatological and systemic. A thorough history and examination is needed to distinguish different causes of scalp pruritus. Wherever required, relevant investigations must be done to confirm the etiology. The treatment is both symptomatic and disease-specific. To conclude, scalp pruritus must be managed seriously as it can cause significant distress to the patient.

KEY POINTS

- Scalp pruritus is an umbrella term encompassing all dermatological, systemic and psychological diseases
- A good clinical history and examination elucidates the cause in most cases, sometimes scalp pruritus may be idiopathic
- Investigations are indicated for pruritus due to systemic causes
- Symptomatic treatment is given in all depending on the severity of the condition
- Disease-specific treatment is given where cause can be established.

SUGGESTED READING

1. Borda LJ, Wikramanayake TC. Seborrheic dermatitis and dandruff: A comprehensive review. J Clin Investig Dermatol. 2015;3(2).
2. Chiu E, Baker D. Endoscopic brow lift: A retrospective review of 628 consecutive cases over 5 years. Plast Recosntr Surg. 2003;2:628-33.
3. Clark GW, Pope SM, Jaboori KA. Diagnosis and treatment of seborrheic dermatitis. Am Fam Physician. 2015;91:185-90.
4. Contact and Occupational Dermatoses Forum of India. Patch testing [cited 2018 Aug 09]. Available from: http://codfi.org/Medical-Resources/Patch-Testing
5. de Souza Leão Kamamoto C, Sanudo A, Hassun KM, et al. Low-dose oral isotretinoin for moderate to severe seborrhea and seborrheic dermatitis: A randomized comparative trial. Int J Dermatol. 2017;56:80-5.
6. DeAngelis YM, Gemmer CM, Kaczvinsky JR, et al. Three etiologic facets of dandruff and seborrheic dermatitis: *Malassezia* fungi, sebaceous lipids, and individual sensitivity. J Investig Dermatol Symp Proc. 2005;10:295-7.

7. Farrant P, Mowbray M, Sinclair RD. Dermatoses of the scalp. In: Rook's textbook of dermatology 9th Edn. John Wiley & Sons, Ltd. 2016. Oxford. P. 128.1-87.
8. Friis UF, Goosens A, Giménez-Arnau AM, et al. Self-testing for contact allergy to hair dyes-a 5-year follow-up multicentre study. Contact Dermatitis. 2018;78(2):131-8.
9. Hoss D, Segal S. Scalp dysesthesia. Arch Dermatol. 1998;134:327-30.
10. Hurliman E, Groth D, Wendelschafer-Crabb G, et al. Small-fibre neuropathy in a patient with dermatomyositis and severe scalp pruritus. Br J Dermatol. 2017;176:209-11.
11. Huynh M, Sheehan MP, Chung M, et al. Scalp. In: Lewallen R, Clark A, Feldman SR, editors. Clinical Handbook of Contact Dermatitis. Diagnosis and Management by Body Region. Boca Raton: CRC Press; 2014. P. 6-12.
12. Kim TW, Shim WH, Kim JM, et al. Clinical characteristics of pruritus in patients with scalp psoriasis and their relation with intraepidermal nerve fiber density. Ann Dermatol. 2014;26:727-32.
13. Kobayashi M, Ito K, Sugita T, et al. Physiological and microbiological verification of the benefit of hair washing in patients with skin conditions of the scalp. J Cosmet Dermatol. 2016;15:e1-8.
14. Misery L, Sibaud V, Ambronati M, et al. Sensitive scalp: Does this condition exist? An Epidemiological Study. Contact Dermatitis. 2008;58:234-8.
15. Rakowska A, Olszewska M, Rudnicka L. Trichoscopy of scalp dysesthesia. Adv Dermatol Allergol. 2017;34:245-7.
16. Reich A, Me zdrek K, Adamski Z, et al. Itchy hair–trichoknesis: A variant of trichodynia or a new entity? Acta Derm Venereol. 2013;93:591.
17. Schwartz RA, Janusz CA, Janniger CK. Seborrheic dermatitis: An overview. Am Fam Physician. 2006;74:125-30.
18. Shumway NK, Cole E, Fernandez KH. Neurocutaneous disease: Neurocutaneous dysesthesias. J Am Acad Dermatol. 2016;74:215-28.
19. Thorsberry L, English J. Scalp dysetheia related to cervical spine disease. JAMA Dermatol. 2013;149:200-3.
20. Unna PG. Das seborrhoische Ekzem. Monatsschr Prakt Dermatol. 1897;6:827-6.
21. Wahlberg JE, Lindberg M. Patch testing [cited 2018 Aug 09]. Available from: https://link.springer.com/chapter/10.1007/3-540-31301-X_22.
22. Wilkinson M, Orton D. Allergic contact dermatitis. In: Griffiths CEM, Barker J, Bleiker T, Chalmers R, Creamer D. Rook's Textbook Of Dermatology 9th Edn. John Wiley & Sons, Ltd. Oxford. 2016; pp 128.1-87.
23. Zahir A, Kindred C, Blömeke B, et al. Tolerance to a hair dye product containing 2-methoxymethyl-p-phenylene diamine in an ethnically diverse population of p-phenylene diamine-Allergic Individuals. Dermatitis. 2016;27:355-61.

CHAPTER 16

Facial Melanosis

Rashmi Sarkar, Isha Narang, Bhavya Swarnkar

INTRODUCTION

Facial melanoses is a group of heterogenous disorders sharing a common clinical feature of hyperpigmentation of the face and visible cosmetic disfigurement.

Hypermelanotic disorders include melasma which is the most common one and other nonmelasma facial melanoses. Nonmelasma facial melanoses can be brown or blue type of hypermelanoses. Facial melanoses can be also classified as in Flowchart 1.

Pigmentation on face is often visible to others and, therefore, may lead to significant psychosocial consequences. This is leading to increasing dermatological consultations, thus explaining the growing importance of these disorders.

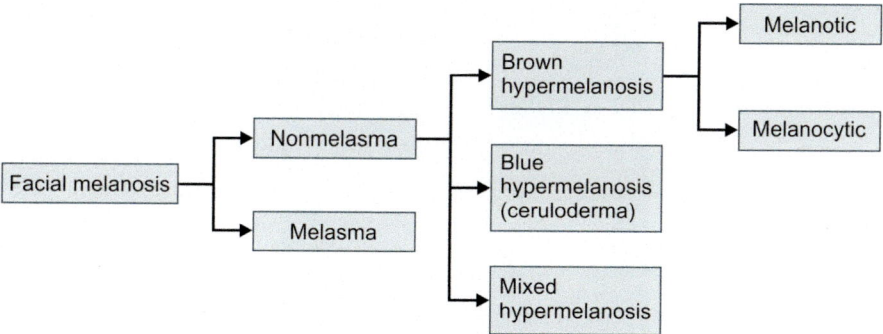

Flowchart 1: Classification of facial melanoses.

CASE 1

A 36-year-old female presented to the dermatology outpatient department (OPD) with a chief complaint of darkening over cheeks bilaterally for 2.5 years months and now has progressed to upper lip and forehead for the last 6 months. There was history of darkening of lesions in summers and on sun exposure. Similar complaints were present in her mother. No history of thyroid disease or oral contraceptives intake. There is no history of onset/aggravation of the lesions postpregnancy.

On examination, vitals, general and systemic examinations were normal.

On mucocutaneous examination, there were irregular brown macules over bilateral malar prominences, the forehead, the nose and the chin. Melasma Area and Severity Index (MASI) score was calculated to be 10 (Figs. 1–3).

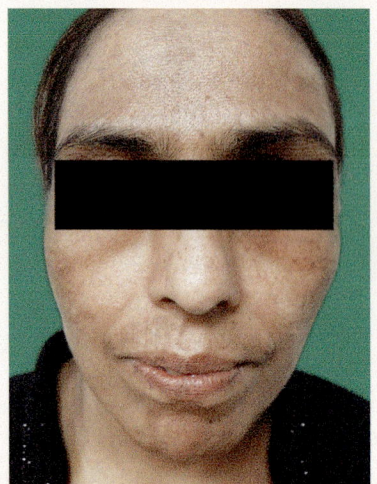

Fig. 1: Melasma (front view).

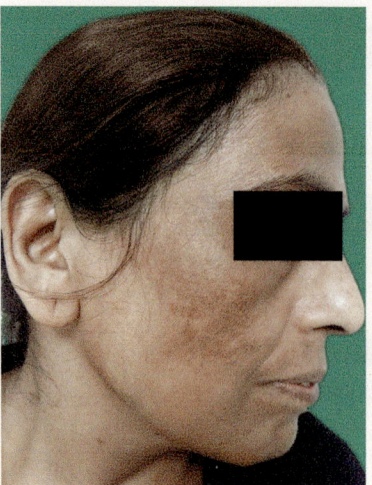

Fig. 2: Melasma (side view).

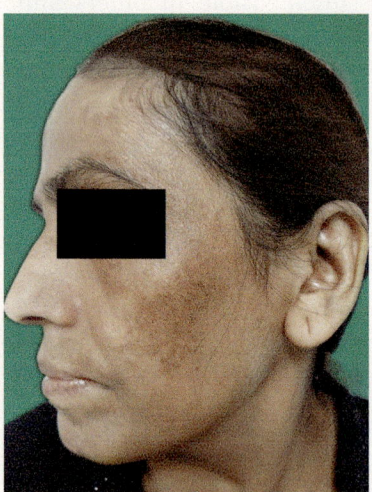

Fig. 3: Melasma (side view).

Investigations: Dermoscopy showed diffuse reticular brown pigmentation with follicular sparing. Wood's lamp examination showed enhancement of contrast.
Thyroid profile and ultrasonography of pelvis were normal.

Treatment: Based on history, examination and investigations the diagnosis of centrofacial type of melasma was made. Patient was emphasized on role of photoprotection (broad spectrum sunscreen, long brimmed hat/cap and parasol) and regular and correct use of sunscreens. She was started on modified Kligman's formula, i.e. 4% hydroquinone, 0.01% fluocinolone acetonide, and 0.05% tretinoin.

Outcome: There was 50% decrease in the MASI score with 12 weeks of therapy. Patient is planned to be put on tretinoin plus hydroquinone/kojic acid or arbutin for maintenance therapy. Other modalities like chemical peeling and laser toning can also be added to act as an adjunct. Importance of sunscreens and photoprotection will be reiterated to the patient.

Case Review in a Nutshell

In any case of facial melanosis presenting to the dermatology OPD, it is imperative to know all the common clinical differentials to reach a correct diagnosis as treatment modalities differ.

For this 36-year-old female presenting to us with hyperpigmentation over forehead, bilateral malar prominences, nose and chin, the following differential diagnoses were kept:
- Melasma
- Riehl's melanosis
- Drug-induced hyperpigmentation
- Acanthosis nigricans (AN)
- Hori nevus
- Exogenous ochronosis.

As there was no history of erythema and pruritus prior to appearance of lesions, pigmented contact dermatitis was thought as a less likely possibility, though patch testing was not performed. There was no history of drug intake [nonsteroidal anti-inflammatory drugs (NSAIDs), phenytoin, antileprosy treatment and griseofulvin] prior to appearance of lesions so drug induced hyperpigmentation was ruled out. As the lesions were nonvelvety to touch and there were no other signs of insulin resistance or AN, possibility of AN was ruled out. Absence of involvement of eyelids and alae of nose made hori nevus as least likely diagnosis. Based on absence of history of topical application of hydroquinone and color of lesions on examination, exogenous ochronosis was also ruled out.

As epidermal type of melasma responds nicely to the therapy, patient was started on triple combination (modified Kligman formula) which is usually first line of therapy. After 3 months of treatment she responded very well with 50% decrease in MASI score.

CASE 2

A 42-year-old female presented with dark colored, slightly itchy patches on her forehead and sides of face for 8 months. No history of any drug intake/summer exacerbation/reddish border surrounding dark colored lesions. There was history of application of hair dye and mustard oil over scalp.

On examination, diffuse hyperpigmented dark-brown to slate-gray macules with no evidence of erythematous border were present over forehead and neck.

> **Investigations:** Dermoscopy showed diffuse brown background, hem-like pattern of pigment, gray-colored dots and globules and perifollicular pigment deposition.
>
> **Treatment:** Patient was advised photoprotection and topical tacrolimus 0.03% local application twice daily.
>
> **Outcome:** After 12 weeks of treatment, there has been 30% decrease in the pigmentation.

■ INTERACTIVE TOPIC REVIEW

Q.1 What are the causes of facial melanoses?

Ans: See Box 1.

BOX 1	Classification of facial melanosis.

Well-defined facial melanoses:
- Melasma
- Erythema dyschromicum perstans (EDP)
- Lichen planus pigmentosus (LPP)
- Poikiloderma of Civatte
- Nevus of Ota
- Riehl's melanosis
- Erythromelanosis follicularis of face and neck (EF)
- Erythrose peribuccale pigmentaire de BROCQ (EPP)

Acquired facial melanoses which also involves face:
- Friction melanosis
- Tar melanosis
- Berloque dermatitis (BD)
- Idiopathic eruptive macular pigmentation
- Postinflammatory hyperpigmentation (PIH)
- Hyperpigmentation secondary to drugs and heavy metals

Miscellaneous:
- Periorbital melanosis
- Exogenous ochronosis
- Acanthosis nigricans
- Macular amyloidosis (MA)
- Addisonian pigmentation

Q2 What are the salient steps in the management of a case of facial melanosis?

Ans: Management of a case of facial melanosis depends largely on the correct diagnosis:
- Finding out the triggering factors like photo exposure, allergens like musk ambrette, hair dyes, fragrances, red kumkum, mustard oil, chronic hydroquinone use, etc.
- Utilizing different diagnostic modalities like dermoscopy, Wood's lamp examination, confocal/fluorescence microscopy, patch testing and histopathology

- Finally specific therapy, counseling regarding nature and prognosis of respective disease and most importantly strict photoprotection to prevent disease exacerbation.

Q.3 What are the clinical pointers toward correct diagnosis in a case of facial melanosis?

Ans: See Table 1.

TABLE 1: Differential diagnosis for facial melanosis and clinical pointers for each.

History	Examination	Investigations	Diagnosis
Sunlight/pregnancy/ovarian tumor/OCPs/hypothyroidism/positive family history	Bilaterally symmetrical hyperpigmented macules in irregular pattern on mostly butterfly area of face	• Dermoscopy—reticular pigmentation-epidermal while pseudoreticular in dermal • Wood's lamp—accentuation-epidermal • Histopathology—normal or increased melanocytes	Melasma
Sunlight/acne vulgaris/dermatitis/pyoderma/trauma	Irregular areas of hyper-pigmentation, extrafacial lesions may be present	–	Postinflammatory hyperpigmentation
Errors of refraction/atopy/family history/fatigue and weakness (anemia)	Variable discoloration varying from brown to black around the eyes	Hemogram	Periorbital hyperpigmentation
Sunlight/family history	Small pigmented spots usually light brown	–	Ephelides
Fragrances/hair dyes/mustard oil	• Usually asymptomatic (can be itchy), diffuse (less commonly reticular or perifollicular) hyper-pigmented slate-gray to brown, black macules present mostly over exposed areas and flexures • Mucous membranes spared	• Patch test • Histopathology—suggestive of lichenoid changes with pigment incontinence	LPP
Radiocontrast dye, cobalt exposure/HIV infection	Asymptomatic, gradually enlarging, persistent, macules of different sizes. In early stage there is an erythematous hue and an elevated dusky border later these lesions eventually become pigmented. Affects face, trunk and limb	• Patch test • Histopathology—along with vacuolar basal cell degeneration, there is perivascular lympho-histiocytic infiltrate at the active border	EDP

Continued

Continued

TABLE 1: Differential diagnosis for facial melanosis and clinical pointers for each.

History	Examination	Investigations	Diagnosis
Cosmetics/dyes/fragrances	Diffuse/patchy or reticular brown to black pigmentation, sometimes with satellite perifollicular hyperpigmented macules and follicular hyperkeratosis	Patch test	Riehl's melanosis
MDT/ATT/phenytoin/griseofulvin/NSAIDs	• Melasma like/diffuse pigmentation • Extrafacial pigmentation can be present	–	Drug induced hyper-pigmentation
Topical steroid abuse/cosmetics	Diffuse dark brown-red pigmentation present symmetrically around the mouth, sparing vermillion border. It may involve forehead, angles of the jaw and temples	–	EPP
Cosmetics	Presence of brownish reticulate pigmentation, telangiectasia and atrophy in irregular, symmetrical pattern on the convexities of cheeks and the sides of the neck, sparing the area under the chin	–	Poikiloderma of Civatte
	Progressive red-brown pigmentation and telangiectasis surmounted with pale, tiny follicular papules from which vellus hairs are lost over preauricular area which may extend to neck	Histopathology—sebaceous glands and hair follicles are enlarged with the follicles containing lamellar horny masses. The overlying flattened epidermis has high melanin content and there is a minimal lymphocytic infiltrate around dilated vessels	EF
Present since birth/puberty	Mottled coalescing blue-gray macules in the dermatomes supplied by trigeminal nerve. Blue sclera	–	Nevus of Ota
Chronic hydroquinone use	<1-mm blue macules in a reticulate pattern. Lesions occur in the hydroquinone treated photoexposed areas	Histopathology—yellowish brown banana-shaped granules in and around collagen bundles. There is presence of giant cells and melanophage rich granulomas	Exogenous ochronosis

Continued

Continued

TABLE 1: Differential diagnosis for facial melanosis and clinical pointers for each.

History	Examination	Investigations	Diagnosis
History of chikungunya fever (fever with severe joint pains)	Brown-black pigmentation, mainly involving the centrofacial area. The lesions can be freckle-like/slate-colored pigmentation/melasma-like pigmentation over the face/periorbital hypermelanosis/a flagellate type of pigmentation on the face and limbs	–	Postchikungunya pigmentation
History of autoimmune diseases/TB	Hyperpigmentation on the photoexposed areas, flexures, palmoplantar creases, areas of repeated friction, the normally pigmented sites (e.g. nipples) and mucous membranes	Serum cortisol/ACTH	Addisonian pigmentation
Weight gain/diabetes/family history	• Hyperpigmented, velvety plaques over body folds, alar creases and less commonly acral parts of body like hands • Obesity	Serum insulin level/blood sugar level and lipid profile	Acanthosis nigricans

(OCPs: oral contraceptive pills; LPP: lichen planus pigmentosus, HIV: human immunodeficiency virus; EDP: erythema dyscromicum perstans; MDT: multidrug therapy; ATT: antitubercular treatment; NSAIDs: nonsteroidal anti-inflammatory drugs; EPP: erythrose peribuccale pigmentaire de BROCQ; EF: erythromelanosis follicularis; TB: tuberculosis; ACTH: adrenocorticotropic hormone.)

Q.4 What is melasma and what are its various types?

Ans: Melasma (Greek: melas-black), formerly known as chloasma taken from the word chloazein (green), is an acquired disorder of pigmentation, occurring most commonly over the face.

It is more prevalent in females and individuals with darker skin types. This is predominantly attributed to ultraviolet (UV) exposure and hormonal influences.

Melasma is a clinical diagnosis consisting of symmetric reticulated hypermelanosis in three predominant facial patterns—malar, centrofacial and mandibular.

On the basis of location of melanin, melasma is classified into:
- Epidermal type: The lesions are light to dark brown and their margins are well defined
- Dermal type: Gray-brown pigmentation occurs and lesional margins are not clearly defined

- Mixed or epidermodermal type: Pigmentation is both epidermal and dermal
- Indeterminate type: This group is composed of unclassifiable melasma (even after Wood's lamp examination), seen especially in dark-skinned individuals.

Three patterns of melasma are seen on the face:
1. Malar: Pigmentation over cheeks and nose
2. Centrofacial: The most common type with hyperpigmentation on forehead, cheeks, nose, upper lip and chin
3. Mandibular: The least frequent pattern with pigmentation over ramus of the mandible.

On the basis of natural history of the lesions, melasma can be of two types:
1. Transient type: This type of melasma disappears within 1 year of withdrawal of hormonal stimulus
2. Persistent type: This persists for more than a year after withdrawal of stimulus (hormones) and is because of the action of UV radiations and other factors.

Q.5 What is the role of laboratory investigations in a case of facial melanosis?

Ans: Keeping in mind the various etiological possibilities in a patient with facial melanosis, the following investigations should be done on a case-to-case basis:
- Wood's lamp examination [type of melasma-epidermal (pigment accentuation)/dermal/mixed]
- Dermoscopy [melasma-epidermal (reticular pigmentation)/dermal (pseudoreticular pigmentation)]
- Histopathology (LPP-lichenoid dermatitis with pigment incontinence)
- Reflectance Confocal Microscopy [melasma-epidermal (cobblestoning and loss of dermal papillary rings at the basal layer)/dermal(bright plump cells in dermis)]
- Patch test (Riehl's melanosis-fragrances/cosmetics).

Q.6 What are the causes of melasma?

Ans:
- Genetic predisposition
- Ultraviolet radiation
- Thyroid disease
- Pregnancy/oral contraceptive pills
- Ovarian tumor
- Drugs such as phenytoin/griseofulvin/NSAIDs.

Q.7 Briefly describe pathogenesis of melasma.

Ans: The pathogenesis of melasma is as follows:
- Sun exposure: Acts as a trigger and exacerbating factor
  - Ultraviolet radiation-induced melanocytosis and melanogenesis
  - Ultraviolet exposure-induced dermal inflammation and fibroblast proliferation and activation may stimulate stem cell factor (SCF) in the dermis, causing melanogenesis.
- Role of dermal factors: Though majorly epidermal disease, but dermal factors are a major cause for persistence and resistance to treatment of melasma

- o Fibroblasts play a major role. Fibroblast derived SCF and cytokines are increased in the lesional skin
- o There is increased vascularization (Increased vascular endothelial growth factor). Melasma with "telangiectatic erythema" is severe in degree and poorly responsive to laser treatments.
- Drugs: NSAIDs, phenytoin, griseofulvin
- Genes related to melanin biosynthesis and melanocyte markers like *TYRP1*, *TYR*, *MITF*, etc. are upregulated
- Wnt pathway modulation genes, genes related to prostaglandin synthesis and fatty acid metabolism are also involved in melasma pathogenesis
- Role of *H19* gene (decreased function in melasma leading to stimulation of melanogenesis and increased melanin transfer from melanocytes to keratinocytes)
- The iNOS (inducible-nitric oxide synthase) and nuclear factor-kappa B pathways have also been found to be involved in melasma pathogenesis
- Lipid metabolism genes, such as, type diacylglycerol o-acyltransferase 2-like 3, peroxisome proliferator-activated receptor-γ coactivator 1-α, peroxisome proliferator-activated receptor-α, β (ALXO 15B) and arachidonate 15-lipoxygenase were found to be downregulated.

Q.8 What are the noninvasive measurement methods of melasma?

Ans:
- Dermoscopy
- Wood's lamp examination
- Reflectance confocal microscopy.

Q.9 What are the oral agents for the treatment of melasma? Also mention their mechanism of action.

Ans: See Table 2.

TABLE 2: Mechanism action of oral agents in melasma.

Oral agent	Mechanism of action
Tranexamic acid	• Inhibits plasminogen pathway, hence inhibition of melanin synthesis • Decreases vascular proliferation
Polypodium leucotomos	• Inhibition of reactive oxygen species, hence reactive melanogenesis
Glutathione	• Inhibition of reactive oxygen species

Q.10 Enumerate chemical peels for the management of melasma.

Ans:
- Glycolic acid (20–70%)
- Mandelic acid (10%)
- Salicylic acid (20–30%)
- Trichloroacetic acid (10–20%).

Q.11 Classify chemical peels.

Ans: See Table 3.

TABLE 3: Classification of chemical peels.

Type	Examples	Depth of penetration into skin
Very superficial	• Glycolic acid (30–50%) • Trichloroacetic acid (10%) • Jessner's solution (1–3 coats) • Salicylic acid (20–30%)	Up to stratum corneum
Superficial	• Glycolic acid (50–70%) • Trichloroacetic acid (10–30%) • Jessner's solution (4–7 coats)	Up to basal layer
Medium	• Glycolic acid (70%) • Trichloroacetic acid (35–50%)	Up to papillary dermis
Deep	• Baker–Gordon 88% phenol • Trichloroacetic acid (>50%)	Up to midreticular dermis

Q.12 What are skin lightening agents?

Ans: Topical treatment for decreasing facial hyperpigmentation is more effective when the pigment is epidermal.
- Hydroquinone (2–5%)
- Azelaic acid (20%)
- Kojic acid (1–4%)
- Retinoids (retinoic acid, isotretinoin, adaplene, etc.)
- Topical steroids, e.g. fluocinolone acetonide
- Glycolic acid gel
- Niacinamide
- Mequinol (2%)
- Arbutin, deoxyarbutin
- Ascorbic acid (5–25%)
- Liquorice derivatives (20%)
- N-acetyl-4-S-cysteaminylphenol (NCAP) (4%)
- Alpha tocopheryl
- Flavonoids like catechin (green tea leaves), ellagic acid (green tea, strawberies, eucalyptus, etc.) and aloesin (aloe vera tree)
- N-acetyl glucosamine, paper mulberry extract, thiotic acid (alpha-lipoic acid) and soybean extract.

Q.13 Classify sunscreens.

Ans: Sunscreens can be topical/systemic. Topical sunscreens can be classified into organic and inorganic.
- Organic: Presented in Table 4.
- Inorganic:
    - Zinc oxide
    - Titanium dioxide
    - Others—kaolin, calamine, iron oxide, red veterinary petrolatum, ichthammol and talc.

TABLE 4: Organic sunscreens.

UVA blockers	UVB blockers	UVA + UVB blockers
Benzophenones (UVB and UVA2 absorbers): • Oxybenzone • Sulisobenzone • Dioxybenzone	Para-aminobenzoic acid derivatives: Padimate O	Ecamsule (Mexoryl SX)
Avobenzone (UVA1 absorber)	Cinnamates: • Octinoxate • Cinoxate	Silatriazole (Mexoryl XL)
Meradimate (UVA2 absorber)	Salicylates: • Octisalate • Homosalate • Trolamine salicylate	Bemotrizinol (Tinosorb S)
	Octocrylene	Bisoctrizole (Tinosorb M)
	Ensulizole	

(UV: ultraviolet)

- Systemic sunscreens:
    o Beta carotene
    o Green tea polyphenols
    o Antimalarials
    o Selenium
    o Ascorbic acid
    o Antihistamines
    o Aspirin, indomethacin
    o Tocopherols (vitamins A, C and E), retinol
    o Corticosteroids
    o Para-aminobenzoic acid.

Q.14 Which sunscreens are to be used and the correct usage of them?

Ans: An ideal sunscreen would be a combination of chemical and physical agents, broad spectrum, substantive, nonirritant, noncomedogenic, hypoallergenic, cosmetically elegant and cost-effective.

Sunscreens are to be applied in adequate amount to all sun exposed areas (in a concentration of 2 mg/cm^2), and allowed to dry for 15–30 minutes before exposure to sun. It should be reapplied every 2 hours, and after vigorous activity, toweling, excessive perspiration or swimming.

"Teaspoon rule" to be used:
- 3 mL (slightly more than half a teaspoon):
    o For the face and neck
    o For each arm.

- 6 mL (slightly more than a teaspoon)
  - For the chest
  - For the back
  - For each leg.

For intermittent, casual daily use, a sun protection factor-15 (SPF-15) sunscreen is sufficient. For prolonged recreational exposures, an SPF-30 is more desirable.

Q.15 What are the common scoring systems in melasma?

Ans:
- Melasma Area and Severity Index
- Modified MASI
- Melasma Quality of Life scale (MELASQOL)
- Hindi-Melasma Quality of Life scale (Hi-MELASQOL).

Q.16 Mention surgical/laser therapies for treating melasma.

Ans:
- Q-switched NdYAG laser
- Microneedling
- Intense pulsed light
- Radiofrequency
- Fractional laser.

Q.16 What are the differentiating points between LPP and EDP/ashy dermatosais?

Ans: See Table 5.

TABLE 5: Differentiating points between LPP and EDP.

Lichen planus pigmentosus	Erythema dyscromicum perstans/ashy dermatosis
There is a predilection for photoexposed areas and flexures	No predisposition for photoexposed sites
Lesions are usually pruritic	Lesions are nonpruritic
There may be associated features of lichen planus that could be present with involvement of nails and mucous membranes	These features are absent
The pattern of pigmentation can be diffuse/blotchy/perifollicular or reticular	The lesions are mostly symmetrical with polycyclic margin. Residual hypopigmented halo may be present
This is a chronic condition with relapses and remissions	A chronic and insidious condition. Spontaneous resolution may be present in children

CONCLUSION

Since facial melanosis is distressing for a patient. It is of utmost importance to take good history, perform proper physical examination, make judicious use of investigations, and appropriately manage the case.

Proper counseling regarding prognosis and nature of disease is also of great significance as the disease may be affecting emotional status of the individual.

KEY POINTS

- Every patient of facial melanosis should undergo thorough examination and relevant investigations based on differential diagnoses kept
- Characteristic features of disease should be noted carefully to make correct diagnosis
- Based on diagnosis, therapy should be initiated
- Apart from medical/surgical/laser therapy, general measures should be explained in detail like photoprotection.

SUGGESTED READING

1. Baldini E, Odorisio T, Sorrenti S, et al. Vitiligo and autoimmune thyroid disorders. Front Endocrinol (Lausanne) [Internet]. 2017;8:290. Available from: https://www.ncbi.nlm.nih.gov/pmc/articles/PMC5663726
2. Falabella R. Pigmentary disorders in Latin America. Dermatol Clin. 2007;25 (3):419-30, x.
3. Hassan I, Aleem S, Bhat YJ, et al. A clinicoepidemiological study of facial melanosis. Pigment Int. 2015;2:34-40.
4. Kaimal S, Abraham A. Sunscreens. Indian J Dermatol Venereol Leprol. 2011;77:238-43.
5. Khanna N, Rasool S. Facial melanoses: Indian perspective. Indian J Dermatol Venereol Leprol. 2011;77:552-64.
6. Khunger N. Standard guidelines of care for chemical peels. Indian J Dermatol Venereol Leprol. 2008;74:S5-12.
7. Miazek N, Michalek I, Pawlowska-Kisiel M, et al. Pityriasis Alba-common disease, enigmatic entity: Up-to-date review of the literature. Pediatr Dermatol. 2015;32(6):786-91.
8. Molinar VE, Taylor SC, Pandya AG. What's new in objective assessment and treatment of facial hyperpigmentation? Dermatol Clin. 2014;32(2):123-35.
9. Neema S, Jha A. Lichen planus pigmentosus. Pigment Int. 2017;4:48-9.
10. Pichardo R, Vallejos Q, Feldman SR, et al. The prevalence of melasma and its association with quality of life in adult male Latino migrant workers. Int J Dermatol. 2009;48:22-6.
11. Praetorius C, Sturm RA, Steingrimsson E. Sun-induced freckling: ephelides and solar lentigines. Pigment Cell Melanoma Res. 2014;27(3):339-50.
12. Sanchez NP, Pathak MA, Sato S, et al. Melasma: A clinical, light microscopic, ultrastructural, and immunofluorescence study. J Am Acad Dermatol.1981;4(6):698-710.
13. Sarkar R, Arora P, Garg VK, et al. Melasma update. Indian Dermatol Online J 2014;5:426-35.
14. Sharquie KE, Noaimi AA. Gazelle eye like facial melanosis (clinico-histopathological study). Pigmentary Disorders. 2014;1:111.
15. Singh KG. Non-melasma facial melanosis. In: Lahiri K, Chatterjee M, Sarkar R, (Eds). Pigmentary Disorders: A Comprehensive Compendium: Jaypee Brothers, Medical Publishers Pvt. Limited; 2014.

Index

Page numbers followed by '*b*' box; '*f*' figure; '*fc*' flowchart; and '*t*' indicate table respectively.

A

Acantholytic cells 127*f*
  in clumps 123*f*
  multiple 122
Acanthosis nigricans 13, 221, 222
Acid fast bacilli 80
Acne
  rosacea 99
  vulgaris 99
Acquired facial melanoses 222
Acquired immune mediated 82
Acquired immunodeficiency syndrome 32
Acrodermatitis enteropathica 116
Acromegaly 61
Acropustulosis of infancy 116
Actinic keratosis 99, 102
Addison's disease 60, 61, 65
Addisonian pigmentation 222
Adenovirus 176
Adrenocorticotropic hormone 67, 225
Alkali spill 128*f*
Allergic contact dermatitis 125, 135, 208
Alopecia areata 13, 205
  diffuse type of 197, 199
  incognita 199
Alopecia in syphilis, clinical picture of 204
Alpha tocopheryl 228
American Academy of Dermatology 142
Aminexil 203
Amiodarone 64
Amitriptyline 49, 53
Amlexanox oral paste 10
Ammonium lactate 48
Amoebiasis 29
Ampicillin 74
Amyloidosis 82
Anagen effluvium 204
Anagen hair loss 197, 199
  clinical features of 201
Analyte-specific reagents 162
Androgen excess disorders 201
Androgenetic alopecia 199, 204
  in women 200
Aneurysm, rupture of 5
Angiofibroma 99
Angiotensin II inhibitors 54
Angiotensin-converting enzyme inhibitors 54, 142, 200
Anhidrosis 91
Anti-androgens like cyproterone acetate 203
Antibody assay 47
Antidepressants 49, 200
Antihistaminics 49
Anti-inflammatory analgesics 11
Antilipoid immunoglobulin 40
Antimalarials 229
  drugs 26
  like chloroquine 63
Antimicrobial resistant 180
Antinuclear antibody 12, 14, 210
Antipsychotics 54
Antithyroid drugs 200
Antitubercular treatment 225
Apert syndrome 100
Aphthae like oral ulceration 2*f*
Aphthous
  stomatitis 24*f*
  ulcers 4
Apocrine gland 99
Appendages, loss of 91
Apremilast 10
Aprepitant 49, 51
Aquagenic pruritus 45
Arbutin 228
Argyria 64
Arsenic 64, 90
Arthritis 14
Articular
  involvement, management of 11
  manifestations 5
Ascorbic acid 228, 229
Ashy dermatosis 61, 230
Aspirin 229
Atopic dermatitis 55, 208
Autoimmune blistering disease 121
  primary 136
Autoimmune blistering disorders 137*t*, 139*t*
Autoimmune bullous
  dermatosis 76
  disease in children 115
Autoimmune diseases 118
Autoimmune disorders 125

Autoimmune vesiculobullous disorders 128, 130f
Automated regain test 40
Autonomic integrity, testing 85
Autosomal dominant 114
Avobenzone 229
Azathioprine 10, 11, 18, 25, 144
Azelaic acid 228
Azithromycin 40, 163, 164, 168, 169, 181

B

Bacillus Calmette-Guérin vaccination 90
Bacterial
    infection 29, 41
    prostatitis 176
    vaginosis 156, 158, 160f, 160-165, 169
Bacteroides 162
Basal cell carcinoma 30, 99, 102
Basaloid follicular hamartoma syndrome 100
Bazex–Dupré-Christol syndrome 100
Beçhet syndrome 41
Behçet's disease 2, 4, 8, 3f, 30, 32, 33, 34, 36
    case of 8
    clinical features of 2, 7
    cutaneous lesions of 7
    diagnostic criteria for 6
    international criteria for 6t
    neonatal 117
    over tongue in 2
    treatment options in 9
Bell's palsy 90
Benediction sign 85
Benign cephalic pustulosis 113
Benzathine penicillin 40
    single dose of intramuscular 29
Benzophenones 229
Berloque dermatitis 222
Beta carotene 229
Biguanides 54
Biliary
    cirrhosis, primary 62
    occlusion 46
Biomimetic peptides, topical 203
Birt-Hogg-Dubé syndrome 100
Blaschko lines 66
Blister formation, mechanism of 135
Blistering diseases 136
    clinically resemble child abuse 118
Blistering disorders 115
    in children, approach to 117
Blistering distal dactylitis 108
Blisters in children 108t
Bone mineral density 145
Boric acid 164
Bourneville's syndrome 100
Bowen's disease 30
Brain-derived neurotrophic factor 209

Bronze baby syndrome 61
Bronze diabetes 62
Brooke-Spiegler syndrome 100
Bubos 33
Buccal mucosa 2
Bulla and villi formation 127f
Bullous dermatoses 30, 151
    chronic, childhood 119f
Bullous disorder
    chronic, childhood 107
    in children 104
        classify 107
Bullous erythema multiforme 76, 115, 126
Bullous ichthyosiform erythroderma 115
Bullous lichen planus 128
Bullous lupus erythematosus 125, 128
Bullous mastocytosis 116
Bullous pemphigoid 125, 133, 134f, 141
    childhood 118t
    direct immunofluorescence test 140f
Bullous sweet's syndrome 125
Busulfan 64, 65
Butorphanol modulates opioid system 51

C

Caffeine 203, 228
Calcineurin inhibitors 25
Calcinosis cutis 13
Calcitriol 44
Calcium
    acetate 44
    channel blockers 54, 142
Camphor 48
Cancer
    cachexia 61
    cells 54
Candida 160, 161, 162
Candida albicans 157f
Candida glabrata 159
Candida krusei 159
Candida species 159
    presence of 162
Candida tropicalis 159
Candidal vulvovaginitis 156, 158
Canidida albicans 159
Capixyl 203
Captopril 16, 142
Carbamazepine 16, 54, 126, 152
Carcinoid syndrome 46, 61
Card test 85
Cardiovascular manifestations 5
Carotenoids 65
Catastrophic paralysis 87
Cefadroxil 142
Cefixime 164
Ceftriaxone 163, 164

Centers for Disease Control 163, 164, 169, 180
Central nervous system 5, 105, 111
   involvement, management of 11
Centrifugal pattern 74
Cephalocaudal progression 73*f*
Cephalosporins 54
Cerebellopontine angle tumors 90
Cerebral
   abscess 46
   tumor 46
Cervical
   infection 164
   os 167*f*
Cervicitis
   gonococcal 167, 169
   nongonococcal 167
Cetirizine 48
Chancre 36, 37, 38
   atypical manifestations of 39
   in males 38
   primary 33
   redux 39
Chancroid 37
Charcot' joints 91
Charcot-Marie-Tooth neuropathy 82
Chemical
   irritation 176
   peels, classification of 227, 228*t*
Chicken pox 110
Chikungunya 110
   fever 78
   virus 78
Chilblain lupus 19
Chlamydia 158, 160, 162, 165, 178
Chlamydia trachomatis 158, 172
Chlorambucil 54
Chlorhexidine gel 10
Chloromas 34
Chloroquine 25, 26
   blood levels in therapy 26
Chlorpheniramine maleate 48
Cholestatic
   pruritus, causes 52
   pruritus, clinical characteristics of 53
"Christmas" tree pattern 200
Chrysiasis 64
Cicatricial pemphigoid 30, 34
Cimetidine 152
Cinnamates 229
Cinoxate 229
Clindamycin 163, 164
Clofazimine 64
Clotrimazole 163, 164, 169
   vaginal pessaries 157
Clue cells, gram stain for 161
Coalesced herpes lesions 33

Colchicine 10, 11, 107
Collagen vascular conditions 73
Colloid milia 99
Colonoscopy 2
Condoms, use of 32
Connective tissue disorders 199
Contact dermatitis
   common causes of 214
   treatment of 216
Corkscrew motion 39
Corneal ulcers 91
Coronal sulcus 28
Coronary artery lesions 5
Corticosteroids 11
Cowden syndrome 100
Creatine phosphokinase 210
Creutzfeldt-Jakob disease 46
Crohn's disease 30, 31, 32, 41, 194
Crusting over
   neck 122*f*
   scalp 123*f*
Crystallina 112
Cushing syndrome 61, 62
Cutaneous examination 34, 44
Cutaneous horn 99
Cutaneous leishmaniasis 185
Cutaneous lesions 3
Cutaneous lupus erythematosus 12
   acute 22, 23*f*
      treatment of 25
   classification of 12
   clinical features 17
   histopathology and types of 17
   subacute 21, 22*f*
      clinical features 22
      drugs causing 21
      etiology 21
Cutaneous sarcoidosis
   clinical variants of 191
   management of 192
Cutaneous sensation 43
Cutaneous T-cell lymphoma 151
Cutaneous tuberculosis
   classification of 186
   classify 186
   diagnosis of 187, 188
   drug resistance 188
   suspected case of 187
   treatment regimen for 189
Cutaneous vascular disease 13
Cyclophosphamide 25, 144
Cyclosporine 10, 11
Cystic mastitis 204
Cytomegalovirus 29
Cytoplasmic antineutrophil cytoplasmic
   antibodies 9

D

Dactinomycin 64
Dandruff 212
Dapsone 10, 18, 25, 107, 144
Deep dermis 65
Deep fungal infection 185
Deep tendon reflexes 83
Deformity 91
Degos disease-like lesions 13
Dehydroepiandrosterone 16
Dengue
  fever 78
  virus 78
Deoxyarbutin 228
Dermal hyperpigmentation 60
  differential diagnosis of 60
Dermal papillae 138*f*
Dermatitis 151
Dermatitis herpetiformis 24, 125, 133*f*, 136, 138*f*, 141
  direct immunofluorescence 140*f*
Dermatological
  causes 61
  diseases 45
    symptom of 43
  disorders 43
Dermatomyositis 208
Dermatosis papulosa nigra 99
Dermis 59
  superficial 65
Dexamethasone-azathioprine pulse 144
Dexamethasone-cyclophosphamide pulse 143
Dexamethasone-methotrexate pulse 144
Dexamethasone mucosal paste 10
Diabetic neuropathy 208
Dicloxacillin 107
Diffuse alopecias, trichoscopic features 204
Diffuse dermal melanosis 63
Diffuse hair loss 196
  case of 201
  common type of 198
  differential diagnosis of 199
  hormonal profile 201
  important points for history taking 201
  laboratory investigations 202
  measures for managing 203
  scalp biopsy in 202
Diffuse hyperpigmentation 57, 65*t*, 67
  approach to 66*fc*
  causes of 61*t*
  patient with 64, 65
Diffuse telogen hair loss 199
  identify 200
  triggers of 199
Dioxybenzone 229
Diphtheria 90
Disability 91
Discoid lupus erythematosus 17
  disseminated 17
  histopathology 18
  hypertrophic 19
  immunopathology 18
  mucosal 19
  prognosis 18
  treatment of 18
Discoid rash 14
Disseminated disease 105
Donovan bodies 35, 38
Donovanosis 37, 38
Double stranded deoxyribonucleic acid 9
Down-regulate T-cell activity 25
Doxepin 49, 50, 55
Doxycycline 40, 163, 169, 181
Drug induced
  disorders 125
  hyperpigmentation 221
  pemphigus 142
Drugs and toxins 61, 63
Drugs like minocycline 65
Dyshidrosiform pemphigus 142
Dyshidrotic dermatitis 125, 135

E

Eccrine
  gland 99
  hidrocystoma 99
Eczema herpeticum 127*f*
Egawa's test 85
Electron microscopy 134
  role for 136
Electrophysiological testing 85
Emotional stress 199
Endocrine
  and metabolic disease 46
  causes 61
Endomyocardial fibrosis 5
Enzyme-linked immunosorbent assay 36, 138, 161
Eosinophil cationic protein 209
Eosinophil-derived neurotoxin 209
Eosinophilic pustular folliculitis 7, 117
Epidermal hyperpigmentation 60
Epidermis 59, 184*f*
  ballooning degeneration of 38
  fishnet appearance of 123*f*
  severe sloughing of 150
Epidermolysis bullosa 114, 121
Epidermolysis bullosa acquisita 115, 117, 125
  childhood and adult 118*t*
Epithelioid cell granulomas 184*f*
Epstein–Barr virus 25, 29, 30, 176
Erosive lichen planus 31
Erythema dyschromicum perstans 58, 61, 225, 230

Erythema multiforme 30, 75, 136
   cases of 135
   like lesions 4
   major 125
Erythema
   nodosum leprosum 93
   over trunk 150*f*
   toxicum neonatorum 112
Erythematous 88*f*
   annular plaques 190*f*
   infiltrated plaques 194*f*
   papules, differentials for 99
Erythroderma 149, 154
   clinical features of drug-induced 152
   common causes of 151
   complications of 153, 153*t*
   different causes of 150
   drugs causing 152
   laboratory findings 153
   manage case of 153
   nail changes seen 152
   occur in neonates 151
   systemic manifestations of 153, 153*t*
   triggering factors of 152
Erythromelanosis follicularis 225
Erythromycin 164
Ethambutol 189
Ethylene glycol 90
Eumelanin and pheomelanin, difference 60*t*
European Dermatology Forum Guidelines, 2015 143
Exogenous ochronosis 221, 222

F

Face
   colored papules on 100
   pigmentation on 58*f*
Facial melanosis 219
   causes of 222
   classification of 219, 222
   correct diagnosis 223
   differential diagnosis 223, 223*t*
   management of case of 222
   role of laboratory investigations 226
Facial nerve palsy, causes of 90, 90*f*, 91
Familial progressive hyperpigmentation 61
Felty's syndrome 61
Female pattern hair loss 197
Fetal varicella 109
Fever 32
Fever and rash with child 72, 73
   approach to patient 77*fc*
   causes of 75
      acute onset of 75*b*
      subacute onset of 75*b*
   classification of 76*t*
   history taking 73*b*
   infectious and noninfectious causes of 75
   management of 76
   signs indicative of 74*t*
   subacute onset of 75
Fever and rash with neonate, causes of 75
Fexofenadine 48
Fibrous papule of nose 99
Flavonoids like catechin 228
Fluconazole 157, 164
Fluorescent treponemal antibody-absorption 35, 40
Fluvoxamine 49, 55
Folic acid deficiency 61
Follicular mucinosis 99
Follman's
   balanitis 39
   sign 85
Fungal infection 110

G

Gabapentin 49
Gardnerella 162
   vaginalis 160, 162
Gastrointestinal involvement, management of 11
Gastrointestinal manifestations 5
Gelatin capsule 164
Gene amplification techniques 88
Genetic susceptibility 15
Genital herpes 158
Genital ulcer 3, 28
   approach to 35*fc*
   atypical manifestations of 38*t*
   case of 30
   causes of 29
      infectious 29
      noninfectious 29
   diagnosis 34
      culture 36
      direct examination 34
      other tests 36
      serological tests 36
   disease 40, 41
Genodermatoses 114
Giant congenital melanocytic nevus 61
Giemsa stain 35
Glans penis 38
Glucose-6-phosphate dehydrogenase 134
Glutathione 227
Glycolic acid gel 228
Gold 64
Gonococcal infection, disseminated 180
Gonococcal isolate surveillance project 180
Gonococcal urethritis 172, 179
   cases of 176, 177
   complications of 180
   pathomechanism of 177

Gonococcus 158, 162
Gonorrhea 156, 158, 163, 164, 167f, 178
Granuloma
    annulare 193
        clinical variants of 194
        histological patterns 194
    classified histologically 185
    faciale 99, 102
    histopathological classification of 186t
    inguinale 29, 33, 35
    type of 186
Granulomatous
    disorders 183, 194
        differential diagnoses 185
    periorificial dermatitis 192
    rosacea 192
Green tea polyphenols 229
Grover's disease 128, 135
Grzybowski syndrome 100
Guillain-Barré syndrome 90

H

Hailey–Hailey disease 125, 127, 127f, 135
Hair
    bonding and weaving 203
    care procedures 200
    cycle, normal 198
    dust 203
    dye dermatitis 215
        etiology of 215
        investigation to confirm 215
        patient prevent 217
        test for 216
    follicle mesenchyme 99
    loss, pattern 203
    prosthesis-like wigs 203
    spray 203
    transplantation 203
HAIR-AN syndrome 203
Hair-pull test 202
Hamartomas 99
Hand foot mouth disease 110
Handicap 91
Head and neck tumors 90
Headache 5
Healing erosions 129f
    pemphigus vulgaris 124f
Hemangioma 99
Hematologic disorder 14
Hematoxylin and eosin examination 134
Hemifacial microsomia 90
Hemochromatosis 46, 61, 62
Hemophilus species 176
Hemorrhagic
    crusts 129f
    fevers in childhood 77
Henoch–Schönlein purpura 73, 76

Heparin 200
Hepatolenticular degeneration 62
Hereditary motor 82
Herpes genitalis 38
Herpes simplex in older children 109
Herpes simplex virus 35, 111, 176
Herpes zoster 29, 110, 111f
    left side of chest 127f
Histamine 4 receptor 208
Histamine test 85
Hodgkin's disease 55, 151
Homosalate 229
Homosexual males 38
Honeycomb pattern 86
Hori nevus 221
Hormonal therapy 203
Hormones, influence of 66
Human immunodeficiency virus 47, 199, 225
    coinfection 38
    infection 28, 32, 46, 151
Human leukocyte antigen 36
Hutchinson lupus 19
Hydantoin derivatives 152
Hydroquinone 228
Hydroxychloroquine 25, 26, 63
    ocular monitoring for 26
Hydroxyzine 48, 55
Hyper IgE syndrome 117
Hypermelanotic disorders 219
Hyperpigmentary disorders, prevalence of 57
Hyperpigmentation secondary to drugs 222
Hyperpigmentation understand by 60
Hyperthyroidism 61, 65
Hypoalbuminemia, care of 154
Hypoesthetic patch 80

I

Idiopathic eruptive macular pigmentation 222
Idiopathic erythroderma 152
Idiopathic facial granulomatous
    disorders 193t
    eruptions 192
Idiopathic thrombocytopenic purpura 77
Ileocecal ulceration 2
Imatinib 64
Imipramine 63
Immune electron microscopy 136
Immune mediated blistering diseases 116t
Immunoadsorption 144
Immunoelectron microscopy 134
Immunofluorescence test 36
    direct 9, 127f, 134, 136
    indirect 134, 136
Immunoglobulin A disease 107
Immunologic disorder 14
Immunological blistering disorders 115
Immunosuppressive adjuvants 144

Impetigo 125
Incontinentia pigmenti 114
   hyperpigmented stage of 61
Increments 143
Indomethacin 229
Infections 61
Infectious
   granulomatous dermatoses 185
   mononucleosis 76
Infective disorders 108*t*
Inflammatory
   blistering disorders 115
   bowel disease 7, 199
   demyelinating polyneuropathy 82
   dermatoses 30, 31
   diseases 45, 125
   disorders 99
   infiltrate, moderate degree of 184
Infliximab 11
Insect-bite hypersensitivity 113
Insulin 44
Intercellular edema 135
Interferon alpha 10
Interferon-gamma release assays 187
International Contact Dermatitis Research Group 216*f*
Intertriginous fissures 127*f*
Intracardiac thrombosis 5
Intracellular
   diplococci, gram-negative 168*f*
   edema, ballooning due to 135
   gram-negative diplococci 176
Intraepidermal blisters 135
Intraepidermal neutrophilic 142
Intraneural synovial tumor 82
Intrauterine herpes 109
Intravaginal clotrimazole 167
Iron 64
   deficiency anemia 46
Iron oxide 228
Irritant contact dermatitis 125, 128*f*
Isoniazid 16, 189
Isotretinoin 10
Itch
   chronic 43
   treat different causes of 48
Itching 43
Itraconazole 164

J

Jaundice 44
Joint pain 1, 8, 103
Joint symptoms 1
Juvenile dermatomyositis 75, 76
Juvenile rheumatoid arthritis 76
   systemic onset 75

K

Kala azar 61
Kaolin 228
Kaposi's sarcoma 100
Kawasaki disease 76
Kayser–Fleischer ring 62
Keratinization disorders 151
Keratoacanthoma 99
Kojic acid 228

L

Labia
   inner aspect of 39
   outer aspect of 39
Lacy white reticulate 33
Langerhans cell histiocytosis 116
Langhans giant cells 190*f*
Laugier–Hunziker syndrome 61, 63
Lead 64
Leg ulcers 13
Leiner's disease 151
Leishman stain 35
Leishmaniasis 29, 89, 98, 100
Lepromatous pole 86
Leprosy 82, 84
   cardinal signs of 93
   classical lesion of 89
   clinical assessment of 93
   diagnostic tests for 87
   examined in 83, 84
   facial lesions of 89
   WHO, disability grading 94, 94*t*
Lesions heal 3
Leukemia 32
Leukemia cutis 61
Leukocytoclastic vasculitis 3, 7
Levofloxacin 164
Lichen planopilaris 209*f*
Lichen planus pigmentosus 58, 61, 66, 225, 230
   associated disorders with 69
   inversus 67
   investigations required for 69
   predisposing factors of 65
   treatment of 69
   variants of 66
Lichen sclerosus et atrophicus 30, 31
Linear IgA disease 140*f*
Lipoid proteinosis 117
Liquorice derivatives 228
Lithium 152
Livedo reticularis 13
Liver disease, chronic 208
Loratadine 48
Lupus erythematosus 23*f*, 24
   nonspecific lesions 13

oral involvement in 23
profundus 20
specific skin disease 12
tumidus 21
   clinical features 21
   histopathologic findings 21
   immunologic abnormalities 21
   significance 21
   treatment 21
Lupus hair loss 13
Lupus miliaris disseminatus faciei 99, 192
Lupus pernio 191
Lupus vulgaris 102, 185
  clinical variants of 187
  complications of 187
Lyme disease 83, 90
Lymph node 47
  examination 32
Lymphogranuloma venereum 29, 33, 35-38
Lymphoma 32, 46, 61, 99
Lymphoproliferative disorders 199
Lymphoreticular malignancies 127

M

Macrolides 54
Macular amyloidosis 222
Maculopapular rash on face 73*f*
MAGIC syndrome 6, 9
Magnetic resonance imaging 86
Malabsorption syndrome 61, 62
Malaise 44
Malar rash 14
Malaria 61
Malassezia 212, 213
Malignancies 61
Malignant neoplasm 30
Mastocytosis 46
Maternal antibodies 115
Measles virus 78
Meatal stenosis 31
Medical disorders 199
Medical Research Council Scale 81
Melanin 59
  chemical composition of 60
  compounds 65*t*
  types of 60
Melanocyte-stimulating hormone 60
Melasma 220*f*
  causes of 226
  common scoring systems in 230
  epidermal type of 221
  management of 227
  measurement methods of 227
  mechanism action of 227, 227*t*
  pathogenesis of 226

  therapies for treating 230
  treatment of 227
  types of 225
Meningococcal septicemia 73
Meningococcemia 75
Menthol 48
Mepacrine 63
Mequinol 228
Meradimate 229
Metals 63, 64
Metastatic melanomas 61
Methotrexate 11, 18, 25, 64, 144
Methyldopa 16
Metoclopramide 164
Metronidazole 54, 167, 169, 181
Miconazole 163, 169
Micro-immunofluorescence test 36
Microneedling 203
Micropigmentation 203
Milia 99
Miliaria rubra 113
Mimic sarcoidosis clinically 192
Minocycline 16
  induced type 3 pigmentation 64
Minoxidil 203
Mirtazapine 49, 50, 53
Mitral valve prolapse 5
Mobiluncus species 160
Möbius syndrome 90
Molecular methods 88
Monilethrix 204
Mononeuritis multiplex 86
Morbilliform 45
Morphology, basis of 76
Motor
  examination 83
  integrity, testing 84
Moxifloxacin 181
Mucha-Habermann disease 125
Mucocutaneous disease 105
Mucocutaneous lesions, management of 9
Mucocutaneous, myriad of 1
Mucosal inflammation 5
Mueller-Hinton agar 36
Muir-Torre syndrome 100
Muscles, wasting of 91
Mycobacterium leprae 80
Mycophenolate mofetil 18, 25, 107, 144
Mycoplasma 158, 160-162
Mycoplasma cervicitis 165
Mycoplasma species 172
Mycosis fungoides 61
Myelofibrosis 46
Myeloma 46
Myotonic dystrophica 90

Index | 241

N

Nalfurafine 49, 51
Naloxone 51, 49
Naltrexone 53, 55
National AIDS Control Organisation 158
Necrobiosis lipoidica 98
Necrobiotic granulomas
    classification of 193
    Lynch and Barrett, classification of 193*t*
Necrobiotic xanthogranuloma 98*f*
    diagnosis of 98
Neisseria gonorrhoeae 172
Nelson syndrome 61, 62, 65
Neonatal
    acne 113
    and systemic lupus erythematosus 76
    candidiasis 75
    erythroderma 75
    herpes simplex 75
    lupus erythematosus 75, 115
    pemphigus 115
    pustular melanosis 112
    varicella 75, 110
Nerve
    biopsy 86
    conduction study 85
    damage
        clinically 84
        methods to examine 85
    enlargement 86
    examination of 83
    function impairment 91
        manage to patient 91
        risk factors for 90
    growth factor 208
    infiltration 82
    multiple 80
    palpation of 84
    single 80
    thickness, grading of 84*t*
Neural leprosy 81, 86
    pure 80
Neuritis
    acute 86
    chronic 86
    recurrent 87
Neurofibroma 82
Neurokinin-1 receptor antagonist 51
Neurological deficit, complications due to 90
Neurological disorder 14
Neurological manifestations 5
Neurolymphomatosis 82
Neuropathic disorders 83
    clinical approach to 83
Neuropathic pain, chronic 87
Neuropathy, development of 80
Neurotransmitter gamma-aminobutyric acid 50
Neutrophilic
    infiltrate 7
    microabscess 138
    vascular reaction 7
Neutrophils forming 138
Niacinamide 228
Niemann–Pick disease 63
Nonbullous ichthyosiform erythroderma 151
Nongonococcal
    cervicitis 156, 160, 163, 164
    urethritis 179
Nonmelanin compounds 65*t*
Nonparenchymal brain disease 6
Nonscarring alopecia 13
Nonsteroidal anti-inflammatory drugs 54, 225
Nontreponemal test 36, 40
Northern blot analysis 134
Norwegian scabies 151
Nose sign 152
Nuclear factor of activated T-cells 25
Nucleic acid amplification test 161, 162, 178
Nutritional causes 61
Nylon monofilament testing 85

O

Octinoxate 229
Octisalate 229
Ocular manifestations 4
Ofloxacin 164
Ophthalmological examination 34
Opioid agonists 51
Oral contraceptive pills 225
Oral corticosteroids, short course of 25
Oral lesions, management of 144
Oral mucosal 32
Oral ulcer 1, 2, 8, 14, 24*f*, 123*f*
    lesions 1
    recurrent painful 1
Organ failure, multiple 62
Organic sunscreens 229*t*
Orofacial granulomatosis 194
Oschner's clasp 85
Oxybenzone 229
Oxygenated hemoglobin 59

P

Paclitaxel 54
Paget's disease 30
Pain, chronic 43
Painless palatal erosion 23*f*
Panniculitis 20
Papules
    black 100
    blue 100
    brown 100

on face, differentials for white-colored 102*fc*
purple 100
white 100
yellowish 100
Papulonodular lesions of face 96-103
case of 102
causes of 98
dermoscopic findings of 100
surface of 100
syndromes associated with 100
Para-aminobenzoic acid 229
Paraneoplastic autoimmune multiorgan syndrome 142
Paraneoplastic pemphigus 142
Paraneoplastic pruritus 50, 54
treated 54
Parasite
disease 46
infestation 111
Parenchymal brain disease 6
Parotid cancer 90
Paroxetine 49, 53, 55
Parvovirus B19 78
Patch test 216
disadvantages of 216
results 216*t*
Pathergy test 6
Paucibacillary multidrug therapy 81
Pearls, string of 117
Pediatric bullous pemphigoid 117
Pediculosis, treatment of 211
Peli incarniti 99
Pellagra 61
Pemphigoid gestationis 115, 141
Pemphigus
classical types 138
clinical practice 138
different types of 138
foliaceus 115, 133*f*
group of disorders 145
herpetiformis 142
neonatorum 115
nonclassical types 142
Pemphigus vulgaris 115, 141
British Guidelines, 2017 143
flaccid bullae of 122*f*
treatment regimens for 143*t*
Pen test 85
Penis, shaft of 29
Per speculum examination 165
Perianal erythema 108
Periocular crusting 122*f*
Perioral dermatitis 99
Periorbital melanosis 222
Peripheral nerve 84
thickening 82
causes of 82
important conditions 82*t*
trunks 84
Peripheral nervous system 5
Peripheral neuropathy 50
Peripheral sensations 83
Periungual telangiectasia 13
Peutz–Jegher syndrome 61, 62
Pharynx and tonsils 2
Phenol 48
group 142
Phenothiazines like chlorpromazine 63
Phenylbutazone 152
Phenytoin 54
Pheochromocytoma 61
Phimosis 176
Photophobia, complained of 1
Photoprotection 25
Photosensitivity 14
Photosensitizer 66
Phthiriasis 29
Phytophotodermatitis 58, 61
Pimecrolimus 10, 25
Plaques on glabella 194*f*
Plasmapheresis, British guidelines only 144
Platelet-rich plasma therapy 203
Polycystic ovary syndrome 204
Polycythemia vera 46
Polymerase chain reaction 9, 35, 88, 111, 134, 188
Polymorphic light eruption 125, 128
Polypodium leucotomos 227
Porphyria cutanea tarda 65, 125, 129*f*, 136
Potassium hydroxide 210
mount 35
smear 134
Prednisolone 10, 81, 143, 144
Pregabalin 49, 55
Pregnancy, cholestasis of 46
Pregnant woman, examining of 166
Prevotella 162
Prevotella species 160
Procapi, topical 203
Propylthiouracil 16
Pruritic popular
eruption 55
lesions 34
Pruritus 43
causes of 45
evaluate case of 46
in human immunodeficiency virus infected 55
management 47
nonpharmacologic measures 47
pathogenesis 52
pathophysiology of 45
role of phototherapy in treatment of 51
systemic
causes of 46*b*

drugs for 48
  topical therapy of 47
  treated 47
Pseudo-bubo-groove sign 33
Pseudochancre redux 39
Pseudoepitheliomatous hyperplasia 38
Pseudohyphae 35, 157*f*
Pseudomembrane 2
Pseudomonas 29
Pseudomonas species 108
Psoriasis 55, 152, 208
Psoriatic erythroderma, clinical clues to diagnose 152
Psudomonas infection 108
Psychogenic diseases 46
Psychogenic scalp pruritus, causes of 209
Psychosocial stress 57
Psychosomatic scalp 209
Pulmonary arterial aneurysms 5
Purpura fulminans 76
Purulent discharge 167*f*
Pyoderma gangrenosum 4, 6, 31
Pyoderma, secondary 112*f*
Pyrazinamide 189

Q

Q switch laser 69
Quality of life 43
Queyrat, erythroplasia of 30
Quinacrine 25, 26, 63
Quinine 63
Quinolones 54

R

Ramsay Hunt syndrome 90
Rapid plasma reagin 111
Rapid plasma reagin card test 40
Raynaud's phenomenon 13, 18, 34
Rebamipide 10
Rectal examination 34
Red veterinary petrolatum 228
Refsum's disease 82
Reiter's disease 30
Relationship to partner/s 32
Renal disorder 14
  acute 52,
  chronic 62, 208
Renal pruritus 52
  clinical characteristics of 52
Resorcinol 48
Retinoids 18, 228
Rheumatic fever 76
Rheumatoid
  nodules 13
  vasculitis 193
Ridley-Jopling classification 93

Riehl's melanosis 58, 59, 61, 221, 222
Rifampicin 54, 142, 189
Rituximab 144
Rombo syndrome 100
Rubella virus 78

S

Sabouraud's dextrose agar 36
SAHA syndrome 204
Salazopyrine 11
Salicylates 229
Salmonella 29
Sarcoidal granulomas, histopathology 192
Sarcoidosis 99, 102
  advise to patient 192
  systemic
    involvement in 191*t*
    manifestations of 191
Scabies 29, 55, 112*f*
Scalp dermatitis, common causes of 215*t*
Scalp dysesthesias 209
Scalp hair grows in cycles 198
Scalp pruritus 207
  causes of 208
  complications of 210
  etiologies of 208, 209
  investigations in 210, 210*t*
  pathogenesis of 208
  treatment of 211
  with diseased skin 210
Schwannoma 82
Sclerodactyly 13
Scleroderma 61, 63
Sclerodermoid changes 128
Sclerosing cholangitis 46
Sclerosis, systemic 46
Scrotal ulceration 3*f*
Sebaceoma 99
Sebaceous
  adenoma 99
  gland 99
  hyperplasia 99, 101
Seborrheic
  dermatitis 55, 208, 212*f*
    eyebrows 213*f*
    nasolabial folds 213*f*
    pathogenesis of 212
    rate increased in 213
    treatment of 214
    underlying conditions 213
  keratosis 99, 101
  sites, common 213
Sebum excretion 213
Secnidazole 164
Segmental necrotizing granulomatous neuritis 87
Selective serotonin reuptake inhibitors 49, 50, 54

Selenium 229
Senile pruritus 53
    management of 53
Sensory
    integrity, testing 85
    nerves, anesthesia of 48
    neuropathy
        onset of 82
        types 1 and 3 82
Septicemia 75
Serodiagnostic test 87
Serositis 14
Sertraline 49, 50, 53, 55
Serum alanine transaminase 105
Serum sickness syndrome 76
Sex
    hormones 16, 54
    partners, treatment of 181
    worker, commercial 28
Sexually transmitted disease 28, 156
    ulcers 36
        presentation of 38
        features of 37
Sexually transmitted infection 31, 38, 41, 172
    causes 176
    infectious causes 29
    management of 41
Sexually transmitted urethritis 172
Sézary syndrome 45
Silver 64
Silver nitrate 10
Sjögren syndrome 46
Skin
    biopsy of intact blister 123*f*
    colored nodules on face 101*fc*
    diseases 43
    failure, acute 153
    lesions 43, 54
        absence of 86
    lightening agents 228
    normal color 59
    pathergy testing 6
Solid tumors 46
Spongiosis 135
Squamous cell carcinoma 30, 99
Staphylococcal scalded skin syndrome 75, 76, 125, 126
Staphylococcus 29
Starch iodine test 85
Steatocystoma 96, 97
Steven–Johnson syndrome 30, 33, 34, 41, 75-77, 125, 176
Streptococcus 29, 108
Subcorneal pustular dermatosis 142
Subepidermal
    blisters 135
    bullae 134*f*

Sucralfate suspension 10
Sulfonamides 54
Sulfonylureas 54
Sulisobenzone 229
Sunscreens
    classify 228
    systemic 229
Sweat test 85
Sweet's syndrome 4, 7, 75
Syndromic management
    advantages 41
    disadvantages of 41
Syphilis 36
    congenital 108
    secondary 199
    serological tests for 40
Syphilitic chancre, diagnosis of 29
Syringocystadenoma papilliferum 99
Syringoma 99
Systemic amyloidosis 199
Systemic disorders 1, 43
Systemic lupus erythematosus 9, 12, 24*f*, 25, 75, 76
    classification of 14*t*
    diagnostic criteria for 13
    drugs implicated in 16*t*
    pathogenesis of 15
Systemic Lupus International Collaborating Clinics 15*t*

T

Tacrolimus 25
Tar melanosis 222
Telogen effluvium 13, 204
    acute 196, 197, 200, 203
    chronic 197, 200
Telogen gravidarum 199
Telogen hair follicle 197*f*
Telogen hair loss 203
    acute 199
    chronic 199
    treatment for 203
Temporal bone fracture 90
Tense bulla left forearm 133
Tetanus 90
Tetracycline 10, 54
Thalidomide 10, 18, 50, 90
Thiopurine methyltransferase, level of activity 145
Thrombophlebitis, superficial 4
Thymol 48
Thyroid disorder 199
Thyrotoxicosis 62
Tinea capitis 211*f*
Tinidazole 164
Tioconazole 163, 169
Titanium dioxide 228

Tocopherols 229
Toluidine red unheated serum test 40
Topical steroids 25
Toxic 90
    epidermal necrolysis 24f, 30, 33, 34, 75, 115, 126
    shock syndrome 76
Toxins 64
Tranexamic acid 227
Transient
    acantholytic dermatosis 125, 128
    blistering disorders in children 112t
    skin disorders, in briefly 111
Trauma, history of 81
Treponema pallidum 29, 39, 108
Treponemal test 36, 40
Triamcinolone acetonide 192
Triamcinolone mucosal cream 10
Trichilemmoma 96, 97, 99
Trichoadenoma 99
Trichodiscoma 99
Trichodynia 208
Trichoepithelioma 96, 99
Trichoepitheliomas: multiple, affecting face 97f
Trichofolliculoma 99
Trichokinesis 208
Trichomonas 160, 161
    suspect 178
    urethritis, treatment options for 180
    vaginalis 158, 162, 165, 166f, 176, 181
Trichomoniasis 156, 158, 163, 164, 169
Trichoscopy normal 197f
Trichoscopy, role of 211
Triclosan 10
Tricyclic antidepressant 49, 50, 54
Trifluoperazine 63
Trolamine salicylate 229
Trophic ulcer 91
    differential diagnoses of 91
Tropical sprue 62
Tuberculids 189
Tuberculin skin test, role of 187
Tuberculoid
    granulomas 189
    leprosy, borderline 89, 185, 191
    pole 86
Tuberculosis 30, 61, 225
Tumors
    benign 99
    malignant 99
    nerves 82
    premalignant 99
    sheath 82
    skin appendages 99
Tzanck smear 35, 122, 123f, 134

U

Ulcers in oral mucosa 123f
Ulnar nerve 85
Ultrasonography 86
Ultraviolet 51
    radiation 16, 61, 63, 65
    rays protection 25
Universal acquired melanosis 61
Ureaplasma 158, 160
Ureaplasma urealyticum 176
Uremic pruritus 52
Urethral discharge 172, 181
    case 172, 174, 175
    causative organisms of 176
    cause of 176, 176t, 178
    clinical diagnosis of 179
    examine patient 178
    investigations 173, 174, 175, 178
    nonsexually transmitted causes 178
    treatment 173-175
    urethritis manifest without 176
Urethral instrumentation 176
Urethral stricture 176
Urethritis
    criteria to diagnose 180
    manifestations of 179
    point-of-care tests for 176
    recurrent 181
    3-glass test used for 177
Urinary tract infection 176
Urine, reddish-black discoloration of 129f
Ursodeoxycholic acid 53
Urticaria 43, 208
Urticarial vasculitis 76

V

Vagabond disease 61, 62
Vaginal cervical smear 161
Vaginal discharge 156
    abnormal 158
    advice and precautions 165
    alternative treatment regimens 164t
    approach 162
    case of 159
    causing 156
    characteristics of 160
    complications of 165
    etiology of 158, 158t
    examination 156
    in HIV-positive patient 169
    in seropositive 168
    investigations 156, 161t
    point-of-care testing 159
    pregnancy affect 166

symptoms of 159
syndromic management 158, 164t
treatment for 157t, 162, 163, 167t
Vaginitis 158, 164
Valve lesions 5
Varicella 78
  in older children 110
  starts 74
  zoster virus 78, 111
Vascular involvement, management of 11
Venereal disease research laboratory 111, 165
Vesicles and bullae in children 114
Vesicopustular disorders in children, classify 107
Vesicular
  dermatophytosis 125
  tinea 126
Vesiculobullous
  disease, diagnosis of 135
  disorder 135b, 138
    based on inflammatory infiltrate 136b
    electron microscopy for 141t
    enzyme-linked immunosorbent assay for 141
    immune electron microscopy for 141t
    in middle age 121, 125b
  lesions 121
    differential diagnosis of 124
    in children 115, 116
Vesiculopustular disorders
  in children 104
  infective causes of 107
Viral
  disorders 109
  exanthems of childhood 77, 78t
  hemorrhagic fevers 78t
  hepatitis 46
Vitamin
  A deficiency 61
  B12 deficiency 61, 62, 65
  D deficiency 200
Vulvovaginal candidiasis 163, 158, 164
  classified 159
  organisms cause 159

W

Warfarin 200
Wegener's granulomatosis 8, 30, 193
Western blotting 134
Wet mount 161
Whiff test 161
Wilson's disease 62
Wright stain 106
Wrist and foot drop 91

X

Xanthine oxidase inhibitors 54
Xanthoma 99
Xerosis skin 45, 47, 55, 91
Xerotic eczema 53
X-linked dominant disease 114

Z

Zinc
  oxide 228
  sulfate 10
Zoon's balanitis 30, 31, 33
Zosteriform lichen planus pigmentosus 66